Communication Disorders in Multicultural Populations

Butterworth–Heinemann
Series in Communication Disorders

Charlena M. Seymour, Ph.D., Series Editor

Battle, D.E. *Communication Disorders in Multicultural Populations* (1993)

Battle, D.E. *Communication Disorders in Multicultural Populations*, Second Edition (1998)

Battle, D.E. *Communication Disorders in Multicultural Populations*, Third Edition (2002)

Billeaud, F.P. *Communication Disorders in Infants and Toddlers: Assessment and Intervention* (1993)

Billeaud, F.P. *Communication Disorders in Infants and Toddlers: Assessment and Intervention*, Second Edition (1998)

Huntley, R.A. & Helfer, K.S. *Communication in Later Life* (1995)

Kricos, P.B. & Lesner, S.A. *Hearing Care for the Older Adult: Audiologic Rehabilitation* (1995)

Maxon, A.B. & Brackett, D. *The Hearing-Impaired Child: Infancy Through High School Years* (1992)

Velleman, S.L. *Making Phonology Functional: What Do I Do First?* (1998)

Wall, L.G. *Hearing for the Speech-Language Pathologist and Health Care Professional* (1995)

Wallace, G.L. *Adult Aphasia Rehabilitation* (1996)

Communication Disorders in Multicultural Populations

Third Edition

Dolores E. Battle, Ph.D.

Professor of Speech-Language Pathology and Senior Advisor to the President for Equity and Campus Diversity, Buffalo State College (State University of New York), Buffalo

With 20 Contributing Authors

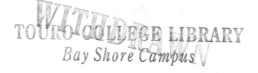
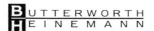
BUTTERWORTH
HEINEMANN

Boston Oxford Auckland Johannesburg Melbourne New Delhi

Every effort has been made to ensure that the drug dosage schedules within this text are accurate and conform to standards accepted at time of publication. However, as treatment recommendations vary in the light of continuing research and clinical experience, the reader is advised to verify drug dosage schedules herein with information found on product information sheets. This is especially true in cases of new or infrequently used drugs.

 Recognizing the importance of preserving what has been written, Butterworth–Heinemann prints its books on acid-free paper whenever possible.

Library of Congress Cataloging-in-Publication Data

Communication disorders in multicultural populations / Dolores E. Battle, with 20 contributing authors.—3rd ed.
　　p. cm.
　Includes bibliographical references and index.
　ISBN 0-7506-7323-0
　　1. Communicative disorders—United States. 2. Transcultural medical care—United States. 3. Multiculturalism—United States. I. Battle, Dolores E.

　RC423 .C6425 2001
　616.85'5—dc21

2001037681

British Library Cataloguing-in-Publication Data
A catalogue record for this book is available from the British Library.

The publisher offers special discounts on bulk orders of this book. For information, please contact:

Manager of Special Sales
Butterworth–Heinemann
225 Wildwood Avenue
Woburn, MA 01801-2041
Tel: 781-904-2500
Fax: 781-904-2620

For information on all Butterworth–Heinemann publications available, contact our World Wide Web home page at: http://www.bh.com

10 9 8 7 6 5 4 3 2 1

Printed in the United States of America

In memory of
William A. Matthews, Jr.
March 3, 1916 – March 22, 2001

Contents

Contributing Authors

Zenobia Bagli, Ph.D.
Professor and Chair, Department of Communicative Disorders, Jackson State University, Jackson, Mississippi

Dolores E. Battle, Ph.D.
Professor of Speech-Language Pathology and Senior Advisor to the President for Equity and Campus Diversity, Buffalo State College (State University of New York), Buffalo

Li-Rong Lilly Cheng, Ph.D.
Professor, Department of Communicative Disorders, San Diego State University, San Diego

Thomas A. Crowe, Ph.D.
Interim Dean, School of Applied Sciences and Professional Studies, University of Mississippi, University; Chair and Professor, Department of Communicative Disorders, University of Mississippi; Director, Center for Speech and Hearing Research, University of Mississippi

Priscilla Nellum Davis, Ph.D.
Professor of Audiology and Speech Pathology, University of Arkansas for Medical Sciences, and University of Arkansas at Little Rock, Little Rock

Glenda DeJarnette, Ph.D.
Associate Professor, Department of Communication Disorders, Southern Connecticut State University, New Haven

Betholyn Gentry, Ph.D.
Professor of Audiology and Speech Pathology, University of Arkansas for Medical Sciences, and University of Arkansas at Little Rock, Little Rock

Theodore J. Glattke, Ph.D.
Professor, Department of Speech and Hearing Sciences, University of Arizona, Tucson; Professor, Department of Surgery, University Medical Center, University of Arizona

R. Wayne Holland, Ed.D., C.C.C.-S.L.P.
President and Chief Operating Officer, Lakeshore Communication Disorders, Inc., St. Clair Shores, Michigan

Pamela Hubbard-Wiley, Ph.D.
President and Director, Los Angeles Speech and Language Therapy Center, Inc., Culver City, California

Aquiles Iglesias, Ph.D.
Professor, Department of Communication Sciences, Temple University, Philadelphia

Rudolph S. Jackson, M.B.A., Ph.D.
Associate Executive Director, Commission on Colleges, Southern Association of Colleges and Schools, Atlanta

Hortencia Ramirez Kayser, Ph.D.
Professor of Speech-Language Pathology, New Mexico State University, Las Cruces

Tommie L. Robinson, Jr., Ph.D.
Assistant Professor of Pediatrics, George Washington University School of Medicine, Washington, D.C.; Director, Scottish Rite Center for Childhood Language Disorders, Hearing and Speech Center, Children's National Medical Center, Washington, D.C.

Diane M. Scott, Ph.D.
Chair and Associate Professor, Department of Communication Disorders, North Carolina Central University, Durham

Sandra L. Terrell, Ph.D.
Professor of Speech and Hearing Sciences and Associate Dean, Toulouse School of Graduate Studies, University of North Texas, Denton

John D. Tonkovich, Ph.D., C.C.C.-S.L.P./A.
Associate Professor, Department of Special Education, Eastern Michigan University, Ypsilanti; Private Practice, Speech-Language Pathology, Shelby Township, Michigan

Christine Begay Vining, M.S., C.C.C.-S.L.P.
Senior Speech-Language Pathologist, Early Childhood Evaluation Program, Center for Development and Disability, University of New Mexico, Albuquerque

Carol Westby, Ph.D.
Professor, Department of Communicative Disorders and Sciences, Wichita State University, Wichita, Kansas; Research Associate, Center for Family and Community Partnerships, University of New Mexico, Albuquerque

Toya A. Wyatt, Ph.D.
Associate Professor, Department of Speech Communication, California State University, Fullerton

Introduction

It has been 10 years since the first edition of this text was published. The past decade has made us all aware of the many changes and advances we have made in the age of technology. Not only has technology changed the way we do business, learn, and communicate with each other, it has made us all aware of how small the world has become. What was new just a few years ago is obsolete today. The IBM 286 computer I used to prepare the first edition of this text is obsolete. We use hand-held wireless computers to send instant messages to any place in the world and even to people circling the globe in outer space. Technology and the changing global economy have made the need to communicate effectively and efficiently more important. An era of relative world peace has lead to more movement to and from countries around the world. Changes in computer technology have overshadowed the changes that have occurred in the demographics of the United States in the last decade.

The 2000 Census showed that the diversity of the United States continued to increase through the 1990s. People continued to immigrate to the United States from Europe, Asia, and Central and South America. The 2000 Census, however, showed changes in the countries of origin of those coming to the United States. In the 1990s, the leading countries of origin of people immigrating to the United States were the countries of Central and South America and Asia. Immigration from Mexico led all other countries of origin of immigrants to the United States, accounting for more than 25 percent of all immigration to the United States in the 1990s. Other leading countries of origin included the Dominican Republic, Haiti, Jamaica, and the countries of Central America such as El Salvador. Immigration from the Asian and Pacific areas also continued in the 1990s. The Philippines led all other Asian Pacific countries in immigration followed by immigration from Vietnam, China, and India. Immigration from the countries of the former Soviet Union accounted for nearly 40% of all immigration from the countries of Europe in the 1990s. This was followed by immigration from Poland. Taken together, immigration from the former Soviet Union and Poland accounted for more than 50% of all immigration from European countries in the 1990s.

By 2000, the U.S. population had grown to more than 272 million people. The 2000 Census collected data using a different model than used in the past. The Statistical Policy Directive No. 15 changed the categories that were used in the 2000 Census from those used in previous reports. According to the directive, the basic racial categories are American Indian or Alaskan Native, Asian or Pacific Islander, black, and white. The directive identifies Hispanic origin as an ethnicity. The concept of race was provided by self-identification by respondents (i.e., the individual's perception of his or her racial identity). The concept was not intended to reflect any biological or anthropological definition. Recognizing the difference between race and ethnicity and that many residents were multiracial, the data was collected to allow persons to identify themselves by race and ethnicity. The differences between the 2000 Census data and that of previous censuses affect the comparability of data for certain racial groups and American Indian tribal groups.

Analysis of the resident population by race showed that 75.1% of the resident population were white; 12.3% were black or African American; 3.6% were Asian or Pacific Islanders; 0.1% were American Indian, Eskimo, or Aleut; 0.2% were Native Hawaiian; 2.4% were two or more races; and 5.5% were identified as other (U.S. Bureau of the Census, 2000). The ethnic composition of the country showed that 87.5% were non-Hispanic, and 12.5% of the residents of the country were identified as Hispanic (U.S. Bureau of the Census, 2000).

The changes in the countries of origin of new arrivals to this country have increased the cultural diversity of the United States. In 1989, Cole (1989) projected that if the growth rates among those from non-European countries continued at the present rate, the minority groups would become the majority and the majority will become the minority. That projection has indeed occurred in many cities and at least one state. In San Antonio, more than half of the residents are of Hispanic origin. In California, whites are no longer the majority; persons from Asian and Pacific Islander countries and persons of Hispanic origin make up more than half of the resident population, particularly in the larger metropolitan areas of Los Angeles and Fresno (U.S. Bureau of the Census, 2000). The changes have increased the need for speech-language pathologists to understand the communication and communication disorders of multicultural populations.

Although it is easy to focus on the identification of racial and ethnic groups and to assume homogeneity (special characteristics of each which distinguish that group from others), the challenge for service providers is to recognize both the overwhelming similarity among racial and ethnic groups, as well as the individual differences or heterogeneity within any group and among its members. The Human Genome Project has helped us understand the vast similarity among all humans.

Any attempt to generalize statements or attributes to all members of an identified group fails to recognize individual differences in life history, personal experiences, personal values, or personal beliefs. Although it is easy to make statements such as American Indians do X, to do so would fail to recognize the heterogeneity among American Indians. Even among whites, there are differences between persons who can trace their family roots to the descendants from England from those who are recent immigrants from the Ukraine or Portugal. Third-generation Asians from Japan have very different life stories than recent immigrants from Laos. Immigrants from the African countries of Egypt and Somalia cannot be regarded as a homogeneous group of African immigrants. Within any group, differences of age, gender, socioeconomic status, educational level, and personal motivations make it imperative that the service providers not lose sight of the individual as they learn about cultural groups.

We must not assume that the many cultures coexisting in our society will assimilate into one melting pot. Indeed, it is this country's multicultural character that is one of its great strengths. We are one people under the law, yet we are so diverse in so many ways. As the population continues to become increasingly diverse with respect to culture, language, values, and beliefs, speech-language and hearing professions will increasingly be called on to provide services to individuals and families from a wide variety of cultures, each with their own normative behaviors, learning styles, social beliefs, and world views. It is important that speech-language pathologists and audiologists be familiar not only with the cultures of the individuals they serve, but also of the individual within the culture. It is important to use treatment approaches that are appropriate to the individual regardless of the cultural or ethnic background of the client.

This text provides a framework for speech-language pathologists and audiologists to develop an understanding of the many issues related to the provision of clinical services to individuals from various cultures and of various linguistic backgrounds.

Speech, language, and communication are embedded in culture; therefore, one cannot understand communication by a group without a thorough understanding of the cultural factors related to the group's communication. However, one cannot understand the communication of the individual without recognizing that communication is largely defined by the individual within the context of the individual's personal history. These factors are linked to the historical, geographic, social, and political histories that bind the individual to the group as well as distinguish the individual from the group. Understanding of individuals within a culture implies a fully developed sense of the complex web of meanings, perceptions, actions, symbols, and adaptations that make individuals and cultural groups who they are. To understand and serve clients from diverse cultural backgrounds, it is important to understand the relationship between the individuals and their culture and communication and communication disorders. Recognizing this relationship will facilitate cross-cultural communication and improve the quality of service to all people. This is the premise on which this text is built.

The authors in Part I of this text provide an overview of the major cultural groups in the United States, with particular reference to the factors that have had an impact on the assessment and treatment of communication disorders. The authors are leading experts in the study of communication disorders in their particular culture. Each presents a survey of the major cultural characteristics of the particular group, including speech and language variables, and the implications for assessment and intervention. The text begins with a chapter that stresses that the United States has always been a culturally diverse nation and shows how political and economic factors influenced the nation's development and the perceptions of its peoples. It develops concepts of barriers to assimilation and acculturation in relation to the United States' historical past as well as the present. The remainder of Part I focuses on the major cultural groups in contemporary America and the implications for assessment and intervention for those of the culture. Sandra L. Terrell and Rudolph S. Jackson provide a comprehensive overview of African American culture and African American English with new material on access to health care and prevalence of disease related to communication disorders in African American groups. Li-Rong Lilly Cheng provides an extensive survey of Asian and Pacific Islander cultures, their language behaviors, and the issues involved in their assimilation and acculturation in the United States. The chapter recognizes the progress and changes that have occurred among Asian Pacific Islanders in the past decade. The next chapter on the Middle Eastern and Arab cultures provides valuable insight into diversity within Arab cultures and the implications for clinical services for people from this predominantly Muslim area. Carol Westby and Christine Begay Vining bring their considerable expertise in understanding American Indian cultures, communication, and communication disorders. Aquiles Iglesias discusses Latino cultures and the cultural and linguistic factors that affect the assessment and treatment of communication disorders among those from diverse Latino cultures in Central and South America as well as the Caribbean region.

Part II addresses bilingual language development and specific communication disorders in culturally and linguistically diverse populations. Hortencia Ramirez Kayser provides a comprehensive review of bilingual language development and clinical services for persons learning English as a second language. This chapter is new to this edition and is important given the major increase in persons from non-English speaking countries coming to the country. John D. Tonkovich discusses cultural factors related to neurogenic disorders, including dysphagia, alternative augmentative communication, acquired immunodeficiency syndrome, neonatal crack cocaine exposure, and traumatic brain injury in various cultural groups. Tommie L. Robinson, Jr., and Thomas A. Crowe present a new approach to the role of culture in the assessment and treatment of dysfluency, including multicultural approaches to counseling. The current research findings of the assessment and treatment of voice disorders in various cultural groups are presented by R. Wayne Holland and Glenda DeJarnette.

Part II continues with two chapters that discuss hearing disorders and deafness. Diane M. Scott presents a comprehensive review of racial and ethnic diversity in hearing disorders, including new information from the Human Genome Project related to hearing disorders and the implications for auditory assessment. Zenobia Bagli continues the presentation of advancements in audiology through a chapter on deafness, which provides cultural implications of cochlear implants in the Deaf culture in culturally and linguistically diverse populations. The bicultural interface between the Deaf culture and the cultures of the racially and ethnically diverse are presented for their impact on aural rehabilitation.

The text contains two chapters devoted to clinical issues. Toya A. Wyatt adds her expertise for the chapter on assessment of communication disorders in diverse cultures. Priscilla Nellum Davis and Betholyn Gentry, who have knowledge and experience with clients in the southeastern parts of the United States, have collaborated with Pamela Hubbard-Wiley, from culturally diverse California, to provide guidelines and resources for successful intervention, including World Wide Web sites that contain cultural and clinical information. New to this edition is a chapter on the issues related to multicultural and ethnographic research by Theodore J. Glattke. The chapter discusses the challenges of conducting research on cultural groups, as well as presenting challenges and needs for future research.

Understanding another culture is a continuous and not a discrete process. This text introduces the reader to the variety of issues related to culture and communication disorders and the need to become a culturally competent clinician. It is intended to be a catalyst to encourage professionals to learn more about the clients they serve. Because the Unites States is a cultural mosaic, cultural knowledge will greatly facilitate cultural literacy. Cultural literacy requires systematic study to come to a level of cognitive consciousness. Cultural competence requires systematic study of individuals, including the impact that their culture and linguistic background have on clinical service. Cultural competence involves far more than an understanding of language form and dialectical considerations. It involves understanding all dimensions of culture and communication and how they impact on the individual. Because culture permeates every dimension of communication, the culturally competent clinician understands that most, if not all, truths are merely perceptions of truth viewed through the prism of culture. Learning to provide clinical services in a multicultural environment recognizes that every clinical encounter is a multicultural encounter. The cultural variables of the clinician and those of the client and the family are usually different. Interacting with individuals from cultures different from one's own involves far more than simply learning culture-specific information, which constitutes, at best, general cultural tendencies and, at worst, cultural stereotypes (e.g., "It is an African American tradition to . . .," or "Japanese people are offended by . . .," or "Navajo children are required to . . ."). Instead, it involves establishing a framework for systematically analyzing similarities and differences that can serve as a template through which to conduct ethnographic clinical inquiries.

I conclude by proposing several "dos" and "don'ts" to consider when treating individuals with a consideration of their cultural background. The list is not meant to be all-inclusive, nor will all items be important for all groups in all circumstances. The items are meant to challenge the thinking of clinicians as they strive to become culturally competent clinicians.

1. When providing clinical service to all individuals, it is important to consider one's own personal cultural beliefs, attitudes, and values and to be aware that they contribute to and are a major factor in the multicultural, cross-cultural clinical encounter.

2. When communicating with individuals, learn the name of the individual cultural or geographic group as assigned by its members, and use it. For example, use *Colombian* to describe a person from Colombia, not *Hispanic* or *Latino*. Use *Japanese* to refer to an individual from Japan, not *Asian*. Use *Nigerian* to describe an individual from Nigeria, not *African*. Adherence to this simple rule will help the clinician to recognize heterogeneity among groups and to show respect for the individual regardless of cultural background. It will also help to reduce the dilemma faced in trying to decide whether to refer to a group as black or African American, Latino or Hispanic, Asian or Oriental, American Indian or Native American, or white or Caucasian.

3. Do not use generic terms as substitutes or synonyms for more descriptive racial or ethnic terms. For example, avoid using *minority* to refer to African Americans, *bilingual* to refer to Latinos or Hispanics, or *culturally diverse*

or *multicultural* to refer to individuals. In some areas, such as in Washington, D.C., African Americans are not minorities. The term *minority* means less than 50%, referring to a numerical entity, but using the term denigrates the importance of the numerical minority groups to society. The term *bilingual* does not explain the language use of the individual. One can be bilingual English-French, or English-Russian, or Spanish-American Sign Language. The term *multicultural* refers to societies, not to individuals. In another way of thinking, all individuals are multicultural, because we all are members of several cultural groups, including those defined by race, ethnicity, social class, gender, sexual orientation, geographic and life history, and so on. In this respect, we are all multicultural. Surely, the term does not only refer to non-white non-Europeans.

4. Be aware of words, images, and situations that suggest that all or most members of a racial or ethnic group are the same without taking into account intragroup variations related to factors such as gender, age, socioeconomic status, and education. Do not assume that all African Americans speak African American English. Do not assume that standard English is spoken by all white Americans or only by white Americans. Do not assume that all Asian Americans or Latinos share the same beliefs and cultural patterns. People with Caribbean roots, for example, have a different social and political history from people whose ancestors were brought to this country in captivity from Africa or from Mexico.

5. Be aware that some terms have questionable or negative racial, ethnic, or socioeconomic connotations, such as *culturally deprived*, *at risk*, *minority*, and *culturally disadvantaged*. Such terms suggest that European Americans are the standard by which all else should be judged and are thus racist and ethnocentric. Do not assume that poverty is the exclusive characteristic of any one cultural group.

6. Avoid using unnecessary qualifiers, clichés, and color-symbolic language that reinforce racial and ethnic stereotypes, such as the "articulate black student," "Chinese fire drill," "Chinese auction," "Indian giver," "white lie," "black sheep," and "yellow journalism."

7. Be aware of the nonverbal sources of miscommunication between people from different cultural groups. These include such nonverbal factors as the role of touch during conversation, distance between speakers, appropriate topics of conversations, and styles of greeting behavior. Many of the sources of miscommunication between those from different cultural groups are not related to the particular words that are used or the phonologic or syntactic contrasts that exist between two languages but are more deeply rooted in misunderstandings in role definition, communication style, and a lack of appreciation of the relation between culture and language.

8. Be aware of verbal sources of miscommunication while communicating. Verbal miscommunication goes beyond phonologic contrasts and reaches to the very roots of the communication between individuals in cultures. The importance of the individual in relation to the group, for example, is an important cultural distinction that several authors discuss in this volume.

Every professional must accept the challenges to acquire new attitudes toward cultural diversity and to learn more about cross-cultural communication. If you are ready to commit yourself to an understanding of the issues before you in the changing face of America, and if you are open to finding new ways to function in a profession that is changing, I applaud you. It is critical to continue to develop the understandings and skills to function as a professional in a world sure to continue to change in the years ahead. It is through a better understanding of many cultures that we can better understand communication and communication disorders in a world that will never remain the same.

Dolores E. Battle, Ph.D.

References

Cole L. E. (1989). *E pluribus unum*: Multicultural imperatives for the 1990's and beyond. *ASHA 31*(9), 65–70.

U.S. Bureau of the Census. (2000). *Statistical abstract of the United States* (120th ed.). Washington, DC: U.S. Bureau of the Census.

I

Cultural Diversity: Implications for Speech-Language Pathologists and Audiologists

1

Communication Disorders in a Multicultural Society

Dolores E. Battle

Culture is about the behavior, beliefs, and values of a group of people who are brought together by their commonality. More important, culture is the lens through which one perceives and interprets the world (Vecoli, 1995). It is the filter through which all that one does must pass before entering the collective conscious. Religion, language, customs, traditions, and values are but some of the components of culture. Speech, language, and communication are embedded in culture. Edward T. Hall (1959) said, "Culture is communication. Communication is culture." Culture can be viewed as a system of competencies shared in broad design and deeper principles and varying among individuals. Its specificities are what an individual knows, believes, and thinks about his or her world. Culture is a theory of what one believes his or her fellows know, believe, and mean. It is more than a collection of symbols fit together by the analyst. It is a system of knowledge sharpened and constrained by the way the human brain acquires, organizes, and creates internal models of reality (Keesling, 1974). Culture provides a system of knowledge that allows people of a cultural group to know how to communicate with one another.

The relationship between communication and culture is reciprocal: Culture and communication influence each other (Keesling, 1974). Therefore, one cannot understand communication by a group of individuals without a thorough understanding of the ethnographic and cultural factors related to communication in that group. These factors are intricately embedded in the historic, geographic, social, and political history, which bind a group, give it a sense of peoplehood, and give it ethnic identity.

Because the roots of communication are embedded in culture, it is logical to assume that one cannot study communication or communication disorders without reference to the cultural, historical, or societal basis for the communication style or language used by the members of the ethnic or cultural group. The social rules of discourse and narratives (e.g., topic selection, who selects the topic, who initiates the conversation, who ends the conversation, distancing, eye gaze, and sense making) are culturally determined. Who speaks to whom, when, where, and about what must be understood in the context of the culture of both partners in the communicative event if the clinician is to determine the presence or absence of a communication disorder.

Communication behavior and the perception of what constitutes a communication disorder within a particular group are the products of cultural values, perceptions, attitudes, and history. These factors must be considered when determining the communication competence of a particular person within a group. For example, reluctance to speak and failure to initiate a conversation or use a particular narrative style can be appropriate to one culture but inappropriate to another. The impact of a voice disorder can be different for speakers of tonal languages than for speakers of nontonal languages. Expectations of the benefits of rehabilitation for the effects of stroke or traumatic brain injury can also differ across cultural groups.

The terms *race* and *ethnicity* are often used interchangeably; however, they have different meanings. *Ethnicity* refers to a shared culture that forms the basis for a sense of peoplehood based on the consciousness of a common past. For example, African American is considered a race, but Hispanic is considered an ethnicity. Hispanics can be of any race. Race, language, and ancestral customs constitute the major expressions of ethnicity in the United States. Ethnicity is not passed genetically from generation to generation. Rather, ethnicity is constructed and reconstructed in response to particular historical circumstances and changes. In its most intimate form, an ethnic group can be based on face-to-face relationships and political realities that mobilize its members into political self-determination. Joined by the aspirations for political self-determination, ethnicity is used to identify groups or communities that are differentiated by religious, racial, or cultural characteristics and that possess a sense of peoplehood.

Ethnography refers to the fully developed sense of the meaning of a culture and the complex manner in which one comes to understand the intricacies of the culture. The ethnographic understanding of a culture implies a fully developed sense of the complex web of meanings, perceptions, actions, symbols, and adaptations that make a people who they are.

Race refers to the biologic and anatomic attributes and functions, such as skin color, facial features, and hair texture. Two people can be of the same race but differ widely in cultural identity, personal history, and their view of the world. For example, a Korean child reared in a Korean family will have Korean cultural values; however, a Korean child adopted at birth by an African American family has the biologic and genetic characteristics attributed to his or her genetic ancestors but has the cultural values imparted by the adoptive parents.

In the 2000 U.S. Census, the racial groups were identified as white, American Indian or Alaska Native, Black, Asian, or Pacific Islander. In addition, a group called *multiracial* was included. Hispanic was identified as an ethnicity. Individuals were identified as Hispanic or non-Hispanic. The term *Hispanic* was used to identify persons who speak Spanish. Many Hispanic persons prefer the use of the term *Latino* to refer to their origin in the countries of Central and South America. This distinguished them from persons who are identified only by the language that they speak. Although both terms are used, the term *Latino* is preferred.

Culture is a term that implies the implicit and explicit behavior in a variety of areas. Explicit cultural behaviors are visible to the world and include observable features of dress, language, food preferences, customs, and lifestyle. Explicit behaviors are readily visible and are often used to identify the cultural group to observers. These behaviors are the focus of "culture-of-the-month" activities and programs. Implicit cultural variables are those factors that are not easily depicted and observed. They include such factors as age and gender roles within families, child-rearing practices, religious and spiritual beliefs, educational values, fears and attitudes, values and perceptions, and exposure to and adoption of other cultural norms. Implicit cultural values are beneath the surface, relatively invisible; however, they shape the fiber of those who identify as a member of a cultural group.

Multicultural is used to describe a society characterized by a diversity of cultures with varieties of religions, language, customs, traditions, and values. It is used to describe a society in which people from diverse racial and ethnic backgrounds and socioeconomic groups live and work together to create a mosaic composed of individuals that work together to form a rich whole. It also includes the cultures defined by socioeconomic class, gender, sexual orientation, ability level versus disability, and other variables that define persons as individuals. The term is used to describe a society in which each individual is respected and valued for their contribution to the whole. It is important to realize that the multicultural society is a diverse society of individuals who belong to many different cultural groups. All individuals have a group identity and an individual identity. This includes the clinician and client and members of the family. All persons seeking clinical services are to be considered as individuals with individual cultural and ethnic values. All persons providing clinical services are also individuals with individual cultural and ethnic values. The clinically competent clinician works to bring the persons in the clinical situation into harmony with each other so that the most appropriate clinical services can be provided.

Stereotyping results from the overestimation of association between group membership and individual behavior (Gudykunst & Nishida, 1984). Stereotyping occurs when a person ascribes the collective characteristics associated with a particular group to every member of that group, discounting individual characteristics. Cultural competency requires that clinicians avoid developing stereotypes and keep the individual at the forefront of any clinical encounter.

Becoming a Multicultural Society in America: History of Immigration in America, 1500–1990

From its beginning, the United States has been a complex ethnic mosaic with a wide variety of communities differentiated by culture, race, religion, and language. The process of peopling this continent has been a story of cultural diversity brought about by immigration. Even the original American Indians walked across a land bridge from Siberia thousands of years ago. Thousands of years later, in 1500, the more than 4.5 million inhabitants of America were divided into hundreds of tribes, each with distinctive cultures, religions, and languages (Vecoli, 1995).

Americans are immigrants or the descendants of immigrants. Immigration into America has been a long and continuous process. Although many early settlers came primarily from the European countries seeking political and religious freedom, others earned their passage to the New World by signing on as indentured servants or sailors. They brought with them the ideals and values that formed the foundation of the social, educational, economic, and political systems of the United States. They were held together by shared political beliefs, principles, and practices that were common in Northern Europe. These common beliefs were melded to form the founding principles of the United States.

As the United States grew in economic strength, inexpensive labor became necessary, particularly in the rich farming areas of the Southern colonies and states. By the end of the eighteenth century, some 600,000 Europeans and Africans were recruited or enslaved and transported to the United States, where they contributed to the economic growth of the country.

When the first census was taken in 1790, the United States was already a nation of many cultures. Almost 19% of Americans were of African ancestry; 12% were Scottish and Scotch-Irish; and smaller amounts were German, French, Irish, Welsh, and Sephardic Jews (Vecoli, 1995). The census did not include American Indians or Hispanics. Those counted as citizens of the United States comprised only 48% of the total population of the country.

To preserve the ideals on which the nation was founded, the Naturalization Act of 1790 was passed. It specified that citizenship in the United States was open to "any alien, being a free white person," thus excluding from citizenship of the country those who were not white and those who were enslaved.

First Wave of Immigration: 1841–1890

Immigrants are persons admitted for legal permanent residence in the United States. It includes persons who have entered the country as refugees. After the passing of the Naturalization Act of 1790, population growth in the United States, other than by natural increase, came primarily through three massive waves of immigration. During the first wave of documented immigration to the United States, which included the gold rush period of the 1850s, many Europeans came in search of a better economic opportunity. During this period, almost 15 million immigrants arrived, including 4 million immigrants from Germany after the failure of social reform, 3 million each from Ireland and Britain as a result of the potato famine of 1847, and 1 million from Scandinavia who were seeking land available through the Homestead Act. American capitalism became dependent on the rural workers of Europe, French Canada, Mexico, and Asia to support its factories and mines (Vecoli, 1995; Morrison & Zabusky, 1980). During this period, there was the first major surge in immigration from Asia. During the gold rush in the early 1850s, Chinese came to the country to work in the mines. As mining became less lucrative, the Chinese opened their own businesses and found employment in other areas, such as working on the railroad. From the 1870s to the early 1880s, the number of persons from China increased from 63,000 to nearly 180,000.

By 1882, some Americans became concerned that the newcomers would pose a danger to "American" values and institutions. The slow evolution of a national policy on immigration resulted in a series of laws that progressively restricted immigration or reduced the rights of those who were new to the country (Morrison & Zabusky, 1980). For example, the Chinese Exclusion Act of 1882 denied immigration to Chinese laborers and barred Chinese from acquiring citizenship. In addition, immigration laws established qualitative health and moral standards by excluding criminals, prostitutes, "lunatics," "idiots," and paupers from immigrating to the United States. As a result of these policies, the Chinese population in the United States had dropped to the 1870 levels.

Second Wave of Immigration: 1891–1920

The second wave of immigration occurred during the industrial revolution, when Europe was experiencing extreme poverty and political oppression. This wave brought an additional 18 million immigrants to the United States, including more than 4 million from Italy, 3.6 million from Austria-Hungary, and 3 million from Russia (Vecoli, 1995). Overpopulation in Scandinavia, resulting unemployment, and a desire for freedom led to a significant increase in immigration from Sweden and Norway during this period. They relocated in the states of the Midwest, especially Illinois, Minnesota, Michigan, Iowa, and Wisconsin. Nearly one-fifth of all Swedish immigrants settled in Minnesota.

In addition to the European immigration during this period, a large number of Asians, primarily from China and Japan, and persons from Greece and the Middle East also entered the United States. The early Greek and Arab immigrants were mostly young men from rural agricultural areas who came to America for economic opportunities. The Arabs were primarily from the areas known today as Lebanon, Syria, and Turkey. Between 1900 and 1935, nearly 10% of the Mexican population, approximately 1 million persons, immigrated north to the United States. The new peoples had language, culture, social institutions, customs, and a collective experience that differed significantly from that of European immigrant groups.

The concerns about the differences between Asians and Europeans culminated in the Immigration Acts of 1921 and 1924. These acts denied entry to aliens ineligible for citizenship (i.e., those who were not deemed white) and established national quota systems designed to reduce the number of Southern and Eastern Europeans entering the country and to bar Asians entirely. The laws attempted to freeze the biologic and ethnic identity of the American people by reducing the influence from those not like the early immigrants who had gained political and economic power in the country.

The time between 1920 and 1945 marked a hiatus in immigration due to restrictive immigration policies, economic depression, and the effects of two world wars. Immigration after World War II reflected political unrest in Europe and the Middle East. Immigrants from Jordan, Egypt, Lebanon, Iraq, and Syria were Palestinian refugees who fled from Israel when it was declared a state.

The postwar era brought a modest influx of immigrants, followed by a new surge of subsequent changes in laws and immigration policy. After World War II, the need for migrant farm workers encouraged more than 1 million persons from Mexico to come to the United States. This has continued such that persons from Mexico have been the largest group of immigrants to the United States for the past 30 years. In addition, approximately 20,000 Russians and other displaced individuals immigrated to the United States immediately after World War II (Magocsi, 1995). Although many Jews leaving Russia after the war were granted permission only to go to Israel, many hoped to go to the United States. Of the nearly 3 million Americans who identified themselves as wholly or partially Russian in the 1990 Census, nearly 44% resided in the Northeast (Magocsi, 1995). By 1985, nearly 300,000 Russian Jews had reached the United States and settled in the major cities of the Northeast (Magocsi, 1995). Turkish, Croatian, and Serbian immigration also increased after World War II, including professionals such as engineers and physicians seeking better job opportunities.

Third Wave of Immigration: 1965–1990

Abhorring the racism of Nazism and stirred by the valor that the Asian Americans and African Americans showed in the fight to protect the freedom of America during World War II and the Korean War, the nation changed the way it thought about race and equality. A combination of international politics and democratic idealism resulted in the elimination of racial restrictions from American immigration and naturalization policies. The Civil Rights movement in the 1960s and the enactment of the Civil Rights Act of 1964 created a belief of democratic idealism. The Immigration and Nationality Act of 1965 removed the national origin quotas and opened the United States to immigration from throughout the world by regional quotas. The unexpected consequence of the 1965 act was the beginning of the third wave of immigration. Not only did the total number of immigrants increase steadily to 1 million or more arriving each year, but also the countries of origin changed from being primarily European countries to those of Asia and Latin America (Vecoli, 1995). Each year, 170,000 people were allowed to immigrate to the country from the Eastern Hemisphere, and 120,000 people were allowed to immigrate to the country from the Western Hemisphere.

The Refugee Act of 1980 provided a uniform admission procedure for refugees of all countries. It removed the geographic origin quotas, established an annual general quota of immigration at 270,000, and gave preferences to the family members of American citizens and resident aliens, skilled workers, and refugees. The Immigration Reform and Control Act of 1986 allowed illegal immigrants who had been in the United States since January 1982 and those who had been employed in agricultural work for seasonal work to become temporary and then permanent residents of the United States.

The third wave of immigration differs from the previous two waves, because the major countries of origin of the immigrants have changed. During the first two waves of immigration, almost 90% of the immigrants originated from Europe. During the 1980s, however, only 12% of the 7.3 million immigrants originated from European countries. Nearly 85% of the immigrants in the 1980s came from Asia and Latin America, with Mexico and

China having the largest numbers of immigrants, respectively. More than 1.6 million people came from Mexico, another 4.5 million came from Central and South America and the Caribbean, and more than 2.8 million came from Asia (U.S. Bureau of the Census, 1996). Immigrants from Asia and the Pacific Island nations were well educated, with 70–80% having completed at least a high school education and approximately 50% having advanced degrees. More than 71% of the recent immigrants from the West African countries of Nigeria, Egypt, Senegal, and Ethiopia have at least a high school education, and 25% have college degrees. Although most of these immigrants are underemployed (i.e., employed in positions of lower income levels than expected based on their education) when they arrive, increased fluency in English and increased immersion into the American culture appear to greatly increase their economic success (U.S. Bureau of the Census, 1996).

There was a significant increase of people immigrating to the United States from the Southeast Asian countries and Pacific Islands in the post–Korean War era of the 1970s and the post–Vietnam War era of the early 1980s. Many immigrants from Vietnam and Cambodia who came to the country as impoverished "boat people" had spent many years in refugee camps and did not have viable educations or technological skills before moving to the United States (Galens et al., 1995). Poor fluency in English and low education levels have hampered economic development of some immigrants from Southeast Asia and the Pacific Islands, with many continuing to live below poverty levels.

Immigrants in the late 1980s and the 1990s from Europe, Asia, Central and South America, and the Caribbean came to the United States seeking refuge from political and economic difficulties in their home countries. Between 1980 and 1990, the Hispanic population in the United States grew by 36%, with major countries of origin being Mexico, Haiti, the Dominican Republic, and Cuba (U.S. Bureau of the Census, 1996).

Immigration in the 1990s

The Immigration Act of 1990 established a major numerical limits and preferences system regulating legal immigration. Preferences were given to family-sponsored and employment-based immigrants. As a result, immigration into the United States continued through the 1990s. In the 2000 U.S. Census (U.S. Bureau of the Census, 2000), the U.S. population increased by 13.2% between 1990 and 2000. As shown in Table 1-1, the growth in the white population was only 3.4%, whereas the growth in other racial/ethnic groups was many times that rate. The growth in the population was largely due to significant increases in immigration of nonwhite racial/

Table 1-1 Population Growth in the United States 1990–2000

	1990	*2000*	*Percent Change*
White	188,128,296	194,552,774	+3.4
Black	29,986,060	34,658,190	+15.6
Hispanic	22,354,059	35,305,818	+57.9
Native American	1,959,234	2,475,956	+26.4
Asian/Pacific Islander	7,273,662	10,641,833	+46.3
Multiracial	(not an option)	6,826,228	—

Source: Adapted from U.S. Bureau of the Census. (2000). *Statistical abstract of the United States* (122th ed.). Washington, DC: U.S. Bureau of the Census.

ethnic minority groups. Care must be taken in comparing 1990 and 2000 census data, because the 2000 census was the first census to allow people to identify themselves as multiracial. However, general trends and patterns were consistent overall.

Between 1991 and 1998, more than 7.6 million people immigrated to the United States. The immigrants came from Europe, Asia, North America, South America, and Africa. There were more than 1 million immigrants from Europe, with the largest group coming from the former Soviet Union. There were more than 2.4 million immigrants from Asia, with the largest groups coming from the Philippines, China, Vietnam, and India. There were more than 344,000 immigrants from South America and more than 200,000 from Africa. By far, the largest groups of immigrants were from the countries of North America, including Central America and the Caribbean area. More than 2.7 million immigrants came to the country from this area, with nearly 2 million coming from Mexico alone (U.S. Bureau of the Census, 2000).

In addition to the documented legal immigrants to the United States, there are many undocumented or illegal immigrants. Immigration Services estimates that approximately 3.5–4.0 million undocumented immigrants are residents in the country. A large number of undocumented immigrants who enter the country illegally are from Mexico; however, many undocumented immigrants have origins in El Salvador, Guatemala, Canada, Haiti, Poland, and the Philippines (Fernandez & Robinson, 1994). The overwhelming majority of legal immigrants in 1994 settled in California and New York (27,379 and 20,892, respectively). Many also settled in Texas, Washington, Illinois, Florida, Pennsylvania, Massachusetts, Georgia, and Michigan (U.S. Bureau of the Census, 1996).

In addition to those illegally crossing the borders, a large number of undocumented immigrants who enter the country as students, tourists, or temporary workers simply stay in the country after their visas have expired. More than 250,000 Chinese intellectuals, scientists, and engineers have come to the United States for advanced degrees and have stayed after their visas expired or have applied for alien resident status. The result of the dramatic increase in immigration shows considerable diversity in the demographic makeup of America.

Population Projections

National estimates of population growth provide a compelling glimpse of the face of the new America. It is estimated that the increase in immigration will continue well into the twenty-first century. If middle population estimates of population changes between 1995 and 2020 are used, then the U.S. population will increase by 8.5% from 1995 to 2020 (U.S. Bureau of the Census, 1996). It is projected that by 2020, the white population will increase by 2.4%; however, the African American population will increase by 11.9%, the American-Indian population by 13.1%, the Asian and Pacific Islander population by 26.4%, and the Hispanic/Latino population by 26.4% by 2020 (U.S. Bureau of the Census, 1996).

First- and second-generation immigrant children are the fastest growing segment of the U.S. population younger than age 15 years (Fix & Zimmerman, 1993). Between 1990 and 1999, the U.S. Census counted 9 million foreign-born persons in the United States (U.S. Bureau of the Census, 2000), including 266,000 under the age of 5 years. Adding second-generation immigrants to that total boosts the number of immigrant children and children of immigrants to more than 5 million. The total school-age population is expected to grow by more than 20%, from 34 million in 1990 to 42 million in 2010 (Fix & Passel, 1994). It is estimated that the children of new immigrants will account for more than half of this growth. The number of children of immigrants is expected to rise to 9 million in 2010, representing 22% of the school-age population (Fix & Passel, 1994).

Acculturation and Assimilation

Models of Assimilation

Tens of millions of immigrants with differing cultures have been incorporated into American society by the processes of acculturation and assimilation. *Acculturation* is the process by which newcomers assume

American cultural attributes, such as the English language, cultural norms, behaviors, and values. *Assimilation* is the process of their incorporation into the social and cultural networks of the host society, including work, place of residence, leisure activities, and family. It refers to the process of giving up one's culture and taking on the characteristics of another. Primarily, three models of assimilation and acculturation have been used to explain cultural diversity in America.

Anglo-Conformity Model

The Anglo-conformity model of acculturation and assimilation has been favored through much of the history of this country. Convinced of their cultural and biologic superiority, early Americans passed laws restricting immigration and citizenship to those from Western Europe. Nonwhite people were expected to abandon their distinctive cultural, religious, and linguistic values and practices and conform to the American model. The "American way" was considered the "only" way. Immigrants strove to adopt as much of the American culture as possible so that they could gain the economic and political benefits of being "American." The immigrants believed that the sooner they assimilated into the American culture, the sooner and easier they could share in the riches of America. In their eagerness to become Americans, they rejected or altered family names and the languages and customs of the "old country" (Morrison & Zabusky, 1980).

Melting Pot Model

A competing model of acculturation and assimilation, the melting pot model is a process whereby, inasmuch as possible, the elements of culture brought by the immigrants are transmuted into a new American culture that embodies cultural variants. The result is an amalgam of the varied cultures and peoples in which no single culture is dominant and all blend into a rich whole. The melting pot ideology provided a rationale for the more liberal immigration policies in the late 1960s. The policy came under attack, however, as the determination of the ethnic groups to retain their individual identity, traditions, and customs increased.

Cultural-Pluralism Model

The cultural-pluralism model has been offered as an alternative to the melting pot model in the 1990s. It has been viewed as an internal attitude that predisposes but does not make compulsory the display of ethnic identification in interactions. In the cultural-pluralism model, it is valued and accepted to maintain ethnic identity. Although sharing a common American citizenship and loyalty, ethnic groups maintain and foster their particular languages, customs, and cultural values. Cultural pluralism recognizes diversity within the nation.

Levels of Adaptation and Assimilation

The independent variable in the process of acculturation and assimilation is the determination or willingness of the immigrants to assume the culture of America. The degree of adaptation and assimilation varies with each individual and with each group of immigrants. For example, the early immigrants in the first two waves of immigration, influenced by the immigration and naturalization policies of the time, made great efforts to acculturate and assimilate into the fabric of America. The level of assimilation is an important factor to consider in understanding clients and their families. Cheng and Butler (1993) describe six levels of adaptation and assimilation that affect culturally and linguistically diverse immigrants.

At the first level, reaffirmation, the people reject the new culture and attempt to maintain or revive native cultural traditions. Chain migrations and preferences in immigration policies allow relatives and friends to group for mutual assistance. They maintain their customary ways by establishing churches, societies, and newspapers and build institutions and communities that reflect and retain their cultural values and language.

At the second level, people attempt to synthesize a selective combination of cultural aspects of both cultures. For example, they may accept the dress and food of the new culture but retain the native view of health care and education. Through selective assimilation and adaptation, immigrants take from the American culture what they need to survive and keep traditional cultural beliefs and practices that they value. Although many may gradually adapt the parts of the American culture they chose, many hold dear the culture and language of their ancestors. Rather than shed old country customs, the new immigrants may enroll their children in "cultural schools." Cultural schools ensure that children do not forget the customs of the past.

Such schools allow children to adopt ancestral names and to continue speaking their native language in the home, thus ensuring that America remains a culturally pluralistic country.

At the third level, withdrawal, people may reject and withdraw from their native culture or the new culture because of cultural conflict. People who reject their native culture become isolated from their cultural peers and do not maintain relationships with individuals other than immediate family members. People who withdraw from the new culture do not learn the language or culture of the new country. Depending on the level of assimilation, these people may experience loneliness and fear when attempts are made to engage in activities and associations to increase adaptation to the new culture.

People at the constructive-marginality level tentatively accept the two cultures but do not fully integrate into either one. They may believe that they do not belong in either culture and may not be sure of which cultural rule or language to use in a situation.

The biculturalism level refers to the full involvement of both cultures. Bicultural individuals retain fluency in the native language and obtain fluency in the new language. They are equally comfortable functioning in either culture and can switch between the cultures with relative ease.

At the compensatory adaptation level, people become thoroughly mainstreamed into the new culture, rejecting and avoiding identification with the native culture and language. Young adolescents and young adults at this level reject any knowledge of the native country and try to be as American as possible. They are anxious to learn the new language and cultural expectations as quickly and as thoroughly as possible. They may enroll in accent-reduction programs to remove any trace of their native language in their newly adopted language.

Barriers to Assimilation and Acculturation

There are several barriers to assimilation and acculturation, even for those who intend to be fully assimilated into the American mainstream. Many immigrants experience only limited acculturation and practically no assimilation in their lifetimes. Among the factors that affect the process of acculturation and assimilation are circumstances of immigration, race and ethnicity, class, gender, and the character of community.

Voluntary immigrants, involuntary immigrants, and refugees differ in their circumstances of immigration. Voluntary immigrants are usually prepared for the move, psychologically motivated, and willing to accept the linguistic and cultural changes required to succeed in the new country. Involuntary immigrants, such as those brought to this country in slavery, were resistant to their new circumstances and suffered social and political isolation from the political mainstream that hampered their attempts at assimilation. Refugees, on the other hand, are forced to leave their country because of adverse domestic, social, or political conditions. Preparation for the move is limited, and many enter the country without knowledge of the language or culture of the receiving country. Like involuntary immigrants, they may have been separated from their families and may have spent days or years in unpleasant circumstances before having access to the benefits of the receiving country. As a result, the effects of culture shock are more pervasive on refugees than on voluntary immigrants. Thus, refugees usually achieve low levels of assimilation into the receiving country, do not become proficient in English, and live in ethnic enclaves for longer periods of time (Ima & Keogh, 1995).

Race, especially skin color, has been a dominant factor in barriers to assimilation and acculturation for Asians, Hispanics, African Americans, and Native Americans. Among the important factors limiting acculturation and assimilation is the willingness of the dominant culture to accept those perceived as different. Because it is relatively easy to identify those who differ from the mainstream white individuals by race and skin color, it has been relatively more difficult for African Americans and some Asian Americans to assimilate into the American mainstream.

Other factors also affect acculturation and assimilation. Differences in religious practices—particularly those that require dress codes and religious observances that differ from the Christian mainstream and language—have been construed as barriers to assimilation and acculturation. Social class, dictated largely by economic factors, has also limited interactions among different ethnic groups and has limited assimilation and acculturation along class and ethnic lines. Traditional roles for women in various ethnic groups have restricted the acculturation and assimilation experience for some women.

The density of the population and the location of the immigrant communities influence the rate and character of incorporation of some immigrants into the mainstream culture. Most immigrants live in densely populated areas of California, Texas, New York, Florida, New Jersey, and Illinois (Fix & Zimmerman, 1993; U.S. Bureau of the Census, 1996). Seventy-eight percent of all recent immigrant children attend school in just five states—California, Florida, Illinois, New York, and Texas—with 45% attending school in California (Board on Children and Families, 1995). Concentration of immigrants in communities in urban cities of the Northeast and in isolated communities of the South and Midwest limits contact between immigrants and mainstream Americans and tends to inhibit the processes of acculturation and assimilation. It can be assumed that adults who remain at home or are employed within the community are more likely to hold customs, language, values, and beliefs of the country of origin than children who attend school or adults who are employed outside the community.

The children and grandchildren of immigrants retain fewer of the ancestral cultural values than their ancestors do. This is largely owing to attendance in public schools and the interaction with children from other cultures. The language of the home is often lost or does not keep pace with the growing language skills necessary for academic achievement. Although some second- and third-generation immigrants choose to abandon their ancestral customs and traditions, many retain a sense of identity and affiliation with their ethnic group through family and community ties.

The models for assimilation and acculturation have come into question in recent years. As the United States enters the twenty-first century, its future as an ethnically plural society is questioned. There is need for a new paradigm that encompasses the faith of all Americans by embracing them in their many diversities.

Cultural Diversity in a New America

The three waves of immigration, the adoption of the cultural-pluralism model, and the barriers to acculturation and assimilation have resulted in an America that is culturally and linguistically diverse. The 1990 U.S. Census report on ancestry identified more than 215 ancestral groups in response to the question "What is your ancestry of ethnic origin?" (Vecoli, 1995; U.S. Bureau of the Census, 1990). The largest ancestral groups reported were, in order of magnitude, German, Irish, English, and African American. Each of these groups contained more than 20 million people (Vecoli, 1995). Groups reporting more than 6 million people were Italian, Mexican, French, Polish, Native American, Dutch, and Scotch-Irish groups; another 28 groups reported more than 1 million each. The rich complexity of diversity in America is marked by the plethora of groups that reported fewer than 1 million members each, including Hmong, Maltese, Honduran, Carpatho-Rusyns, Nigerian, and Egyptian groups (U.S. Bureau of the Census, 1990).

Religious Diversity

The importance of religious diversity to the founding of the United States is shown in the guarantee of religious freedom in the First Amendment to the Constitution. Many early settlers came to the country in search of religious freedom. They were primarily Protestants of many denominations and sects. Groups who came for religious freedom were Irish, German, Italian, Eastern European, and, more recently, Hispanic Roman Catholics. The Slavic Christian and Jewish immigrants from Central and Eastern Europe established Judaism and orthodoxy as major religious bodies. As a result of Middle East and African immigration, as well as the conversion of many African Americans, there are currently more than 4–5 million Muslims in the United States (Barrett et al., 2001). In addition, there are 5.6 millions persons who practice Judaism, 2.4 million Buddhists, and 1 million Hindus. In addition, there are more than 28,000 persons who practice Baháĺ

Faith, making them the eleventh largest religion in the country, and more than 47,000 who practice American Indian religions (Kosman & Seymour, 1990). Each religion has its own beliefs and practices that affect the identification of communication disorders and the delivery of services to those with communication disorders.

All cultural or ethnic groups have definable implicit characteristics in universal categories of behavior, including views toward education and health care. Many of these beliefs are embedded in religion. Health care in Western or European cultures is based on germ theory (i.e., the theory that a disease or disorder is caused by a germ or a physical malady within the body). To restore health, one must destroy the germ or repair malfunction of the body. For example, by the study of genetics, European medicine hopes to identify the gene related to certain disorders and, by controlling or altering the genetic structure, control the emergence of the disorder. Also, by attempting to identify a specific virus that causes a disease, scientists hope to develop vaccines to control or a medicine to cure the disease. If one can identify the germs or viruses causing or related to the disease, then one can control the disease or effect a cure. Those who hold this view of medicine are more likely to seek medical care through medicine or rehabilitation.

Non-European and, often, Eastern views of health care see a connection between illness and internal forces. People who have this point of view believe that health is the result of physical or spiritual harmony with nature and that illness and disease are the result of spiritual or internal disharmony. Eastern medicine and health care is intended to restore harmony. Those with this belief are more likely to seek relief through prayer, incantations, or religious ceremony than through medicine, rehabilitation, or therapy.

Other cultural groups see disease as the result of a specific punishment for an ill deed or religious failing. People with these beliefs are more likely to accept a disorder or illness as a burden that they are obligated to bear. These people do not usually seek assistance from a person who does not share their cultural beliefs (Cole, 1989).

Linguistic Diversity

According to data from the 1990 Census, there are 26 languages other than English spoken at home by nearly 32 million people 5 years of age and older in the United States (U.S. Bureau of the Census, 1996). As shown in Table 1-2, more than 17 million people in the United States speak Spanish at home. Other languages spoken at home by more than 1 million residents include French, German, Italian, and Chinese. Many other languages are spoken by fewer than 1 million residents and include Tagalog, Polish, Korean,

Table 1-2   Languages Spoken at Home by People 5 Years of Age and Older

Language	Number of Speakers (in Thousands)	Language	Number of Speakers (in Thousands)
Speak only English	198,601	Hindi (Urdu)	331
Spanish	17,339	Russian	242
French	1,702	Yiddish	213
German	1,547	Thai (Laotian)	206
Italian	1,309	Persian	202
Chinese	1,249	French Creole	188
Tagalog	843	Armenian	150
Polish	430	Navaho	149
Korean	626	Hungarian	148
Vietnamese	507	Hebrew	144
Portuguese	430	Dutch	143
Japanese	428	Mon-Khmer	127
Greek	388	Gujarathi	102
Arabic	355		

Vietnamese, Portuguese, Japanese, Greek, Arabic, Hindi, Russian, Yiddish, Thai, Persian, and French Creole (U.S. Bureau of the Census, 2000).

The U.S. Bureau of the Census (1990) estimated that 1.8 million school-age children live in households in which no one older than age 14 years speaks English well. Although these figures are not restricted to immigrant children, they contribute to the number of children who are identified as limited English proficient.

As shown in Table 1-3, the number of people who speak English "less than well" increases with age from 37.8% of school-age children to 47.2% for those older than 65 years of age (U.S. Bureau of the Census, 1996). The same pattern is shown for those who speak Asian languages at home. This has implications for the assessment and intervention of older Americans who are at greater risk for neurologic disease and hearing impairment.

Communication Disorders in a Multicultural Society

The need for speech-language pathologists and audiologists to understand communication disorders in a multicultural society was recognized soon after the passing of the Civil Rights Act in 1964. There was a grow-

Table 1-3   People 5 Years of Age and Older Who Speak a Language Other Than English at Home and Those Who Speak English Less Than "Very Well"

Age Group and Language Spoken at Home	Number of People Who Speak the Language (in Thousands)	Percent Who Speak English Less Than "Very Well"
5 Yrs old and older		
Speak only English	198,601	—
Speak Spanish (or Creole)	17,345	47.9
Speak Asian/PI language	4,472	54.1
Speak a language other than English, Asian/PI, or Spanish	10,028	32.4
5–17 Yrs old		
Speak only English	39,020	—
Speak Spanish (or Creole)	4,168	39.3
Speak Asian/PI language	816	44.2
Speak a language other than English, Spanish, or Asian/PI	1,340	29.2
18–64 Yrs old		
Speak only English	153,908	—
Speak Spanish (or Creole)	12,121	49.6
Speak Asian/PI language	3,301	54.7
Speak a language other than English, Asian/PI, or Spanish	6,286	31.4
65 Yrs and older		
Speak only English	27,381	—
Speak Spanish (or Creole)	1,057	62.3
Speak Asian/PI language	355	72.0
Speak a language other than English, Asian/PI, or Spanish	2,402	36.9

PI = Pacific Islander.
Source: Adapted from U.S. Bureau of the Census. (1990). *Statistical abstract of the United States: 1995 (115th ed.). No. 57: Persons speaking a language other than English at home by age and language: 1990* (pp. 53). Washington, DC: U.S. Bureau of the Census.

ing concern that African American children who spoke African American English were being inappropriately classified as having speech-language disorders. Speech-language pathologists and sociolinguists began the study of communication disorders in multicultural populations in response to the need for understanding the linguistic skills of African American children in schools. In recognition of the growing concern, the American Speech-Language-Hearing Association (ASHA) adopted a position paper on social dialects (ASHA, 1983) that recognized that any dialect of English was a legitimate form of the language and that dialect was not to be considered a pathologic form of English.

Although initially the concern was for African Americans, the need to study cultural diversity in communication disorders grew in direct relationship to the third wave of U.S. immigration, the non-European cultural origins of the new immigrants, and the changes in acculturation and assimilation patterns of the new immigrants.

Not only did the increase in immigration population that began in the 1970s continue into the 1980s and 1990s, but the new immigrants were also more diverse than before, arriving from a broad spectrum of countries encompassing a range of linguistic variables and increasingly non-European cultural backgrounds. Concerns about cultural and linguistic diversity that once were directed at African American children were related to other ethnic minority groups. In 1985, ASHA published *Clinical management of communicatively handicapped minority language populations* in recognition of the need to address the needs of those from various cultural and linguistic backgrounds in speech-language and hearing programs (ASHA, 1985).

Communication Disorders in Culturally Diverse Populations

There are few reliable data on the general prevalence or incidence of communication disorders among culturally and linguistically diverse populations in the United States. Estimates are based on projections from data based on the mainstream population. The National Health Interview Survey indicates that there is a greater prevalence of communication disorders among racial and ethnic minorities than among white individuals (Benson & Marano, 1994). ASHA estimates that 10% of the U.S. population has a disorder of speech, hearing, or language unrelated to the ability to speak English as a native language (Cole, 1989). If the prevalence of communication disorders among racial and ethnic minorities is consistent with that of the general population, then it is estimated that 6.2 million culturally and linguistically diverse Americans have a communication disorder.

Diversity among Children in Special Education

In 1999, 38% of students enrolled in public elementary and secondary schools in the United States were African American, Hispanic, Asian/Pacific Islander, or American Indian/Alaskan Native (National Center for Education Statistics, 2001). It was projected that between 1995 and

Table 1-4   Race/Ethnicity of Preschool Children Receiving Special Education and of the General Preschool Population, 1998–1999

	General Population (%)	Special Education Population (%)
White (non-Hispanic)	63.3	68.9
Hispanic	17.2	12.0
Black (non-Hispanic)	15.8	15.7
Asian/Pacific Islander	4.2	2.0
American Indian	0.9	1.3

Source: Adapted from U.S. Office of Special Education Programs. (2000). *Twenty-Second Annual Report to Congress on the Implementation of IDEA*. Washington, DC: U.S. Department of Education.

2005 there would be a 30% increase in Hispanic/Latino children and a nearly 40% increase among Asian/Pacific Islander children enrolled in the public schools (Office of Special Education Programs, 2000). The Individuals with Disabilities Education Act (IDEA) Amendments of 1997 required that the states report by race and ethnicity the number of preschool and school-aged children served. Data were collected in five categories: American Indian, Asian/Pacific Islander, Black (non-Hispanic), Hispanic, and white (non-Hispanic). The disparities in race/ethnicity distribution of the population of students served by IDEA and the general population of students are shown in Tables 1-2 and 1-3. The data reported for 1998–1999 indicate that the racial/ethnic distribution of the general preschool population versus the special education preschool population was, on average, generally comparable (Table 1-4). However, Hispanic and Asian/Pacific Islander preschool children were slightly underrepresented in the special education preschool population. Conversely, white non-Hispanic children were slightly overrepresented among preschool children receiving special education and related services.

The race and ethnicity distribution of the population of students served under IDEA and the general population of students aged 6–21 years also showed some disparities (Table 1-5). In general, Asian/Pacific Islander and white students were underrepresented in the special education population, whereas African American and American Indian students were overrepresented. Hispanic students were the only group that was represented at the rate comparable to its representation in the general population.

Asian/Pacific Islander students represent 3.8% of the general population; however, students receiving special education services in all disability categories represent only 1.7% of the population. This percentage varies by disability area. In the areas of hearing impairment (4.6%), autism (4.7%), and

Table 1-5   Percentage of Students Ages 6–21 Years Served by Disability and Race/Ethnicity in the 1998–1999 School Year

Disability	*American Indian*	*Asian/ Pacific Islander*	*Black (Non-Hispanic)*	*Hispanic*	*White (Non-Hispanic)*
Learning disabilities	1.4	1.4	18.3	15.8	63.0
Speech-language impairment	1.2	2.4	16.5	11.6	68.3
Mental retardation	1.1	1.7	34.3	88.9	54.1
Emotional disturbance	1.1	1.0	26.4	9.8	61.6
Multiple disabilities	1.4	2.3	19.3	10.9	66.1
Hearing impairment	1.4	4.6	16.8	16.3	66.0
Orthopedic impairment	0.8	3.0	14.6	14.4	67.2
Other health impairment	1.0	1.3	14.1	7.8	75.8
Visual impairment	1.3	3.0	14.8	11.4	69.5
Autism	0.7	4.7	20.9	9.4	64.4
Deaf-blindness	1.8	11.3	11.5	12.1	63.3
Traumatic brain injury	1.6	2.3	15.9	10.0	70.2
Developmental delay	0.5	1.1	33.7	4.0	60.8
All disabilities	1.3	1.7	20.2	13.2	63.6
Resident population	1.0	3.8	14.8	14.2	66.2

Source: Adapted from Office of Special Education Programs. (2000). *Twenty-Second Annual Report to Congress on the Implementation of IDEA.* Washington, DC: U.S. Department of Education.

deaf-blindness (11.2%), the representation of the Asian/Pacific Islander students is greater than their representation in the general population.

Black (non-Hispanic) students account for 14.8% of the general population of children aged 6 through 21 years; however, they represent 20.2% of the children receiving special education in all disabilities. In 10 of the 13 disability categories, African American (non-Hispanic) children equaled or exceeded their representation in the general population. The representation of African American students in mental retardation (34.3%) and developmental delay (33.7%) categories was more than twice the national population estimates.

Hispanic students in special education (13.2%) were generally similar to their representation in the general population (14.2%). However, they were overrepresented in three categories: specific learning disabilities (15.8%), hearing impairment (16.3%), and orthopedic impairments (14.4%).

American Indian students represent 1% of the general population and 1.3% of the children receiving special education services. They exceeded the national average in nine disability categories, reaching the largest percentages in deaf-blindness (1.8%) and traumatic brain injury (1.6%).

White (non-Hispanic) students made up the smaller percentage of special education (63.6%) than in the general population (66.2%). However, they are overrepresented in five disability categories: speech-language impairments (68.3%), orthopedic impairments (67.2%), other health impairments (75.8%), visual impairments (69.5%), and traumatic brain injury (70.2%).

Common causes given for the disproportionate representation of African Americans and Hispanics in special education include (1) poverty, (2) cultural bias in referral and assessment, and (3) unique factors related to race and ethnicity. Reschly (1996) and Wagner and Blackorg (1996) implicate poverty and the lack of access to health care caused by poverty with resulting low birth weight as factors that affect a population's representation in special education programs. More than 30% of the children with disabilities live in households in which the annual income (in 1986 dollars) was less than $25,000 (Office of Special Education Programs, 2000). According to the U.S. Department of Health and Human Services (1985), economically disadvantaged children are more predisposed to disorders related to environmental, teratogenic, nutritional, and traumatic factors than other groups. For example, exposure to carbon monoxide and other chemicals and pesticides found in the air, paint, soil, and plumbing of older homes often located in poverty areas has teratogenic effects on the neurologic functions of young children.

The incidence of neurologic impairments, some of which lead to communication disorders, due to the absorption of lead has been found to be higher in nonwhite children than in white children (National Center for Health Statistics, 1994). In addition, although some people from ethnic minority communities have the same types of communication disorders as those in the dominant population, incidences, causes, and effects can be different, indicating different approaches to treatment. For example, African Americans succumb to stroke 306 times more often than white individuals, and strokes occur in African Americans at an earlier age (Singletary, 1993). Although 11% of the deaths among white Americans are from stroke, 13% of the deaths among African Americans are from stroke (U.S. Department of Health and Human Services, 1985). Death rates from hemorrhage, thrombosis, and embolism (the major types of strokes) are higher for African Americans than for white individuals (Singletary, 1993). This is thought to be related to increases in hypertension, differences in diet, and lack of access to health care.

Access to Health Care

Access to health care and health insurance is a critical issue for the immigrant population in the United States. This issue affects the physical and mental well-being of families, as well as the ability to adapt to the culture of the United States. For many immigrants, especially children, the immigration process itself is an event of extraordinary stress. Immigrants are often torn by conflicting social and cultural demands while trying to adapt to an unfamiliar and sometimes hostile and discriminatory environment with limited or no use of the English language. In addition, undocumented immigrants deal with the stress or fear of deportation and separation from family members.

For some immigrants, health worsens in the United States. A study of aggregate data across all immigrant groups found that on virtually every measure of health status, immigrants who had lived in the United States 5 years or less were healthier than those who had lived in the United States more than 10 years (Rumbaut, 1995). The findings were explained by a number of factors, including (1) existing physical conditions that were masked during the early years after immigration, (2) deterioration of health due to limited access to health care, and (3) socioeconomic factors. The data point to the importance of identifying conditions under which immigrants do well and those that produce negative health outcomes. Among the factors to consider are family networks and social supports, relationships within families, the effect of mobility on children's lives, segmented assimilation into different kinds of contexts, and cultural medical practices from the country of origin.

Rumbaut (1995) found that generation effects and length-of-residence effects have confirmed associations between these variables and health. For example, difficult pregnancies, low birth weight, and infant mortality increased among Hispanic populations with subsequent immigrant generations in the United States. In contrast, Indochinese immigrants in San Diego County who appeared to be at risk for poor infant health due to high levels of unemployment, poverty, welfare dependence, and depression were found to have much lower infant mortality rates than the average resident in San Diego County. This was explained by the nearly universal absence of tobacco, alcohol, and drug abuse among Indochinese women, even though they had less access to prenatal care.

Becoming a Clinician in a Multicultural Society and Understanding Cultural Variables

Understanding another culture is a continuous, not discrete, process. Identifying the sources of cultural conflict while providing clinical services to those from cultures different from one's own involves far more than learning about the implicit and explicit variables of a culture. It is important for speech-language pathologists and audiologists to understand the importance of potential sources of cultural conflict in the clinic.

Monocultural assumptions in providing clinical services are not currently relevant. Most literature on communication disorders, intervention, and treatment in multicultural populations assumes that the clinician is a member of the majority culture and that the client is a member of a minority culture. This is a logical conclusion, because less than 5% of the members of the ASHA identify themselves as nonwhite. It is more accurate to take a broad view of the use of the term *multicultural* or *cross-cultural* clinical services. The clinician and the client may differ by culture, racial and ethnic group, sex, age, socioeconomic class, gender, or religion, to name but a few cultural variables that can affect the clinical interaction. The clinician must look to the various parameters of differences, as well as those of similarity, and construct the clinical management program accordingly. Clinicians realize that they must understand their own culture and cultural assumptions, as well as those of the client. Whether there is a cultural conflict must be considered in the interaction. The culturally competent clinician seeks continuous self-assessment regarding cultural differences. The clinician needs knowledge and resources to be competent to provide clinical services in an increasingly culturally diverse world.

In becoming a culturally competent clinician, it is important to consider culture-bound variables and language-communication–bound variables. Culture-bound conceptualizations have many variables. Among the most important in studying communication disorders in the multicultural society is the importance of individuals and groups in the culture, power and distance, time orientation, and several dimensions of verbal and nonverbal communication.

Individualism and Collectivism

Individualism emphasizes the individual. In collectivism, on the other hand, group goals have precedence over individual goals. Individuals from individualistic cultures are supposed to look after themselves and their immediate family. Individuals from cultures of collectivism look after the needs of the entire group in their social network. Although individualism and collectivism exist in every culture in varying degrees, cultures in which individualism tends to predominate include but are not limited to the European countries. Cultures in which collectivism tends to predominate include but are not limited to Arab, African, Asian, and Hispanic cultures (Brislin, 1994). Individualism and collectivism play an important role in clinical encounters. These factors affect the client's willingness to establish individual goals and expectations for the individual or the family or group.

The Power-Distance Variable

The power-distance variable focuses on the social relationships between people of different statuses (i.e., superiors and subordinates). This can extend to relationships between men and women. People from high power-distance cultures do not question the orders or suggestions of superiors. On the other hand, people in low power-distance cultures do not necessarily accept superiors' orders. When the clinician and the client are from two different systems, misunderstanding in making and following clinical recommendations is possible.

Time Orientation

Time orientation differs across cultures. When the culture is long-term and future oriented, the establishing of long-term goals and priorities is highly valued. When the focus of the culture is on the past, the establishment of long-term goals is not as relevant as preserving the present and the establishment of short-term, more readily attainable goals. Western cultures are more often oriented toward the future. Many non-Western cultures are focused on the past, as shown by their respect for elders and ancestors.

Nonverbal and Verbal Communication Styles

Language and communication styles are highly correlated with race, culture, and ethnicity. All ethnic groups have communication styles that have major implications for clinical services. These language differences have verbal and nonverbal dimensions.

Nonverbal Communication Styles

In nonverbal communication, information is transmitted by means other than words. This can involve many behaviors, including proxemics, kinesics, eye contact, paralanguage, silence, and directness. Proxemics, or the use of personal space and conversational distance in communication, differs across cultures. Kinesics, or the use of body movements (e.g., facial expressions, smiling, head positioning and nodding, hand shaking, and eye contact), has also been shown to differ across cultures (Battle, 1997). In addition, paralanguage variables such as silence, loudness, inflection, and stress vary across cultures and can affect the clinical relationship.

Verbal Communication Styles

Verbal communication can also vary across cultures. In addition to the barriers created by differences in the linguistic contrasts between the languages of the client and the clinician, differences in word meanings can affect the clinical encounter. The meanings of words such as *bad* or *normal* can vary across cultures. Pragmatics, or the way language is used in greeting, taking compliments, and more ritualized social rules, can affect the clinical encounter. Social distance can also affect the role that the individuals play in the communication process. In Western cultures, conversation tends to be horizontal, with each person in the communication event having equal responsibility and freedom within the conversation. In non-Western cultures, patterns of communication tend to be vertical, with conversation flowing from those of higher prestige to those of lower prestige (Battle, 1997; Sue & Sue, 1990).

Conclusion

In becoming a culturally competent clinician, it is important to develop an awareness of the beliefs and attitudes held by the clinician and by the clients. Multicultural awareness is not an end in itself. It is, rather, a means of increasing a clinician's power, energy, and freedom of choice in a multicultural world (Pedersen, 1988; Lynch & Hanson, 1998). Clinicians need to become culturally aware of their own values and beliefs before they can adjust to the value system of others. Clinicians should understand and value the differences that exist among clients and should develop an awareness of the cultural, verbal, and nonverbal factors that influence the clinical situation.

In developing a cultural awareness, the clinician should ask, "What can I do to serve this client in a culturally appropriate manner?" and "How can I best serve this client according to his or her cultural, as well as clinical, needs?"

Clinicians must develop an understanding of the sociopolitical systems operating in the United States and an understanding of the sociopolitical history faced by the client. This knowledge helps the clinician understand the institutional and historical barriers that affect the client as a member of a particular group. This knowledge can also help the clinician understand the client's response to treatment and interaction in the clinical situation.

Finally, clinicians in a multicultural society must develop skills in interacting with clients from a variety of cultures with myriad cultural and linguistic variables, none of which is the same for different clients (Lynch & Hanson, 1998). Clinicians should be able to send and receive verbal and nonverbal messages appropriately in each culturally different context.

References

American Speech-Language-Hearing Association. (1985). Clinical management of communicatively handicapped minority language populations. *ASHA, 26*(1), 55–57.

American Speech-Language-Hearing Association. (1983). Social dialects: A position paper. *ASHA, 25*(1), 23–24.

Barrett, D., Kurian, G. T., & Johnson, T. M. (2001). *World Christian encyclopedia: A comparative survey of churches and religions* (AD 30–AD 220). London: Oxford University Press.

Battle, D. (1997). Multicultural considerations in counseling communicatively disordered persons and their families. In T. Crowe (Ed.), *Applications of counseling in speech-language pathology and audiology* (pp. 118–144). Baltimore: Williams & Wilkins.

Benson, C. A., & Marano, A. (1994). *Current estimates from the national health interview survey* (United States Vital Health Statistics Series 16 No. 173). Washington, DC: National Center for Health Statistics.

Board on Children and Families. (1995). Immigrant children and their families: issues for research and policy. In R. E. Behrman (Ed.), *The future of children: Critical issues for children and youths* (Vol. 5) (pp. 72–89). Los Angeles: The Center for the Future of Children, The David and Lucille Packard Foundation.

Brislin, R. W. (1994). *Intercultural training: An introduction.* Thousand Oaks, CA: Sage.

Cheng, L., & Butler, K. (1993, March). *Difficult discourse: Designing connections to deflect language impairment.* Paper presented at the annual meeting of the California Speech-Language-Hearing Association, Palm Springs, CA.

Cole, L. (1989). *E pluribus unum*: Multicultural imperatives for the 1990's and beyond. *American Speech-Language-Hearing Association, 31*(2), 65–70.

Fernandez, E. W., & Robinson, J. G. (1994). *Illustrative ranges of the distribution of undocumented immigrants by state.* Technical working paper no. 8 in U.S. Bureau of the Census. Statistical yearbook annual. Washington, DC: U.S. Immigration and Naturalization Service.

Fix, M., & Passel, J. (1994). *Immigration and immigrants: Setting the record straight.* Washington, DC: Urban Institute.

Fix, M., & Zimmerman, W. (1993). *Educating immigrant children.* Washington, DC: Urban Institute.

Galens, S., Sheets, A., & Young, R. V. (1995). *Gale encyclopedia of multicultural America.* New York: Gale Research, Inc.

Gudykunst, W. B., & Nishida, T. (1984). Individual and cultural influences on understanding reduction. Communication Monographs, 51, 23–26.

Hall, E. T. (1959). *The silent language.* New York: Doubleday.

Ima, K., & Keogh, P-E. (1995). "The crying father" and "My father doesn't love me": Selected observations and reflections on Southeast Asians and special education. In L. L. Cheng (Ed.), *Integrating language and learning for inclusion: An Asian-Pacific focus* (pp. 149–177). San Diego: Singular Publishing.

Keesling, R. (1974). Theories of culture. *Annual Review of Anthropology, 3,* 73–97.

Kosman, B. A., & Seymour, P. L. (1990). *National Survey of Religious Identification (NSRI).* New York: Graduate School of the City University of New York.

Lynch, E. W., & Hanson, M. J. (Eds.). (1998). *Developing cross-cultural competence: A guide for working with young children and their families* (2nd ed.). Baltimore: Brookes.

Magocsi, P. R. (1995). Russian Americans. In J. Galens, A. Sheets, & R. V. Young (Eds.), *Gale encyclopedia of multicultural America* (pp. 1159–1170). New York: Gale Research, Inc.

Morrison, J., & Zabusky, C. F. (1980). *American mosaic: The immigrant experience in the words of those who lived it.* New York: E. P. Dutton.

National Center for Education Statistics. (2001). *Racial/ethnic distribution of public school students.* Washington, DC: United States Department of Education.

National Center for Health Statistics. (1994). *Healthy United States, 1993.* Hyattsville, MD: Public Health Service.

Office of Special Education Programs. (2000). *22nd Annual Report to Congress on the Implementation of IDEA.* Washington, DC: Office of Special Education and Rehabilitative Services.

Pedersen, P. (1988). *A handbook for developing multicultural awareness.* Alexandria, VA: American Association for Counseling and Development.

Reschly, D. J. (1996). Identification and assessment of students with disabilities. In *The future of children: Special education for children with disabilities* (Vol. 6) (pp. 40–53). Los Angeles: The Center for the Future of Children, The David and Lucille Packard Foundation.

Rumbaut, R. G. (1995). A legacy of war: Refugees from Vietnam, Laos, and Cambodia. In S. Pedraza & R. G. Rumbault (Eds.), *Origins and destinies: Immigration, race, and ethnicity in America* (pp. 583–621). Belmont, CA: Wadsworth.

Singletary, J. (1993). *The Black health guide to stroke.* New York: Holt.

Sue, D. W., & Sue, D. (1990). *Counseling the culturally different.* New York: Wiley.

U.S. Bureau of the Census. (1990). *Statistical abstract of the United States* (110th ed.). Washington, DC: U.S. Bureau of the Census.

U.S. Bureau of the Census. (1996). *Statistical abstract of the United States* (116th ed.). Washington, DC: U.S. Bureau of the Census.

U.S. Bureau of the Census. (2000). *Statistical abstract of the United States* (120th ed.). Washington, DC: U.S. Bureau of the Census.

U.S. Department of Health and Human Services. (1985). *Report of the secretary's task force on black and minority health* (Vol. 1). *Executive Summary* (Pub. No. 491-313/44706). Washington, DC: U.S. Department of Health and Human Services.

U.S. Office of Special Education Programs. (2000). *Twenty-Second Annual Report to Congress on the Implementation of IDEA.* Washington, DC: U.S. Department of Education.

Vecoli, R. J. (1995). Introduction. In J. Galens, A. Sheets, & R. V. Young (Eds.), *Gale encyclopedia of multicultural America* (pp. xxi–xxvii). New York: Gale Research.

Wagner, M., & Blackorg, J. (1996). Transition from high school to work or college: How special education students fare. In R. E. Behrman (Ed.), *The future of children: Special education for children with disabilities* (Vol. 6) (pp. 103–120). Los Angeles: The Center for the Future of Children, The David and Lucille Packard Foundation.

Additional Resources

Cheng, L. (1995). *Integrating language and learning for inclusion: An Asian-Pacific focus.* San Diego: Singular Publishing.

2

African Americans in the Americas

Sandra L. Terrell and Rudolph S. Jackson

A Brief History of Africans in the Americas

The history of people of African descent in the Americas can be traced to the largest involuntary migration movement in modern times. From the sixteenth to the nineteenth centuries, nearly 40 million people from the countries of West Africa were forced to leave their homelands and were sold into slavery. More than 20 million Africans were brought to the New World, the countries of Central and South America, the Caribbean, and North America.

As many as 80% of the inhabitants of the Caribbean countries of Jamaica, Haiti, the Dominican Republic, the Bahamas, and Barbados descended from countries in West Africa. Although they share the common history of slavery, they took on the cultural roots of the British Empire, which controlled the area during the period of slavery. The British influence remains in the area and can be seen in the customs, models of education, and language and dialects used in the countries once dominated by the British Empire. Many of the Caribbean countries speak a dialect of English. Some speak Spanish, German, and French. In Haiti, because of the control of the island by the French, the people speak a dialect of French and English.

The people of African descent in South America and the Caribbean share a heritage of life in the Americas different from that of those in North America (Willis, 1992). Many Caribbean people of African descent made a second migration to North America in search of educational and economic opportunities and freedom from political oppression.

The Caribbean descendants of Africa and new African immigrants share a common genealogical root with African Americans, but the history of the Africans who were brought to the United States in slavery is different. This distinction is necessary as speech-language pathologists and audiologists come to understand the cultural parameters associated with service delivery to African Americans. It is important to understand that the material that follows cannot be applied uniformly to those in America who appear to have an African heritage. It is important that the speech-language pathologist and audiologist identify the ancestral root of the client to determine the specific psychological, cultural, and linguistic variables that impact service delivery for that client.

African Americans are currently the largest racial minority group in the United States (U.S. Bureau of the Census, 2000). The more than 35 million blacks in the United States are largely descended from West Africa. The history of slavery of Africans in America has not only involved economic conditions, but also sociocultural and psychological factors that influence speech and language. Additionally, the vestiges of slavery in the United States have resulted in disparities in the delivery of health care among African Americans, including delivery of speech-language, audiology, and related health care services. This chapter focuses on several of these variables that are important for clinical assessment, intervention, and general access to health care services.

Cultural Variables among African Americans

African American Music

Music has long played an important role in the life of African American people. Music developed by African American people, especially jazz and blues, is one of America's greatest artistic contributions to world culture (Jones, 1963). Butcher (1964) identified three types of African American music—Negro folk music—including original work songs, the blues, and jazz, a direct descendant of the blues. The first African immigrants to North America brought their native music with them. The "work songs" that were sung in the fields in Africa became "sorrow songs" in America. Negro spirituals developed from the work songs. Spirituals expressed messages such as the hell of hard trials and great tribulations; wanderings in some lonesome valley or down some unknown road; or being a long way from home, with a brother, sister, father, mother, wife, husband, or child sold, dead, or gone. The words often contained cleverly coded messages that had one meaning for slave owners but a different meaning for other slaves. For example, spirituals such as "Steal Away, Steal Away Home: I Ain't Got Long to Stay Here" and "The Old Ship of Zion, Get on Board" were thought by slave owners to be songs of prayer; however, slaves heard underlying messages. Depending on when, where, and by whom the songs were sung, the songs reflected the intent of a slave to run away to freedom or were a sign to indicate the location of the next station in the Underground Railroad (a secret pathway the slaves followed from South to North). For example, "Down by the Riverside" was used to tell those wishing to escape slavery to meet at a specified time by the river.

After the Civil War and the abolition of slavery, African American music adapted to a different set of circumstances. The blues were typically a simple, frank, and honest portrayal of conditions at the time. They expressed love, family life, or general dissatisfaction with a cold and trouble-filled world.

An understanding of the importance of African American music to African Americans is critical to clinicians providing services to African American clients. Many professional offices play classical or popular easy-listening music in the clinic waiting room. This music may make African Americans feel uncomfortable and out of place. Better clinical rapport may be obtained if music consistent with the African American culture is played in the waiting room in areas serving African American clients. Because jazz is universally accepted as a part of American culture, it is appropriate in clinic waiting rooms. In addition, when music is used as a part of an intervention program, it is appropriate to use music consistent with the client's culture.

Religion

Religion plays an important role in the lives of many African Americans. The African American church is often the center of social events in the community and is the primary place where pride and self-respect among African Americans have been preserved (Blake & Darling, 2000). Because the church serves an important function in the lives of African Americans, it is not uncommon to hear African Americans express religious themes in clinical settings. In conversations, the client may refer to religious themes such as getting the spirit and seeing visions or hearing voices. He or she may also use biblical quotes and phrases such as "Yes, Lord" and "Amen."

Some African American clergy have a harsh or hoarse vocal quality because of their emotional manner of delivering sermons. They may sometimes deliver 2- or 3-hour-long sermons on a given Sunday. The African American preacher is likely to be resistant to treatment recommendations that call for complete vocal rest for a period of time, as this is in direct conflict with his or her "calling" to preach. Gospel singers also may have voice problems related to singing, using untrained voices in spiritual and emotional gospel song. Clinicians should provide treatment for African American preachers and gospel singers in a manner that is sensitive to the spiritual and emotional nature of the African American religious tradition. That is, they should provide treatment and vocal techniques that will ensure vocal health while preserving the ability to deliver sermons and music in a manner consistent with cultural tradition.

Names

African Americans regard their names as extremely important. Names for children are selected with great care. The chosen name often reflects the person or characteristics the family wishes to reflect or some social value, such as faith, hope, or chastity.

When Africans first experienced the involuntary immigration to America, they were frequently stripped of their given African names and given simple to pronounce, one- or two-syllable names. Slaves often took the last names of their owners. Many African Americans still carry these last names. Terrell, for example, was the name of a Georgia plantation owner. Some slaves adopted names such as Freeman or Newman that expressed their newly acquired freedom. Others took on the names of important historical figures, such as Washington and Jefferson.

During slavery and long afterward, white individuals rarely addressed African Americans by their last names. Regardless of status or age, African Americans were called by their first name or were simply addressed as "boy," "girl," "uncle," or "aunt." The African Americans used a variety of tactics to counteract this practice. Some gave their children first names of formal address, such as Miss, Princess, Duke, General, and Mister. The slave owners then had little choice but to use these titles when talking to or calling them. Use of terms such as "boy" or "girl" to address an African American is considered culturally offensive. Like their ancestors, African American parents today take great care in selecting names for their children. Some African American parents give their children African names such as LaShawn, Shemeika, Shurtjhana, Latifa, Tanzania, Ivanna Samal, Amani Shama, and Elon Jahdal. Many of these names have important meanings, and, as the child grows, the parents share these meanings with the child.

African American adults resent the use of their first names by clinicians and consider it a presumptuous practice. Clinicians should always address adult clients by the surname until and unless given permission to use the given name. They should also use their own title and surname with all clients, regardless of age, because the use of title and surname is a sign of respect.

It is insulting to an African American child for an adult who is not a member of the child's family or circle of close friends to use a nickname or diminutive form of the child's name. Clinicians should never reduce Shemeika to Mikky or Deborah to Debbie, even if this is the name the child's parents and friends use. Clinicians should always ask the client (or parent) the name of preference and learn how to pronounce and spell the name correctly. To do otherwise is perceived as "calling the person out of his or her name" (an insult) that can negatively affect the clinical service-delivery process.

Health

There are several diseases that are particularly related to speech, language, and hearing disorders among African Americans. These diseases include sickle cell disease, stroke, and lead poisoning.

Sickle Cell Anemia

Sickle cell disease, also referred to as *sickle cell anemia*, is a genetic disorder that affects a number of racial groups, but it primarily occurs among persons of African ancestry. Sickle cell disease results in a misshapen sickle-shape to the normally round red blood cells. The clumping of these cells in the veins and capillaries results in blockages in vital organs of the body, producing pain and in some instances, stroke with resulting aphasia. The clumping can also occur within the *stria vascularis*, resulting in sensorineural hearing loss that can become progressively permanent with successive sickle cell crises. (See Chapter 11 for a more comprehensive discussion of sickle cell disease and hearing loss.)

In addition to stroke and hearing loss, sickle cell disease may impact speech and language development. Children with sickle cell disease often experience severe pain and anemia. The anemia occurs because the spleen destroys the abnormal, sickled red blood cells faster than the body can produce new cells. Because red blood cells carry oxygen within the body, the activity of the spleen causes a deficiency in the number of these cells, thus resulting in anemia and accompanying fatigue. Children who are affected by pain and fatigue may not be able to concentrate on their work in school or have a short attention span.

Stroke

Stroke, also referred to as *cardiovascular accident*, can result in speech and language disorders. Traditional soul food that is high in saturated fat and cholesterol, high-blood pressure, heart disease, and

cultural challenges associated with low socioeconomic status may contribute to a high occurrence of stroke with accompanying aphasia among
African American populations. Because of access to health care as well as
cultural beliefs of caring for one's own, African Americans do not receive
rehabilitation for aphasia and other results of stoke at the same rates as
other racial groups. Those that do begin treatment may not continue, as
termination rates among African Americans are nearly double that of
whites. Higher termination rates of African American clients may result
from perceptions of culturally inappropriate intervention, insensitivity to
the needs of the client and family, as well as suspicion of racial discrimination (Sue & Sue, 1990). Chapter 8 provides more information on stroke
in African American groups.

Lead Poisoning

Lead poisoning primarily affects children from 1 to 11 years
of age who live in homes and neighborhoods in which lead can be
ingested. Children who reside in homes with lead pipes and lead-based
paint and in neighborhoods that surround lead-smelting factories (that
may or may not have been dismantled) are of particular risk for lead poisoning when they ingest food and liquids prepared with water from lead
pipes, eat chips of lead paint, play in soil contaminated with lead from
factories, and breathe lead-contaminated dust particles. Because these
homes and neighborhoods are primarily urban and socioeconomically
low, lead poisoning is not strictly an African American issue but is an
issue of heterogeneity, potentially affecting anyone who resides in areas
in which lead is present.

According to the Department of Health and Human Services (2000),
there is no safe level of lead. However, the Health Department considers
lead poisoning to have occurred when the blood lead level (BLL) in a person
is greater than 10 µg per dL of blood. This is commonly referred to simply
as "10." As the BLL rises, the potential for serious developmental problems
increases. For BLLs above 15, most states require the health department in
that state to take action to remove the risk and to provide appropriate
treatment. A BLL above 70 could result in seizure, profound disability, or
death. Children who are 1 to 2 years of age are at greatest risk for lead poisoning because of their propensity to put anything into their mouths.
These young children, due to their developing nervous systems, also have
an increased susceptibility to the adverse effects of lead (Needleman &
Bellinger, 1991).

Lead is a toxic substance that can damage the nervous, circulatory, respiratory, and reproductive systems. In adults, lead poisoning can result in

fatigue, memory loss, loss of appetite, headaches, dizziness, and other symptoms. In children, lead poisoning can cause learning disabilities, lowered intelligence quotients or mental retardation, poor attention span, or other neurologic deficits. Speech, language, and reading deficits such as auditory processing difficulties and delayed speech development are also potential effects of lead poisoning among children (Campbell et. al., 1995; Pueschels, Linakis, & Anderson,1996).

There are a variety of diseases such as stroke and heart disease that are related to speech, language, and hearing disorders among African Americans. Along with the prevalence of certain diseases among African Americans, there are disparities in access to health care delivery as a function of disproportionate representation in lower socioeconomic levels by African Americans (Andrulis, 1998). Clinicians should be aware of the wide variations in health issues between racial and ethnic groups in this country.

African American English

The language used by African Americans is a cultural factor by which African Americans identify with one another. Language systems have been and continue to be dynamic forces of the culture, constantly evolving to interconnect present with past communicative styles and to create new ones (Goodenough, 1999).

A number of linguistic dialects are spoken among African Americans in the United States. Gullah is spoken by those living on islands off the coasts of South Carolina and Georgia. There are also various Creole dialects such as Jamaican Creole and dialects spoken by people who immigrated to the United States from the Caribbean countries. However, the most prominent linguistic system associated with African Americans is known as *African American English* (AAE).

AAE is a dialect of Standard American English (SAE). Over the years, it has been known by several names, reflecting the evolving racial name identification and the shifts in focus of the field of linguistics from structuralism during the 1950s and 1960s, to semantics in the 1970s, to pragmatics in the 1980s. The term *nonstandard Negro English* was used during the 1950s and early 1960s. The term *Black English* was used in the 1970s and 1980s (Dillard, 1973; Williams & Wolfram, 1976). Since the 1990s, the terms *AAE* or *African American Vernacular English* have been used. The term *Ebonics* was introduced by Williams (1975) during the 1970s to reflect the fusion of *ebony* and *phonics* and has reemerged in recent years.

AAE is a systematic, rule-governed, phonologic, grammatical, syntactic, semantic, and pragmatic system of language. Although AAE is different from SAE, it maintains enough similarity to SAE to be considered a dialect of American English, not a separate language. It includes not only the verbal spoken word but also nonverbal factors, such as body language, use of personal space, body movement, eye contact, narrative sequence, and modes of discourse. AAE patterns are not exclusive to this dialect, as they contain features that are shared by other social and regional dialects, such as Southern English.

Although largely spoken by African Americans, AAE is not spoken by all African Americans. Additionally, African Americans are not the only people who use AAE. Depending on the level and type of socialization with AAE speakers, some white individuals, Hispanics/Latinos, and Asians use AAE. Within the United States, the use of AAE varies from one speaker to the next. Its use is on a continuum that ranges from African Americans who do not use the dialect at all to those who use most AAE features in all communicative contexts (Wyatt, 1991). Age, geographic location, occupation, income, and education are a few factors that have been found to influence the level of usage of AAE among speakers (Labov, 1966; Wyatt, 1991). Furthermore, the extent to which a person identifies with the culture of the speech community has also been found to influence the use of the dialect (Terrell & Terrell, 1981). Individual speakers can also vary their use of the dialect along the continuum, switching codes depending on the communicative context (Washington & Craig, 1998).

Evolution of African American English

There is no empirical evidence that links present-day AAE to West African languages; however, there are several theoretical explanations that attempt to make this connection. One hypothesis proposes that when Europeans and Africans first met on the west coast of Africa during the 1600s, there was a need for a means of communication between the two groups. Europeans and Africans therefore used a reduced, simplified form of English called *pidgin* whenever communication for essential needs was necessary (Haskins & Butts, 1973).

Because the Africans who were brought to this country came from various locations in West Africa, it is highly likely that they did not speak one another's native languages. With no other means to communicate, the slaves began to use pidgin between themselves and when speaking to their masters. With continued use, pidgin developed into an everyday language with rules, inflections, and other systematic linguistic patterns (Burling, 1973; Haskins & Butts, 1973). Gradually, the nature of the pidgin English spoken by the slaves changed in three main ways. First, pidgin became a rule-governed system. African and English words and structures were blended by phonologic, grammatical, syntactic, and semantic rules that provided communicative competence for each speaker of that language (Coleman & Daniel, 2000). Second, this version of English became the primary mode of communication among slaves. Third, as this English variety became the only language used by the members of the slave community, children born into this community acquired this language as their native tongue. When these changes occurred, this English was no longer pidgin but became a type of Creole language.

Some of the English patterns the slaves used were forms learned from their overseers or slave owners. Patterns of AAE such as multiple negation were acceptable forms of SAE during the seventeenth and eighteenth centuries. As English evolved, these patterns became unacceptable. Because of limited contact with their slave owners, the slaves had no way of keeping up with the evolving nature of the language. Their retention of these previously SAE forms therefore resulted in some of the AAE patterns.

The slaves also incorporated sounds, grammatical markings, and vocabulary from their traditional African languages into their English. For example, many West African languages have a tense called the *habitual tense* that implies an activity of a recurring nature. The slaves relegated this habitual tense to the verb *be* when they learned English, because it most closely approximated the habitual tense. The statement "he be going" means "he usually goes" or "he always goes." This linguistic pattern was not only found in the language of the slaves, but also in a feature of AAE and of dialects spoken by many black individuals outside the United States (Haskins & Butts, 1973).

In addition to grammatical features, slaves infused West African words into their English. Some of these African words are incorporated into English and are familiar to many SAE speakers. Words with African origins include *goober, tote, cola, jazz, juke* (as in *jukebox*), and *jive*. The word *john*, meaning the customer of a prostitute, is derived from an African word that is translated as "someone who can be easily exploited." Additionally, the word *okay*, and the sounds "uh-uh" for *no* and "uh-huh" for *yes* are also thought to have West African origins (Burling, 1973).

Linguistic Features of African American English

AAE is a linguistic system and, as such, contains form, content, and use components (Bloom & Lahey, 1978; Lahey, 1988). The following phonologic and morphologic features of AAE were adapted from Williams and Wolfram (1976).

Form
Phonology
In spite of the numerous representations of the phonology of AAE as different from that of SAE, the inventory of phonemes in AAE is very similar

to the inventory in SAE. Every vowel in SAE is present in AAE except for three phonemic diphthongs: /ar/, au, and /ɔɪ/. Every consonant in SAE also occurs in AAE. The phoneme /ð/ is often realized as /d/ in the initial word position such as "dat" for "that", and as /d/ or /v/ in medial and final positions. The /θ/ is often realized as /t/ or /f/; however, /θ/ is realized as /θ/ in the initial position of words (Stockman, 1996). In addition to similarities in the phonetic inventory, AAE and SAE use the same rules for combining phonemes into words. SAE and AAE have the same consonant clusters in initial word position with few exceptions. The cluster /θr/ is reduced to /r/, /ʃr/ is reduced to /sr/, and /str/ is changed to /skr/.

There are three major phonologic rules of AAE from which most of the sound features emanate: (1) silencing or substitution of the medial or final consonant in a word, (2) silencing of unstressed initial phonemes and unstressed initial syllables, and (3) silencing of the final consonant in a consonant cluster occurring at the end of a word.

The first phonologic rule of AAE is the silencing or substitution of the medial or final consonant in a word. The consonants affected by this rule include voiced and voiceless fricatives. For example, the fricative /ð/ is affected, and AAE speakers may say "dey" for *they*, "nofin" for *nothing*, "toof" for *tooth*, and "brovah" for *brother*. The semivowels /r/ and /l/ are also affected. AAE speakers may say "foe" for *four*, "sto'y" for *story*, and "p'otect" for *protect*.

Voiced stops /b/, /d/, and /g/ are generally affected in the final positions of single-syllable words, usually a consonant-vowel-consonant (CVC) combination. In these words, the final voiced stop is pronounced similarly to the consonant's voiceless cognate /p/, /t/, and /k/. In addition, the vowel in CVC words is lengthened. Examples of these changes occur when speakers say "cap" plus the lengthened vowel for *cab*, "but" plus lengthened vowel for *bud*, and "pik" plus the lengthened vowel for *pig*.

The nasals /m/ and /n/ are also affected by this first phonologic rule. Several specific characteristics occur with these nasal consonants. One occurs in CVC-unstressed combinations in a word in which the final consonant in the CVC combination is the /m/ or /n/ (e.g., *mailman*). In these words, the final nasal consonant is silenced, but the quality of nasalization is transferred to the vowel. Some examples of this are "ma" plus the nasalized vowel for *man* and "bu" plus the nasalized vowel for *bun*. This feature is also similar to that which occurs in CVC words such as *pin* and *pen*. In these words, the final nasal consonant /n/ remains intact, but the final consonant nasalizes the adjacent vowels, making these words sound identical.

Other nasalization features in AAE affect the grammatical formulations of the present-progressive verb tense (*-ing*) and the articles *a* and *an*. The *-ing* suffix becomes *-in*, as in "singin" and "runnin." The difference between *a* and *an* also becomes neutralized. In this situation, *a* precedes words that begin with a consonant or a vowel, as in "a apple," "a pear," and "a orange," as opposed to *an apple, a pear,* and *an orange.*

According to Stockman (1996), final consonant silence or absence is most likely to occur under the following conditions:

1. The final consonant is a nasal or a stop (e.g., man, pop).
2. The final consonant or consonant cluster precedes a word that begins with a consonant (e.g., right food, best buy) as opposed to a vowel (e.g., right on, best of).
3. The final consonant occurs in a monomorphemic cluster (e.g., bent) as opposed to a bimorphophonemic cluster (e.g., can't).
4. The final consonant occurs in a word in which contrastive status can be maintained in its absence (e.g., bad, bean).

The second major phonologic rule of AAE is the silencing of unstressed initial phonemes and unstressed initial syllables. Examples of this rule are "bout" for *about,* "cause" for *because,* "matoes" for *tomatoes,* "he uz" for *he was,* and "this un" for *this one.*

The third general rule of AAE is the silencing of the final consonant in a consonant cluster occurring at the end of a word. Examples of this are "des" for *desk,* "min" for *mind,* and "ol" for *old.* This rule also affects the AAE grammatical feature for past tense, as in "miss" for *missed* and "slep" for *slept.* Another feature related to consonant clusters is the use of *skr-* for *str-* in the initial position in words, as in "skring" for *string* and "skreet" for *street.* Additionally, "aks" may be used for *ask.*

Morphologic and Syntactic Features

Unlike the phonologic characteristics, AAE morphologic and syntactic or grammatical features are extensive and cannot be simplified into general rules. However, some of the grammatical features of the dialect affect the past tense of regular verbs (e.g., "cash" for *cashed*) and irregular verbs (e.g., "seen" for *saw* and "done" for *did*). Grammatical features can also affect noun-verb agreement, as in "he walk" (vs. *he walks*). They also affect the future tense of verbs through the use of "gonna" and various reductions of "gonna" (e.g., "I'nga," "I'mon," and "I'ma"). Future verb tense is also affected by the silencing of the contraction "'ll" for *will,* as in "she miss you" for *she'll miss you.*

Other AAE grammatical features include the use of double modals (e.g., "used to couldn't"), the use of "like ta" for *liked to have,* differences in the use of the possessive *'s* morpheme (e.g., "the boy hat" for *the boy's hat*), and differences in the use of the plural morpheme *-s* as in "fifty cent" for *fifty cents.*

Some AAE grammatical features attempt to provide regularity to irregular SAE structures. For example, SAE allows for only one comparative or superlative descriptor within a single noun or verb phrase. For example, only *most beautiful* or *prettier* would be allowed in a single phrase. Although SAE does not permit the use of *more* and *most* with words ending with an *-er* or *-est* suffix, this combination (e.g., most prettiest) is valid in AAE, as well as in several other social dialects. The dialectal formulations of comparatives and superlatives can occur in a variety of combinations, serving to carry the comparative or superlative through the entire phrase. Some examples of normal dialectal formulations in this area include "baddest," "mostest," and "worser."

Negative formulations in AAE also regularize SAE rules. The general logic of negatives within an SAE sentence tells us that two negatives cannot be used together because they negate each other and the sentence becomes positive. In AAE, no such philosophical rule exists. Rather, AAE follows the rules for use of negatives that are present in other languages. In Spanish, for example, the negative is carried throughout the sentence. This means that if the sentence is to be negative, every place in the sentence that can be negated is negated. This same rule applies in AAE, resulting in the normal dialectal feature of multiple negation. Some examples of this feature are "He didn't do nothing," "Couldn't nobody do it?" "Nobody didn't do it," and "Ain't no cat can't get in no coop."

Regularization also extends to reflexive pronouns, in which the suffix-*self* can be added to all personal pronouns. The rules used to formulate the first and second person reflexive pronouns *myself* and *yourself* can be extended to the third person, as in "hisself" and "theirself."

Some AAE grammatical forms reflect a feature of hypercorrection. This generally means that the speaker has overgeneralized a grammatical morpheme to an irregular word that already reflects the function of that morpheme. In all cases of hypercorrection, the speaker does not have sufficient knowledge of the SAE rule for the use of a morpheme. Hypercorrected forms are mostly used by older adult dialectal speakers who have realized that they need a more standard language system but do not have a consistent standard English model to imitate. Hypercorrected forms occur in the areas of third person subject-verb agreement (e.g., "I walks," "you walks," and "the children walks"); in pluralization (e.g., "two childrens," "five mens," and "three deers"); and in the use of the possessive morpheme *'s* (e.g., "John's Taylor car").

The use of the word *even* as an intensifying adverb is also an AAE grammatical feature. When this word is spoken in a sentence with an intensifying function, it generally stands out from the rest of the sentence context by a more intense loudness level and its prosodic pattern. When used this way, *even* carries a meaning of finality—that is, there is nothing greater or nothing left to be said about the topic of the sentence. For example, consider a scenario in which a husband enters the house and asks his wife where their son is. The wife responds that the boy is outside but that he'll be in soon for dinner. The husband asks again 10 minutes later, and the wife responds as before. After 5 more minutes have elapsed, the husband asks again, but this time the wife has become irritated and does not want to be asked the same question anymore. She tells him, "I done tol' you he be home for dinner. Don' *even* aks me no more." *Even* is a final, definitive statement on a subject. For example, a child may comment, "I didn't *even* know what that teacher be talkin' about."

Other AAE grammatical features occur in the following areas:

- Pronominal apposition
- "*My brother he* bigger than you."
- Demonstratives
- "I want some of *them* candies."
- "I like *these here* pants better than *them there* ones."
- Pronouns
- "*Him* ain't playing." "*Me and her* will go."
- "James got *him* book." "Don't eat that candy 'cause it *mines*."
- "*He* can dress *hisself*." "I got *me* one of those."
- The use of *have* and *do*
- "*I* been here for hours." "He *have* a bike."
- "He *don't* go." "He always *do* silly things."
- Completed aspects with *done*. This construction is used when an action started and was completed at a certain time in the past.
- "I *done* tried."
- Remote time construction with *been*. This construction is used when an action has taken place in the distant past.
- "I *been* had it there for about three years."
- Indirect questions. Indirect questions follow the same rules as those for formulating direct questions.
- "I wonder was he walking."
- "I wonder where was he going."
- Use of *do* for *if*. This feature is related to the indirect question feature: A clause beginning with *if* is reformulated into a direct question format.
- "I ask' Elon *do he want* to play football."

A major grammatical feature of AAE involves variations in the use of the verb *to be*. These use rules are as follows:

- The silencing of *is*, *are*, or both in contracted forms. For example, "*He* a man," "*He* running home," and "*You* good." Dialectal speakers use *is* and *are* in other sentence contexts, such as in tag questions (e.g.,

"*He* not home yet, *is* he?"). Also, some dialectal speakers who use a silenced *are* contraction do not use a silenced *is* contraction. Additionally, this feature extends to contractions of *will be* and *would be* ("*He be* here") and ("*She be* happy").

- Neutralization of subject-verb agreement. This construction occurs in past and present forms of *to be*, but neutralization is more frequent in the past tense. Examples include "*I was* there," "*She was* there," "*You was* there," and "*They was* there." An example of the more infrequently used present tense form is "*They is* here."
- Use of *be* as a main verb for *is*, *are*, or *am*. This rule is a prominent AAE feature. Examples include "I *be* here in the evening" for *I am here in the evening*, "Sometime he *be* busy" for *Sometimes he is busy*, and "They *be* coming" for *They are coming*.
- Use of *be* for habitual tense. In the most prominent feature of AAE, *be* does not specify a tense, but it reflects the African-based habitual tense, which indicates a permanent or consistent quality or condition. For example, the statement "My momma *be* workin' two jobs" means *My mother has been working two jobs for a while*. And the statement, "Don' min' him; he jus' *be* actin' crazy" means *Don't pay any attention to him; acting crazy is his normal tendency*.

Content: Semantic or Lexical Features

Semantics involves the meaning and use of words. These words constitute a cultural vocabulary. The lexicon of speakers of AAE is influenced by geographic, economic, regional, sociopolitical, familiar, religious, and racial factors. This means that the person's lexicon is likely to contain words that are unique to the factors that affect the individual's life. Geographically, for example, a carbonated soft drink is "tonic" in the Boston area, "pop" in Pittsburgh, "Coke" in Dallas, and "soda water" in Gainesville, Florida.

The vocabulary of African Americans can have regional influences as well. A child living in a predominantly African American neighborhood in an area may have a lexicon that is different from that of a child who lives in a rural area. In some cases, the same lexical item symbolizes different referents. For example, to a rural child, the word *hog* is likely to represent a large pig, but to the urban child, *hog* might symbolize a type of large expensive car or motorcycle.

Generation-influenced lexicon plays a large role in the vocabulary used among many African Americans. Each generation appears to have developed its own unique set of words and meanings, often called *slang*. It is unknown why slang is so prominent among African American youth. It may be that the lack of acceptance of African American youth by white youth in social activities has led to the creation of slang words for each generation of young people. Slang, like African American music, may be a means for African American youth to create something that is uniquely theirs—a code with which they can identify themselves as a group, communicate with each other, and feel good about being together. Slang words are always subject to rapid change: New words are added; others become archaic. It could be that new slang words are created to replace words that become popular among mainstream groups. Some examples of generation-influenced lexical items (all of which mean good or great) are "crazy" and "real gone" (1950s); "hep," "bad," and "boss" (1970s); "fresh," "phat," "smokin'," "stompin'," and "walk on it" (1990s); and "representin'," "trippin'," "down with that," "that's straight," and "off the hook" (2001).

Regardless of geographic or regional location, generational influences, or economic status, some words are commonly used and understood by the majority of African Americans but are generally absent from the lexicon of mainstream populations. Some of these words reflect the physical or racial characteristics of African Americans, such as the vocabulary for hair and skin care. Other words reflect activities in African American churches and other African American organizations. A few examples of this cultural vocabulary are "ash" and "ashy" (referring to dry skin); "grease," "to grease," "glycerine," "perm," "relaxer," and "curl" (referring to oil-based preparations for the hair); and "shout" and "get happy" (referring to outward physical and emotional response to overwhelming joy and mercy of God).

Other examples of lexical differences that have occurred in AAE include "true dat" (in agreement), "change up or flip the script" (to change), "dis" (disrespect), "down" (cool or nice), "jettin" (quickly), "get my groove on" (have a good time, dancing, romancing), "get my swirve on" (go out with the opposite sex, dance, and have a good time), "crib" (home or parent), "fly" (good looking), and "chump change" (small change, insignificant). Word usage and definition are not only influenced by geography, region, generation, and economic status but also by the city or neighborhood. The meaning also changes dependent on the user (adult or teen), the context in which it is being used, or both. Even the way a word is pronounced can change its definition (Foster, 1990). Although these are AAE terms that are used in AAE neighborhoods and regions, many are incorporated into SAE because of their use in the lyrics of rap, hip-hop, and other crossover music that is being adopted by mainstream youth.

Differences in form and content areas of language can result in communication failures between speakers of different dialects. Some failures can result from differences in pronunciation, grammar, and vocabulary that create intelligibility problems. In the case of different dialects of a language, the actual linguistic differences can be minor but nevertheless implicated in difficulties in communication and in misunderstandings.

Use: Pragmatic Functions

Just as there are normal systematic phonologic, grammatical, and semantic features of AAE, there are also pragmatic characteristics of the dialect. The rules for communicative interactions used by many African Americans include code switching, call and response, wit and sarcasm, eye contact, and narrative style.

Code Switching

Code switching is a major pragmatic feature of the speech of most, if not all, AAE speakers. Code switching involves the speaker's ability to use the linguistic style (formal or informal), dialect, or language that is most appropriate for a particular communication episode. The language used is based on the age, race, gender, or level of authority of the person with whom one is speaking; the intended use; and the context of the communicative event.

Code switching is used by speakers of AAE when significant changes or decrease in the use of AAE features result in an increased use of SAE (Hester, 1996). In addition to code switching, speakers may engage simultaneously in style shifting, which refers to changes in the use of features that are predominately oral style or literate. In an examination of the narrative variability of AAE-speaking fourth-grade children, Hester (1996) found that the code switching and style shifting among the children varied between narrative tasks (e.g., conversation, story retelling, and story generation). The results of the study imply that clinicians should evaluate an AAE-speaking child's language over a variety of narrative types during the assessment process (Hester, 1996).

Wit and Sarcasm

Wit and sarcasm assume a variety of forms by African Americans. Some statements are actual sarcasm, such as the wife who tells her significantly late–arriving husband, "You sho' got home early." Other forms of wit involve creative, verbal turn-taking games, such as playing the dozens. Playing the dozens is typically played by school-aged African American boys. The objective is for a player to create verbal insults about the opponent's mother that are better than the insults directed at the player about his own mother. The following is an example of a typical playing the dozens verbal interchange:

Player 1:   Yo' momma so ugly the dogcatcher tried to net her.
Player 2:   Oh yea? Yo' momma so ugly, when the dogcatcher got yo' momma and put her in his truck, even the other dogs didn' know the difference.

On the surface, playing the dozens reflects disrespect of the parent. On the contrary, because of the love and respect the players have for their mothers, a young

African American man who can learn to withstand insults about his mother is better prepared to withstand negativism and insults that he will face in the future. It is also an excellent way to develop social and verbal interaction skills.

Eye Contact

Some African Americans are taught as children that eye contact with an adult during a verbal interchange is disrespectful. Some African American adults may therefore find it difficult to speak to those of authority on an eye-to-eye basis. Judging children and adults for not looking at an examiner or other professional may be a violation of the person's cultural rule for eye contact. This is particularly important in the treatment of dysfluency as described in Chapter 9. According to Taylor (1987), African Americans demonstrate attentiveness and respect by using indirect eye contact when they are listeners and direct eye contact when they are speakers. SAE speakers could easily misinterpret the lack of eye contact during listening as inattentive or noncaring behavior.

Narrative Style

Heath (1986) describes four types of narrative styles: (1) patterns used to recount past experiences, (2) patterns used to cast or describe present or future activities or events, (3) patterns used to give accounts of what has been experienced, and (4) fictionalized accounts of storytelling. Despite the variable nature of AAE and the awareness of different narrative styles and genres, investigations of the narratives of AAE have generally been restricted to recounts or narratives of personal experiences (Hester, 1994, 1996). In the 1980s, several investigators studied AAE narratives in terms of oral and literate styles (Collins, 1985; Gee, 1985; Heath, 1982; Michaels & Collins, 1984; Nichols, 1989). In oral language style, meaning is implicit or indirect—that is, it is expressed through the use of idioms, slang, gestures, and changes in voice and pitch in conversations between familiar individuals. In literate language, style meaning is expressed more directly with specific syntactic and morphologic structures as in written language (Olson, 1977; Tannen, 1982; Westby, 1985). Many investigators describe AAE speakers as preferring the oral narrative style because of their relation to the oral tradition of the African ancestry (Baugh, 1983; Erickson, 1984).

Michaels (1981), Nichols (1989), Collins (1985), Gee (1989), and Westby (1985, 1994) are among several investigators who studied the oral-literate distinction in the narratives of young children. By analyzing narratives during sharing-time activities for African American and white kindergarten children, Michaels (1981) found that the narrative style used by the AAE-speaking children differed from that used by speakers of SAE. When a particular topic was discussed, speakers of SAE used patterns that involved a fairly strict adherence to a central topic. For example, when a teacher asks a class to talk about things seen and done at a zoo, each child using SAE contributes something appropriate to that main topic. This reflects a topic-centered narrative style. On the other hand, some speakers of AAE engage in a more topic-associated narrative style. With a topic-associated narrative style, a child's statements are not linked by a central topic but by ideas generated from an immediately preceding statement. For example, when a group of children who use this style of discussion is asked to talk about things seen and done at a zoo, the first child may respond that he saw a lion, the second child comments that she saw a lion on the *Circus of the Stars* television special, and the third child adds that she got scared when the performer almost fell off the high wire. The investigators reported that AAE-speaking children's narrative skills are restricted to a topic-associated oral style (Collins, 1985; Michaels, 1981; Nichols, 1989; Westby, 1985).

More recent investigations, however, have found that AAE-speaking children have more flexible narrative styles than was previously thought. Hyon and Sulzby (1994), Hicks (1991), and Hester (1996) studied the use of narrative by kindergarten and first-grade AAE-speaking children. Hyon and Sulzby (1994) and Champion, Seymour, and Camarata (1995) reported African American children used topic-centered and topic-associating features while telling stories to a familiar adult. Hicks (1991) and Hester (1996) found that children who use AAE are able to shift their narrative style according to different task demands. Regardless of the style preferred by the child, African American children can be expected to tell stories and recount events, as do other children.

Other Pragmatic Functions
TURN-TAKING

Turn-taking rules are somewhat different among African American speakers. In AAE, it is not necessary to wait until the first speaker has completed his or her turn before the next speaker begins. Interruptions are acceptable, and the conversational floor is given to the most assertive and aggressive speaker.

Call and response is an important turn-taking feature of AAE. Call and response is characterized by a choral response to an utterance given by a single person. Largely noticeable within the church and in gospel and rhythm and blues music, call and response is also a feature of conversations among African Americans. There are two specific call-and-response patterns: (1) a statement produced by one person followed by a response by one person and (2) a statement produced by one person followed by responses made by people in a group.

The first type of call and response occurs mostly during a conversational dyad. The response is generally a confirmation or acknowledgment of the speaker's statement. In some instances, the response is confirming (e.g., "I know that's right," "Tell me about it," "You got that right," "Girl, I know what you talkin' 'bout," "Ain't it the truth now," and "Amen"). The response can also acknowledge understanding of the statement or, if the speaker's statement is a request, can answer yes or no (e.g., "You got it, man," "I got you covered," or "Can't fly with that"). Additionally, the response can denote some element of surprise regarding the content of the statement. Examples of this type of response include "Get outta here," "Lawd have mercy," "Lawd Jesus!" "Lawd," "Girl" (pronounced with a lengthened semivowel), "Damn!" "Ooo-hhh, child!" and "Um-um-um."

In some instances, the call-and-response patterns in a dyad are echoic or hyperechoic. The echoic response duplicates or repeats some portion of the speaker's statement, as in the following conversation:

Speaker:	I fixed me some turkey and dressing . . .
Respondent:	Um-um! Turkey and dressing!
Speaker:	And some sweet potato pie.
Respondent:	Potato pie, too? I ain't had no good dinner like that since my wife passed.
Speaker:	Then you better come on here and let me fix you a plate.

A pragmatic feature not previously recognized in literature is the hyper-echoic response. The hyperechoic response is superimposed on top of the first speaker's utterance. It is a confirmation that the listener not only understands the response but also anticipates, predicts, and verbalizes what the speaker's next words will be while the speaker is talking. If the respondent is wrong, the speaker makes the appropriate adjustments. An example of a hyperechoic response pattern follows:

Speaker:	You know I done tried to be fair. But I s'pose you can' teach no ol' . . .
Respondent:	Man nothin' new . . . [anticipating "old man, new tricks"]
Speaker:	Nothin' new. I know that's right! [echoed and confirmed]

The second type of call-and-response pattern is a statement produced by one person followed by responses made by people in a group. It is typically found in church services, rallies, and other situations with a main speaker and an audience. Audience verbal responses in church include "Yea," "Speak the truth, now," "Amen," "Well," "Alright," "Uh-huh," "Hallelujah," "Tell it," and "Preach it." Nonverbal responses to a speaker's statements include hand clapping, head shaking and nodding, hand waving and lifting, standing up, dancing, patting the feet, pointing a finger at the speaker, laughing, and crying. In these situations, the speaker not only looks for the responses but, when the audience is too quiet, also encourages the audience to respond by calling statements such as "Hello?," "Ya'll don' hear me," and "Can I get a witness?"

Call-and-response patterns are considered a beneficial communicative feature among those who use and understand them, because the respondents are providing the speaker with complimentary, confirming, and positive feedback. However, these patterns are subject to misinterpretation by people who are unfamiliar with this aspect of AAE. AAE speakers using normal call-and-response patterns may be judged to be rude, interruptive, and disruptive by those who are not familiar with call-and-response patterns.

TOUCHING

During AAE conversations, approval or agreement is demonstrated nonverbally through touching, such as touching the listener's hand or arm. However, the touching of the hair and patting on the head might be considered an insult by speakers of AAE (Taylor, 1987; Roseberry-McKibbin, 1995).

To summarize, it is important to emphasize that social constraints on language are culturally organized and vary from culture to culture and from subculture to subculture. Competent speakers of a language must observe a wide range of sociocultural norms in verbal interaction. For example, competent speakers must know when it is appropriate to address a person using a title and a last name or a first name, they must make vocabulary choices appropriate for their addressee and the social situation, and they must know how to phrase requests without violating rules of etiquette. In many cases, it is the violation of such norms, rather than grammatical or phonologic norms, that are the sources of communication failures. The clinical setting, as well as other service-delivery settings, is one in which many people can experience what they believe are violations of their privacy. Compound this with cultural differences in beliefs about what is considered private and pragmatically appropriate, and it becomes easy to envision the barriers of self-defense that clients may erect that block the flow of information necessary for optimal service delivery.

Development of African American English

Morphologic and Syntactic Development

Research on the normal acquisition of AAE morphologic and syntactic patterns is scarce. The few data-based studies that have been conducted have largely investigated grammatical features and suggest that, in addition to sharing linguistic features with other dialects, AAE also shares features of normal linguistic development in young children (Blake, 1984; Cole, 1980; Reveron, 1978; Steffensen, 1974; Stockman, 1984, 1986a, 1986b; Stockman & Vaughn-Cooke, 1982).

Blake (1984) and Stockman (1986a) have both shown that the morpho-syntactic development of young children who speak AAE is similar to that of children who use SAE up to the age of 3 years, including the development of the mean length of utterance. Children in homes in which AAE is spoken have a well-developed use of one- and two-word utterances by the age of 18 months, as is observed in home in which SAE is spoken (Blake, 1984; Steffensen, 1974). Their mean length of utterance increases with age at least to the age of 2.5 years, with increments similar to those of children who speak SAE (Blake, 1984; Stockman, 1984).

Research, investigating the development of morphologic features, shows that children in homes in which AAE is spoken acquire early morphologic features in the same pattern as children learning SAE, including features to mark the plural, possessive, past tense, and third-person singular (Blake, 1984; Cole, 1980; Reveron, 1978; Steffensen, 1974; Stockman, 1986a). As with SAE, the morphologic features of AAE involving tense, mood, and aspect markers of the verb phrase, negation, and other morphologic features develop in the later preschool years. At the age of 3 years, children learning AAE have developed the use of well-formed multiword constructions, simple declaratives, and questions, with subject, verb, and object complements and a few complex utterances also appearing (Stockman, 1986a). Elaborated sentences with embedded object complements, negative sentences, and the formation of tag questions appear before the age of 4 years. As children develop through the preschool years, a variety of complex sentences and complex semantic relations are used, including coordinated, subordinate, and relative clause sentences and complex wh- question forms (Craig & Washington, 1995; Washington & Craig, 1994). Thus, through the early preschool years, there is little difference in the development of morphologic and syntactic forms between children learning AAE and SAE. This implies that the linguistic forms of children acquiring SAE and of children acquiring AAE cannot be distinguished until the children reach approximately 3 years of age (Steffensen, 1974).

The features that contrast AAE and SAE generally involve the later-developing forms, which begin to evolve at approximately 4 years of age. Like the continuum of development of SAE forms, it appears that AAE rules are also learned in a developmental sequence and that the frequency with which these rules are used increases with age (Cole, 1980; Reveron, 1978). Social class differences become most pronounced after the age of 4 years (Craig & Washington, 1994; Kovac, 1980; Reveron, 1978; Stockman, 1986a).

Cole (1980) found that AAE-speaking children exhibit the AAE rules for regular past tense, third-person singular, present-tense copula, and remote past (*been*) at the age of 3 years. The AAE features of indefinite article regularization and multiple negation were observed in 4-year-old children. The features of reflexive and pronominal regularization occurred when the children were 5 years of age. Because Cole analyzed only the speech of 3-, 4-, and 5-year-old African American children, it can be assumed that other AAE features do not emerge until after the age of 5 years. If this is the case, it would make identification of language disorders within AAE-speaking children by conventional standardized tests extremely difficult (Stockman, 1986b). AAE forms not used until after 5 years of age include the use of *at* in questions (e.g., "Where my coat at?"), the *go* copula (e.g., "There go my coat."), distributive *be*, first-person future, embedded questions, past tense copula, present copula, and second-person pronouns. Features such as the habitual *be* (e.g., "She be working.") and the use of *what* to mark the relative clause (e.g., "He the one what broke it.") develop at much later ages than the other forms (Cole, 1980). Among the later-emerging contrastive AAE forms is the use of *had* to mark the simple past (e.g., "We had went to the store."), *steady* to mark an intensified continuative marker (e.g., "He steady be mockin' me."), and *come* to express indignation about an event or action (e.g., "He come hollering at me.").

Variables in the required use of certain linguistic forms can cause difficulty in distinguishing development from disorders or delays in morphologic development in AAE. For example, although speakers of AAE are required to use the form of *be* in statements such as "yes, he is," it is not obligatory in "John a boy" (Seymour, 1995; Seymour & Roeper, 1999). The expression of habitual *be* (e.g., "he be working"), as opposed to a temporary condition (e.g., "he working"), does not appear in SAE. The feature is not likely to be observed by speech-language pathologists assessing the development of morphologic features using SAE standards.

Phonologic Development

Because SAE and AAE are dialects of the same language, several phonologic features are shared and are thus noncontrastive. Like the early development of morphology and syntax, the early phoneme development of children learning AAE is not different from that of children learning SAE (Seymour & Ralabate, 1985; Seymour & Seymour, 1981; Steffersen, 1974). The features that contrast AAE and SAE involve sounds and phonologic features that develop after the age of 4 or 5 years. These features include final consonant deletion or weakening, final cluster reduction, unstressed syllable deletion, and interdental fricative substitution involving the final /th/ (Haynes & Moran, 1989; Moran 1993; Seymour & Seymour, 1981; Stockman, 1991, 1995; Stockman & Settle, 1991; Vaughn-Cooke, 1986; Wolfram & Fasold, 1974).

Because standard articulation tests vary in the number of items related to AAE, they have limited usefulness in determining the phonologic performance of children learning AAE (Cole & Taylor, 1990; Washington & Craig, 1992). Care must be taken to distinguish between those features that are contrastive and those that are not contrastive between AAE and SAE. According to Bleile and Wallach (1992), the following features are not contrastive between AAE and SAE and can thus be useful in distinguishing between normal disordered or delayed phonologic development in children learning AAE:

- The use of more than one or two stop errors
- Initial word position errors (with the exception of /b/ for /v/)
- Glide errors in children older than 4 years of age
- More than a few cluster errors (with the exception of final clusters)
- Fricative errors other than /th/

The primary indicators of whether a child who speaks AAE is having difficulty in phonologic development are the ability of those familiar with the dialect to understand the child at 5 years of age and the determination of whether the child is considerably more difficult to understand than his or her age and dialect peers.

Pragmatic Development

Communicative intent and semantic-linguistic functions in children learning AAE develop along the same lines as children learning SAE. Children between the ages of 18 months and 2 years develop the same functions as children learning other languages. These functions include informative, requestive, regulative, imaginative, affective, participative, and attentive functions (Blake, 1984; Bridgeforth, 1984; Stockman, 1986a). According to Vaughn-Cooke and Wright-Harp (1992) and Davis and colleagues (1992–1993), the similarity in the development of linguistic function appears to continue through the preschool years.

Because of the apparent lack of assessment tools that distinguish between normally developing AAE and true disorders, children developing AAE are often assessed using assessment tools that fail to take into account the normal development of the dialect. It is essential that the normal development of features in AAE be considered in the determination of distinction between the least competent child considered to have normal development and development of language in children considered to be delayed-learning AAE (Stockman, 1996).

Reducing Bias in the Clinical Management of African Americans

Nonbiased clinical management is the process of establishing a client's native language, dialect, and culture as the basis on which speech-language and hearing evaluations are conducted and results are interpreted and for which treatment is prescribed. For nonbiased management to occur with an individual client, the speech-language pathologist must discover the normal language patterns and cultural views of that client. Because of the complexity of cultural variables that can affect service delivery, reducing bias in clinical management must go beyond the administration of specific tests and procedures. Instead, it must be an entire process emanating from respect of a client's culture, normal linguistic style, family structure, and beliefs. This process seeks to evaluate communication ability from the client's cultural viewpoint instead of from the morals, values, and standards of language normalcy held by the clinician.

Use of Churches for Preventive and Other Service Delivery

Given the importance of the church in African American culture, churches and other religious groups can be instrumental in providing assistance in gaining access to hard-to-reach and underserved segments of African American communities. Organizations such as black churches provide a channel and entry by which public services can be offered to population groups that otherwise may not be served. Church organizations can offer ways to target health messages and increase awareness of health status, including speech, language, and hearing services, to members of the community. Church groups can help persons in African American communities improve access to services while helping them overcome attitudinal barriers regarding their own health and their perceptions of service providers.

To adequately address the risk factors associated with speech, language, and hearing disorders among African American communities, emphasis should be given to making health a participatory enterprise, one in which African American populations are fully aware of the long-term benefits of regular health screening, including hearing screening. Clinicians should act as "coaches," whose role it is to encourage full involvement of African Americans in their health care, particularly to reduce the occurrence of stroke-related hypertension and other factors associated with communication disorders.

Use of Families for Service Delivery

Assessment and intervention services should be as family centered as possible. African Americans have a variety of family unit types, including two-parent, single-parent, and extended-family systems. In certain economic and familial circumstances, the mother may not be the primary caregiver or know detailed information about the child's speech, language, and cognitive development. In some instances, an alternate caregiver such as the child's grandmother or older sibling may know more about the child than the mother.

Family members should be encouraged to attend evaluation and treatment sessions. This provides an opportunity for the clinician to observe the normal language use and interactions within the family. The clinician can also observe the client interacting with different family members and obtain accurate, naturalistic information on the client's speech and language skills. Existence of code switching can be more readily observed and recorded during these interactions. Additionally, when the testing has been completed, the clinician can use family members to comment on the validity of the evaluation results and recommendations and to determine priorities for therapy, if therapy is warranted. In treatment sessions, family members can learn speech and language facilitation techniques to help the client at home, especially if regular attendance is difficult or services become interrupted.

Family-centered therapy services can also enhance communication between family members as they join forces to help the client. For example, in a case familiar to the author, services were provided to an African American family whose members consisted of a deaf mother who could communicate only in sign language, the hearing father who could not and would not use sign language, the 4-year-old client who had severe receptive and expressive delay, and a toddler daughter who was at high risk for language and speech disorder. All family members came to therapy. During the family-centered treatment, the mother began to teach sign language to the father, and the father began to learn sign language and to speak to his wife so that she could lip-read his words. The parents not only learned how to provide stimulation for their son using both language systems, but they also enhanced communication between each other. An additional benefit was that the daughter's language skills began to improve.

Family involvement not only helps the client's development but also enhances the communication between family members.

Additional Suggestions for Reducing Bias in Intervention

Speech-language pathologists should incorporate the following into the clinical intervention process when treating African Americans:

1. Clinicians should conduct a self-examination of their attitudes and possible bias against African Americans. Because intervention requires a respect for the client's race, ethnicity, and culture, a negative attitude toward African Americans or speakers of AAE could negatively influence the clinical process.

2. The clinician should conduct the intervention program using ethnographic methods—that is, the clinician should serve the client considering the

culture of the client. When ethnographic methods are used as the "umbrella" for all clinical services, clinical services are more culturally relevant.

3. Case history questionnaires, permission forms, and documents authorizing the release of information should be used with care and consideration for the client's understanding of the use of the information. Sending home questionnaires that ask for personal and private information may not be returned and may result in the client and family not continuing to seek clinical services. The number of forms sent can be overwhelming and the content of the forms too complex to be understood. The family may be suspicious of the use of the information, particularly in low-income families with a history of dependence on social services.

Before asking for specific information, the clinician should establish rapport to develop a sense of trust and concern for the client and the family. The purpose of the interview and how the information will be used should be made clear. It should also be made clear who will have access to the information. Appropriate permission to release information forms should be presented at the beginning of the session, even if they are not signed until the interview is completed. The question format should use open-ended questions, rather than closed-ended questions. This will allow the client to provide information relevant to the case without feeling pressure to reveal personal and private information. The clinician should ask questions in one area at a time, using summarizing and transitioning to assure that the information provided has been understood. The following factors by Campbell (1996) are important to consider in conducting ethnographic interviews with African American families:

- Make sure the purpose of the interview is clear.
- The clinician should ask the right question to the right people in the right way (Westby, 1990) to ensure that cultural considerations are made in the interview process.
- The clinician should listen actively and not appear to be judgmental in response to information.

4. The clinician should greet family members and clients using their preferred names. He or she should address African American clients in a formal manner using the appropriate surnames and titles (e.g., Mr. Townsend or Mrs. Howard) until requested to do otherwise. The use of first names by service providers and others who are not family members can be taken as a sign of lack of respect.

5. The clinician should determine the client's dialect before interpreting assessment data. Because the client is an African American does not mean that he or she uses AAE. Not all African Americans are speakers of AAE. To determine if a child is learning AAE, Terrell, Arensberg, & Rosa

(1992) recommended comparing the child's performance with that of the child's parents or primary caregivers, or both. Although there are some differences between adult AAE and child AAE forms, the study supports the use of this procedure as an indicator of whether or not a person is an AAE user.

6. Specific assessment methods should be used to reflect the client's linguistic and cultural orientation. (See Chapter 13 for specific assessment techniques.)

7. Recognize that there may be lay leaders or "natural helpers" in the community whom families seek out for health advice and who are instrumental in encouraging client compliance and willingness to participate in clinical services. These lay leaders may be associated with area churches or social organizations. In cases in which the client and opinion leaders have a common link to a church, the client's participation in health care services is reinforced. Clinicians are urged to use these "client-opinion leader" networks as a way of encouraging communication, compliance, and overall client satisfaction.

8. The clinician should not make assumptions about the goals and desires of the client and family. Although they are disproportionately represented among the low-income or working-class families, African Americans are members of every social class and are in every income level. However, as with all members of low-income families, educational and rehabilitation efforts, such as speech-language and hearing services, may become low-priority items in families in which the basic needs of food, clothing, and housing are not met. This can affect the family's perception of the need for service, the length of time the client stays in treatment, attendance at sessions, and the motivation for full participation in services.

9. The clinician should provide clients with prompts to involve or encourage their clients to have routine health examinations, including screening for hypertension and other health conditions. Involving clients in such beneficial activities is well intentioned, but activities that are not incorporated into the clinical service delivery environment on a regular basis can be overlooked or not discussed with patients during a busy visit schedule. Several clinical settings use simple chart notes or inserts as situation reminders. Other clinicians have included support staff members as part of a comprehensive focus on client well-being. Consistent with this total emphasis on the client, selected staff members may be given the responsibility for suggesting that a particular client participate in preventive care and other health activities as part of a personal care plan.

Standardized Tests

There are several current standardized tests that are culturally fair. Washington and Craig (1999) indicate that the *Peabody Picture Vocabulary*

Test III (Dunn & Dunn, 1997), unlike the previous two versions of the test, is valid for African American children. However, Stockman (2000) cautions clinicians in assuming that better performance of African American children on the test may not be solely due to the changes in standardization and construction of the test but rather to other cultural factors. Auditory processing tests or tests that are dependent on auditory processing methods have been shown to reduce potential bias (Campbell et al., 1997). Additionally, on the horizon is the *Dialect-Sensitive Language Screener* (Seymour et al., 2000). This standardized test, which is currently under development, is being designed as an effective tool to determine dialect versus difference among AAE-speaking children.

Although progress is being made regarding tests that can be used effectively with persons who use AAE, many standardized measures are biased against African Americans in overall testing format and in how items are scored (Taylor & Payne, 1983; Washington, 1996). Therefore, if a clinician chooses to use standardized tests, then the following are several suggestions for strengthening the true meaning of the results:

1. Check the validity of the test. Read the validity data in the test manual to determine whether sufficient numbers of African Americans were represented in the sampling data. If African Americans are represented, check to see whether there are separate norms for AAE speakers. If included at all, the number of African Americans in the standardization sample usually depends on the most recent U.S. Census available to the authors. According to Washington (1996), although African Americans are included in the sample, the test items can still be in SAE form. In addition, because a test includes African Americans in the standardization sample does not mean that the test is sensitive to AAE. Usually there is no information as to whether those in the sample speak AAE or SAE. Thus, the test may only be appropriate for African Americans who speak SAE or for those who have had sufficient exposure to mainstream culture.

2. Analyze the dialectal effect of the test. Before administering a test, analyze each item's stimulus and response for possible dialectal effect. For example, if the correct test response for an item is *two dogs*, then the clinician should predetermine that a normal AAE response to that item is *two dog*. The clinician should prepare a list of these dialectal responses for a test. The clinician can then choose to score the test with dialectal variations counted in as normal responses or to score the test according to the manual's guidelines and interpret the results according to dialectal variations. In every case, the report should indicate how the test was scored. The results cannot be reported according to the published norms; rather, the test results should describe the performance of the client in narrative, explaining the items that the client was able to complete and an approximate equivalent to the normative behavior.

3. Determine the use of AAE or other dialect by the family or primary caregivers. It is inappropriate to assume that all African Americans use AAE or that they use all of the published features of the dialect. Failure to determine the dialect used in the home can result in under- or over identification of a disorder.

4. Modify the testing procedure. Any modification changes the validity and reliability of a test; thus, the original norms are no longer appropriate. Nonetheless, the results may still give a better picture of the client's capabilities. All adaptations should be noted in the evaluation report (Campbell, 1996).

Nonstandardized Procedures

There are a variety of nonstandardized clinical procedures that can be used to obtain a description of client communication behavior. Most involve gathering and analyzing a conversational sample. It is important for clinicians to obtain conversational samples that are truly representative of the client's language skills. The following are several ways that this can be facilitated:

1. Use culturally relevant or familiar objects to stimulate conversation. These items can include pictures of African Americans engaged in culturally relevant activities; photographs of family members; and culturally relevant foods, music, clothing, important persons, and significant African American historical figures, such as Martin Luther King, Jr., or Jackie Robinson. This is particularly important when testing elderly African Americans who may have had limited exposure to mainstream cultural icons.

2. Determine the client's narrative skills. If the client is 4 years old or older, consider reading a short, culturally relevant story to the child and have the child retell the story. This helps to determine the nature of the client's narrative skills, bearing in mind the cultural differences in narrative style. Champion et al. (1999) provide a model for the evaluation of narrative productions by African American children according to content analysis, event analysis, and social and cultural practices. Hester (1996) recommends that the clinician evaluate the child's language over several types of narrative types (e.g., conversation, story retelling, and story generation). Additionally, Hyter and Westby (1996) propose the use of a *Multiple Perspective Analysis Element Checklist and Student Profile* when using oral narratives for assessment. This assessment tool can be used to determine the child's strengths for using perspectives and voices, evaluative statements, and cohesive devices in narrativization. The client's story can also be used to analyze AAE features.

3. Obtain a language sample. Conversational sample analysis should always attempt to identify the dialect that the client uses. AAE use among children is more frequent with language samples taken during picture descriptions than free play (Washington, Craig, & Kushmaul, 1998) and also varies as a function of socioeconomic class and gender. Male children and children from low

socioeconomic backgrounds use more AAE features than women and children from middle socioeconomic homes (Washington & Craig, 1998). Additionally, a seminal study by Seymour, Bland-Stewart, & Green, (1998) indicates that analysis of noncontrastive features of AAE and SAE (i.e., linguistic features that are shared by the two dialects) provides more accuracy in determining dialect difference from disorder than analysis of features that only occur in AAE (i.e., contrastive features). Clinicians should vary language sample contexts and conduct analyses of the language samples that focus on noncontrastive features.

4. Use criterion-referenced testing. In criterion-referenced testing, a client's behavior of items is compared with behaviors determined to be the criteria for acceptable responses. Criterion-referenced measures are most frequently used to set performance levels, such as the 95% criterion for correct production of a phoneme. This technique, however, can also be used for assessment, if clinicians have a way to establish valid referent criteria. One way to establish these valid criteria is to use parent-child comparative analysis (Terrell, Arensberg, & Ross, 1992). This method uses the cultural and linguistic patterns of the parent, caregiver, or person who is the primary language model as the referent criteria. The basic procedure of the parent-child comparative analysis is to administer the same speech and language tests to a parent or caregiver and to the client. The client's speech and language patterns are then compared with the patterns of the parent or caregiver. If the client is a child, then patterns that do not match with those of the caregiver are further compared with normal speech expectations for the child's chronological age via normal language charts. Any divergent speech patterns that remain after this two-step comparative analysis have a high probability of being true disorders. Clinicians may also consider Stockman's *Minimal Competency Core* (1996), which is another criterion-referenced assessment tool.

Additionally, because standardized vocabulary tests may be biased against AAE-speaking children, Stockman (1999) proposes several alternatives to standardized vocabulary testing. These include the use of language processing tasks (e.g., nonword repetition, memory within competing stimuli), the evaluation of "fast word mapping" capabilities (i.e., the ability to process novel words rapidly, as in "John *wugged* the ice"), and the assessment and intervention of semantic fields rather than targeting specific words for evaluation and remediation. In using semantic fields for remediation, the clinician targets words within the same semantic field to facilitate the client's learning of specific new words within that same semantic field (Stockman, 1999).

Intervention

If the assessment results indicate a communication disorder, then intervention may be recommended. According to the *Position paper on social dialects* (American Speech-Language-Hearing Association, 1983), the disorder and not the features of the dialect should be the focus of treatment.

The clinician should be cognizant of the client's preferred learning style and make adaptations in the approach to intervention to accommodate the learning style. Learning style is the process of acquiring new information through the organization, perceptions, processing, manipulation, and recall of information. African Americans often, but not always, prefer a field-dependent learning style, in which they are influenced by their surroundings, including peers and authority figures. A high value is placed on social and interpersonal environments and on group achievement and cooperation. They prefer auditory and kinesthetic techniques (cues) and charismatic teaching. These characteristics indicate that speakers of AAE may prefer to work in a group service-delivery model with peers (Battle & Grantham, 1997; Terrell & Hale, 1992).

Franklin (1992) suggests that an affect-oriented, open, and risk-free environment fosters learning in African American students. Franklin also suggests that African American children demonstrate high proficiency levels with varied stimuli, increased verbal interaction, and modified speaking (using rhythm and intonation). Multisensory stimuli (i.e., oral, print, and visual reinforcements), a varied format, and a faster paced, high-energy atmosphere were also noted as techniques that increased learning.

Acknowledgment

The authors would like to acknowledge the valued contributions to this work by Dr. Nan B. Ratner, Professor and Chair of the Department of Hearing and Speech Sciences, University of Maryland, College Park.

Conclusion

Clinician attitudes toward African Americans and African American attitudes toward clinic and health organizations continue to influence how speech-language services are provided and who seeks care.

The culturally competent clinician views African American clients as they view all clients—as people who differ in age, gender, culture, region, ethnicity, religion, and socioeconomic backgrounds who might or do have a communication disorder. Indeed, clinicians should consider the total person as they design creative, innovative, and appropriate assessment and intervention procedures that can make a true and positive difference in a client's quality of life.

References

American Speech-Language-Hearing Association. (1983). Position paper on social dialects. *ASHA, 25*, 23–25.

Andrulis, D. P. (1998). Access to care is the centerpiece in the elimination of socioeconomic disparities in health. *Annals of Internal Medicine, 129*, 412–416.

Battle, D. E., & Grantham. R. B. (1997). Serving culturally and linguistically diverse students. In P. O'Connell (Ed.), *Speech, language and hearing programs in schools: A guide for students and practitioners* (pp. 345–371). Gaithersburg, MD: Aspen.

Baugh, J. (1983). *Black street speech.* Austin, TX: University of Texas Press.

Blake, W. M., & Darling, C. A. (2000). Quality of life: Perceptions of African Americans. *Journal of Black Studies, 30*(3), 411–427.

Blake, I. K. (1984). *Language development in working-class black children: An examination of form, content, and use.* Doctoral dissertation, Columbia University Teachers College.

Bleile, K., & Wallach, H. (1992). A sociological investigation of the speech of African American preschoolers. *American Journal of Speech-Language Pathology, 1*(2), 54–62.

Bloom, L., & Lahey, M. (1978). *Language development and language disorders.* New York: Wiley.

Bridgeforth, C. (1984). *The development of language functions among black children from working class families.* Paper presented at the presession of the 35th annual Georgetown University Round Table on Language and Linguistics, Georgetown University, Washington, DC.

Burling, R. (1973). *English in black and white.* New York: Holt, Rinehart & Winston.

Butcher, M. J. (1964). *The Negro in American culture.* New York: Knopf.

Campbell, L. (1996). Issues in service delivery to African American children. In A. G. Kamhi, K. E. Pollock, & J. L. Harris (Eds.), *Communication development and disorders in African American children* (pp. 73–94). Baltimore: Brookes.

Campbell, T., Dollaghan, C., Needleman, H., & Janosky, J. (1997). Reducing bias in language assessment: Process dependent measures. *Journal of Speech, Language, and Hearing Research, 40*(3), 519–525.

Campbell, T. F., Needleman, H. L., Reiss, J. A., & Tobin, M. J. (1995, June). *Bone lead level and language processing performance.* Poster session presented at the annual meeting of the Symposium on Research in Child Language disorders, Madison, WI.

Champion, T., Katz, L., Muldrow, R., & Dail, R. (1999). Storytelling and storymaking in an urban preschool classroom: Building bridges from home to school culture. *Topics in Language Disorders, 19,* 52–67.

Champion, T., Seymour, H., & Camarata, S. (1995). Narrative discourse of African American children. *Journal of Narrative and Life History, 5,* 333–352.

Cole, L. (1980). *Developmental analysis of social dialect features in the spontaneous language of preschool black children.* Doctoral dissertation, Northwestern University.

Cole, P., & Taylor, O. (1990). Performance of working-class African American children on three tests of articulation. *Language, Speech, and Hearing Services in Schools, 24,* 171–176.

Coleman, R. R., & Daniel, J. L. (2000). Mediating ebonics. *Journal of Black Studies, 31,* 74–95.

Collins, J. (1985). Some problems and purposes of narratives in educational research. *Journal of Educational Research, 167,* 57–68.

Craig, H. K., & Washington, J. A. (1994). The complex syntax skills of poor, urban, African American preschoolers at school entry. *Language, Speech, and Hearing Services in Schools, 25,* 181–190.

Craig, H. K., & Washington, J. A. (1995). African American English and linguistic complexity in preschool discourse: A second look. *Language, Speech, and Hearing Services in Schools, 26*(1), 87–93.

Davis, P., Williams, J., & Vaughn-Cooke, F. B. (1992–1993). A comparison of lexical development in a child with normal language development and in a child with language delay. *Journal of the National Student Speech-Language Hearing Association, 20,* 63–77.

Dillard, J. L. (1973). Black English: Its history and usage in the United States. New York: Vintage.

Dunn, M. L., & Dunn, M. L. (1997). *Peabody picture vocabulary test-III.* Circle Pines, MN: American Guidance Service.

Erickson, F. (1984). Rhetoric, anecdote, and rhapsody: Cohesion strategies in conversations among black American adolescents. In D. Tannen (Ed.), *Cohesion in spoken and written discourse* (pp. 81–154). Norwood, NJ: Ablex.

Foster, H. L. (1990). *Ribbin' jivin' & playin' the dozens: The persistent dilemma in our schools* (2nd ed.). Williamsville, NY: Herbert L. Foster.

Franklin, M. E. (1992). Culturally sensitive instructional practices for African American learners with disabilities. *Exceptional Children, 59,* 115–122.

Gee, J. (1985). The narrativization of experience in the oral style. *Journal of Education, 167,* 9–35.

Gee, J. (1989). Two styles of narrative construction and their literacy and educational implications. *Discourse Processes, 12,* 263–265.

Goodenough, W. H. (1999). Outline of a framework for a theory of cultural evolution. *Cross-Cultural Research, 33*(1), 84–107.

Haskins, J., & Butts, H. F. (1973). *The psychology of black language.* New York: Barnes & Noble.

Haynes, W., & Moran, M. (1989). A cross-sectional developmental study of final consonant production in Southern black children from preschool through the third grade. *Language, Speech, and Hearing Services in Schools, 20,* 400–406.

Heath, S. B. (1982). What no bedtime story means: Narrative skills at home, at school. *Language in Society, 11,* 49–76.

Heath, S. B. (1986). Taking a cross-cultural look at narratives. *Topics in Language Disorders, 7,* 84–94.

Hester, E. J. (1994). *The relationship between narrative style, dialect, and reading ability of African American children.* Doctoral dissertation, University of Maryland, Baltimore.

Hester, E. J. (1996). Narratives of young African American children. In A. Kamhi, K. E. Pollock, & J. Harris (Eds.), *Communication development and disorders in African American children* (pp. 227–245). Baltimore: Brookes Publishing Co.

Hicks, D. (1991). Kinds of narratives: Genre skills among first graders from two communities. In A. McCabe & C. Peterson (Eds.), *Developing narrative structure* (pp. 55–87). Hillsdale, NJ: Lawrence Erlbaum Associates.

Hyon, S., & Sulzby, E. (1994). African American kindergartner's spoken narratives: Topic associating and topic centered styles. *Linguistics and Education, 6,* 121–152.

Hyter, Y. D., & Westby, C. E. (1996). Using oral narratives to assess communicative competence. In A. G., Kamhi, K. E., Pollock, & J. L., Harris (Eds.). *Communication development and disorders in African American children* (pp. 247–284). Baltimore: Brookes Publishing Co.

Jones, L. (1963). Blues people. New York: Morrow.

Kovac, C. (1980). *Children's acquisition of variable features.* Doctoral dissertation, Georgetown University, Washington, DC.

Labov, W. (1966). *The social stratification of English in New York City.* Washington, DC: Center for Applied Linguistics.

Lahey, M. (1988). *Language disorders and language development.* New York: Macmillan.

Michaels, S. (1981). Sharing time: Children's narrative style and differential access to literacy. *Language in Society, 10,* 423–442.

Michaels, S., & Collins, J. (1984). Oral discourse styles: Classroom interaction and the acquisition of literacy. In D. Tannen (Ed.), *Cohesion in written and spoken discourse* (pp. 219–244). Norwood, NJ: Ablex.

Moran, M. (1993). Final consonant deletion in African American children speaking Black English: A closer look. *Language, Speech, and Hearing Services in Schools, 24,* 161–166.

Needleman, H., & Bellinger, D. (1991). Health effects of low level exposure to lead. *Annual Reviews of Public Health, 12,* 111–140.

Nichols, P. (1989). Storytellin' in Carolina: Continuities and contrasts. *Anthropology and Education, 20*(3), 232–245.

Olson, D. (1977). From utterance to text: The bias of language in speech and writing. *Harvard Educational Review, 47*(3), 257–282.

Peuschels, S. M., Linakis, S. G., & Anderson, A. C. (Eds.) (1996). *Lead poisoning in children.* Baltimore: Brookes Publishing Co.

Reveron, W. W. (1978). *The acquisition of four Black English morphological rules by black preschool children.* Doctoral dissertation, Ohio State University, Columbus, OH.

Roseberry-McKibbin, C. (1995). *Multicultural students with special language needs.* Oceanside, CA: Academic Communication Associates.

Seymour, H. (1995, December). *Theory and practice in evaluating child African American English.* Paper presented at the annual convention of the American Speech-Language-Hearing Association, Orlando, FL.

Seymour, H. N., Bland-Stewart, L., & Green, L. J. (1998). Difference versus deficit in child African American English. *Language, Speech, and Hearing Services in Schools, 29,* 96–108.

Seymour, H. N., deVilliers, J., & Roeper, T. (2000, November). *A dialect-sensitive language screener.* Paper presented at the annual convention of the American Speech-Language-Hearing Association, Washington, DC.

Seymour, H. N. & Roeper, T. (1999). Grammatical acquisition of African American English. In O. L., Taylor, & L., Leonard (Eds.), *Language acquisition across North America: Cross-cultural and cross-linguistic perspectives.* San Diego: Singular Publishing Group.

Seymour, H., & Seymour, C. (1981). Black English and standard American contrasts in communication development of 4- and 5-year-old children. *Journal of Speech and Hearing Disorders, 46,* 276–280.

Seymour, H., & Ralabate, P. (1985). The acquisition of a phonological feature of Black English. *Journal of Communication Disorders, 18,* 139–148.

Steffensen, M. (1974). *The acquisition of Black English.* Doctoral dissertation, University of Illinois, Chicago.

Stockman, I. J. (1984, September). *The development of linguistic norms for nonmainstream populations.* Paper presented at the National Conference for Concerns for Minority Groups in Communication Disorders, Nashville, TN.

Stockman, I. J. (1986a). Language acquisition in culturally diverse populations: The black child as a case study. In O. Taylor (Ed.), *Nature of communication disorders in culturally and linguistically diverse populations* (pp. 117–156). San Diego: College Hill.

Stockman, I. J. (1986b). The development of linguistic norms for nonmainstream populations. In F. H. Bess, B. S. Clark, & H. R. Mitchell (Eds.), *Concerns for minority groups in communication disorders [ASHA reports 16]* (pp. 101–110). Rockville, MD: ASHA.

Stockman, I. (1991, November). *Constraints on final consonant deletion in Black English.* Paper presented at the annual convention of the American Speech-Language-Hearing Association, Atlanta.

Stockman, I. J. (1995, November). *Early morphosyntactic patterns of African American children.* Paper presented at the annual convention of the American Speech-Language-Hearing Association, Orlando, FL.

Stockman, I. J. (1996). The promises and pitfalls of language sample analysis as an assessment tool for linguistic minority children. *Language, Speech, and Hearing Services in Schools, 27*(4), 355–366.

Stockman, I. J. (1999). Semantic development of African American children. In O. L., Taylor & L., Leonard (Eds.) *Language acquisition across North America: Cross-cultural and cross-linguistic perspectives.* San Diego, CA: Singular Publishing Group.

Stockman, I. J. (2000). The new Peabody picture vocabulary test-III: An illusion of unbiased assessment. *Language, Speech, and Hearing Services in Schools, 31*, 340–354.

Stockman, I. J., & Vaughn-Cooke, F. (1982). A re-examination of research on the language of black children: The need for a new framework. *Journal of Education, 164*, 157–172.

Stockman, I. J., & Settle, S. (1991, November). *Initial consonants in young black children's conversational speech.* Poster presented at the annual meeting of the American Speech-Language-Hearing Association, Atlanta.

Sue, D., & Sue, D. F. (1990). *Counseling the culturally different: Theory and practice.* New York: John Wiley & Sons.

Tannen, D. (1982). The oral-literate continuum in discourse. In D. Tannen (Ed.), *Spoken and written language: Exploring orality and literacy* (pp. 1–16). Norwood, NJ: Ablex.

Taylor, O. L. (1987). Clinical practice as a social occasion. In L. C. Cole & V. R. Deal (Eds.), *Communication disorders in multicultural populations.* Unpublished manuscript. Rockville, MD: American Speech-Language-Hearing Association.

Taylor, O. L., & Payne, K. T. (1983). Culturally valid testing: A proactive approach. *Topics in Language Disorders, 3*, 8–20.

Terrell, B. T., & Hale, J. (1992). Serving a multicultural population: Different learning styles. *American Journal of Speech-Language Pathology, 1*, 5–8.

Terrell, F., & Terrell, S. (1981). An inventory to measure cultural mistrust among blacks. *Western Journal of Black Studies, 5,* 180–185.

Terrell, S. L., Arensberg, K., & Rosa, M. (1992). Parent-child comparative analysis: A criterion-referenced method for the nondiscriminatory assessment of a child who spoke a relatively uncommon dialect of English. *Language, Speech, and Hearing Services in Schools, 23,* 34–42.

U.S. Bureau of the Census. (2000). *Statistical abstract of the United States, 2000* (120th ed.). Washington, DC: U.S. Bureau of the Census.

U.S. Department of Health and Human Services. (2000). *Healthy people 2010: Understanding and improving health,* 2nd edition. Washington, DC: Department of Health and Human Services.

Vaughn-Cooke, F. (1986). Lexical diffusion: Evidence from a decreolizing variety of Black English. In M. Montgomery & R. Bailey (Eds.), *Language variety in the South* (pp. 111–130). Tuscaloosa, AL: University of Alabama Press.

Vaughn-Cooke, F., & Wright-Harp, W. (1992). *Lexical development in working-class black children.* National Institutes of Health Grant #RR08005-23.

Washington, J. A. (1996). Issues in assessing the language abilities of African American children. In A. G. Kamhi, K. E. Pollock, & J. L. Harris (Eds.), *Communication development and disorders in African American children* (pp. 35–54). Baltimore: Brookes Publishing Co.

Washington, J., & Craig, H. (1992). Articulation test performance of low-income African American preschoolers with communication impairment. *Language, Speech and Hearing Services in Schools, 22,* 203–207.

Washington, J. A., & Craig, H. K. (1994). Dialectal forms during discourse of urban African American preschoolers living in poverty. *Journal of Speech and Hearing Research, 37,* 816–823.

Washington, J. A., & Craig, H. K. (1998). Socioeconomic status and gender influences on children's dialectal variations. *Journal of Speech, Language, and Hearing Research, 41,* 618–626.

Washington, J. A., & Craig, H. K. (1999). Performances of at-risk, African American preschoolers on the Peabody Picture Vocabulary Test-III. *Language, Speech, and Hearing Services in Schools, 30,* 75–82.

Washington, J. A., Craig, H. K., & Kushmaul, A. J. (1998). Variable use of African American English across two language sampling contexts. *Journal of Speech, Language, and Hearing Research, 41,* 1115–1124.

Westby, C. (1985). Learning to talk—talking to learn: Oral literate language differences. In C. Simon (Ed.), *Communication skills and classroom success* (pp. 181–212). San Diego: College Hill.

Westby, C. E. (1990). Ethnographic interviewing: Asking the right questions to the right people in the right ways. *Journal of Childhood Communication Disorders, 13,* 101–111.

Westby, C. (1994). Multicultural issues. In J. Tomblin, H. Morris, & D. Spriestersbach (Eds.), *Diagnosis in speech-language pathology* (pp. 29–52). San Diego: Singular Publishing Group.

Williams, R. (1975). *Ebonics: The true language of black folks*. St. Louis: Institute of Black Studies.

Williams, R., & Wolfram, W. (1976). *Social dialects: Differences versus disorders*. Rockville, MD: American Speech-Language-Hearing Association.

Willis, W. (1992). Families with African American roots. In E. Lynch & M. J. Hansen (Eds.), *Developing communication competence: A guide for working with young children and their families* (pp. 120–247). Baltimore: Brookes Publishing Co.

Wolfram, W., & Fasold, R. (1974). *The study of social dialects in American English*. Englewood Cliffs, NJ: Prentice Hall.

Wyatt, T. (1991). *Linguistic constraints on copula production in Black English child speech*. Doctoral dissertation, University of Massachusetts, Worcester, MA.

Additional Resources

Barboza, S. (1988). *The African American books of values: Classic moral stories*. New York: Doubleday.

Christian, C. M. (1999). *Black saga: The African American experience, a chronology*. New York: Houghton Mifflin.

Estell, K. (1994). *African America: Portrait of a people*. Detroit: Visible Ink Press.

Johnson, C., & Smith, P. (1998). *Africans in America: America's journey through slavery*. New York: Harcourt Brace & Company.

Smitherman, G. (2000). *Talkin that talk: Language, culture, and education in African America*. New York: Taylor & Francis.

3

□ □ □
□ □ □
□ □ □

Asian and Pacific American Cultures

Li-Rong Lilly Cheng

The purpose of this chapter is to provide a current picture of Asian and Pacific American (APA) cultures and languages. In addition, information for speech-language pathologists (SLPs) on assessment and intervention will also be provided. As a note, while the U.S. Bureau of the Census categorizes Asia to include such countries as Iran, Iraq and other countries of the far Middle East, this text will restrict the discussion of Asian to those in the Far East. Asian countries in the Middle East will be considered in Chapter 6 on Middle Eastern and Arab American Cultures.

APAs originate from Pacific Asia or are descendants of Asian and Pacific Islander immigrants. APA is fast becoming an influential presence in the United States socially, politically, and economically. It is projected that the white population in this nation will decrease from 73.5% to 51.2%, while the Asian and Pacific and Hispanic or Latino population will continue to increase (Baker & Pryor Jones, 1998).

The Asian American school-age population increased more than sixfold from 212,900 in 1960 to almost 1.3 million by 1990. In 1996, there were more than 42 million Asian Americans in the United States (U.S. Bureau of the Census, 2000). By the year 2020, Asian American children in U.S. schools are projected to total approximately 4.4 million. According to the U.S. Bureau of the Census (2000) the largest number of Asian immigrants to the U.S. is the Chinese, second only to the immigrants from Mexico of all immigrant groups.

APAs are extremely diverse in all aspects of their ways of life, including language, culture, religion, attitudes toward education, child rearing practices, and roles within the family. The Asian and Pacific Island cultures,

however, have interacted with and influenced each other for many generations and, therefore, share many similarities. The following information is
presented to provide an understanding of APA to assist the speech-language
pathologist in providing services to this culturally and linguistically diverse
group of people.

Overview of Asian and Pacific American People

APAs have been immigrating to the United States for more
than two centuries, with the first records of arrival of Chinese dating from
1785. Since that time, more than 17 Asian groups have immigrated to the
United States. The most numerous APAs have origins in China (i.e., Taiwan
and the People's Republic of China), Hong Kong, Japan, Korea, India, Vietnam, Cambodia (Kampuchea), Laos, Guam, the Philippines, India, Pakistan,
Bangladesh, Malaysia, Indonesia, Singapore, and Samoa. Since 1975, more
than 1 million refugees from Southeast Asia have settled in the United
States (Jiobu, 1996; U.S. Bureau of the Census, 1995). Each of the countries in
Asia and the Asian Pacific represent an individual and distinct culture with
unique values, beliefs, and worldviews. Each has its own language and dialect, communication behaviors, and style. It is critical that clinicians recognize the heterogeneity of the Asian and Asian Pacific peoples and consider
the unique characteristic of each subgroup, as well as the uniqueness of individuals within the group.

Unlike the earlier immigrants from East Asia, the recent influx represents
a diverse group from Southeast Asia, Hong Kong, China, India, Pakistan,
Malaysia, Indonesia, and other Pacific Rim and Pacific Basin areas. Refugees
and immigrants from Asia and the Pacific Islands come from a variety of historical, social, educational, and political backgrounds. Some are affluent, well-
educated, voluntary immigrants, and some are preliterate refugees. They bring
a variety of financial profiles, languages, folk beliefs, worldviews, religious
beliefs, child-rearing practices, and attitudes toward education, all of which
have a profound impact on speech-language pathology services.

Definitions of Impairments: Role of Culture

A cultural definition of what constitutes an impairment is
dependent on the values of each cultural group. APA folklore is full of the
belief system and spiritualism. The treatment of birth defects, disorders,
and disabilities is influenced by cultural beliefs and by the socioeconomic
status of the individual and the family within a given group (Cheng, 1999;
Gollnick & Chinn, 1990; Strauss, 1990). In all cultures, attitudes toward

disabilities can be traced in part to folk beliefs and superstitions. Many Asian Pacific cultures define the cause of a health-related problem in spiritual terms (Cheng, 1999; Meyerson, 1990; Strauss, 1990). Many Eastern cultures view a disabling condition as the result of wrongdoing of the individuals' ancestors, resulting in guilt and shame. The cause of disabilities is explained through a variety of spiritual or cultural beliefs, or both, such as imbalance of inner forces, bad wind, spoiled foods, gods, demons or spirits, hot or cold forces, or fright. For example, the Chamorro culture views a disability as a gift from God and believes that the person with a disability belongs to everyone in the community and in the extended family. The person with the disability is thus protected and sheltered by the family. For example, many Chinese believe disability is caused by karma (fate). Pakistani may view individuals with a visible disability as a curse and ostracize such an individual from society (Cheng, 1989; Trueba, Cheng, & Ima, 1993). Attitudes toward disabilities are a reflection of current and historical beliefs about the nature of disabilities. All over the world, people use different methods to treat illnesses and diseases, including consulting with a priest, barefoot doctor, herbalist, Qi-Gong specialist, clansman, shaman, elder, or a physician. Among the Hmong, for example, surgical intervention is viewed as invasive and harmful. The Hmong believe that spirits may leave the body once the body is cut open, causing death (Fadiman, 1997). Treatment procedures also vary, ranging from surgical intervention or therapy to acupuncture, message, cao (coin rubbing), gat gio (pinching), giac (placing a very hot cup on the exposed area), steam inhalation, balm application, herbs, inhaling smoke or ashes from burnt incense, or the ingestion of hot or cold foods (Cheng, 1995a).

Child Rearing Practices

Child rearing practices and expectations from children vary widely from culture to culture (Hammer & Weiss, 2000; Heath, 1983; Van Kleeck, 1994; Westby, 1990). There are differences in how parents respond to their children's language, how and who interacts with children, and how parents and families encourage children to initiate and continue a verbal interaction. Differences in the best educational practices must be taken into account as well. Some families understand and support bilingual education; others have no opinion because they believe that schools know best about how to educate their children. Among those families there is also variation about attitudes toward the first and second language and culture, various levels of formal education in the first or second language, or both, as well as expectation for their children (Butler & Cheng, 1996; Cheng, 1998; Heibert, 1991).

Languages

The hundreds of different languages and dialects that are spoken in East and Southeast Asia and the Pacific Islands can be classified into five major families: (1) Malayo-Polynesian (Austronesian), including Chamorro, Ilocano, and Tagalog; (2) Sino-Tibetan, including Thai, Yao, Mandarin, and Cantonese; (3) Austroasiatic, including Khmer, Vietnamese, and Hmong; (4) Papuan, including New Guinean; and (5) Altaic, including Japanese and Korean (Ma, 1985). Additionally, there are 15 major languages in India from four language families: (1) Indo-Aryan, (2) Dravidian, (3) Austroasiatic, and (4) Tibeto-Burman (Shekar & Hegde, 1995).

Folk Beliefs, Religions, and Philosophical Views

The Asian and Pacific populations hold a variety of religious and philosophical beliefs. Major religions and philosophies include Buddhism, Confucianism, Taoism, Shintoism, Animism, and Islam. In addition, because of Western influence, Christianity is also practiced. There are many Catholic churches in the Philippines and across the Pacific Islands. Many Pacific Islanders consider the Bible a major source of inspiration. There are many different Asian and Pacific folk beliefs. Folk beliefs are generally passed down informally through oral history from generation to generation, whereas religious beliefs are generally archived and passed down formally. People vary in their reactions to folk beliefs because of their diverse experience in different levels of education and exposure to Western education cultures. In addition to folk beliefs, many APA practice faith healing; other methods of healing include exercises such as Qi-Gong, over-the-counter drugs, prescription drugs, or a combination of methods. The use of non-Western methods of healing may be difficult for Western physicians to manage in their overall treatment of patients, because they are not always familiar with such methods.

Education

The prevailing views toward education in most Asian and Pacific cultures present challenges for American educators and speech-language pathologists. People from China, Korea, Japan, and Vietnam often view education as the most important goal one can achieve in life. This is due largely to the influence of the teachings and principles of Confucius (Cheng, 1993). They often have different approaches to learning, and these approaches have implications for the strategies Asian students use to learn. The selected examples in Table 3-1 are representative of

Table 3-1   Asian Attitudes toward Learning

Asian Cultural Themes	*Educational Implications*
Education is formal.	Teachers are formal and are expected to lecture.
Teachers are to be highly respected.	Teachers are not to be interrupted. Students are reluctant to ask questions.
Humility is an important virtue.	Students are not to "show off" or volunteer information.
Reading of factual information is studying.	Fiction is not considered serious reading.
It is important to have order and to be obedient.	Students are to sit quietly and listen attentively.
One learns by observation and by memorization.	Rote memory is considered an effective teaching tool.
Pattern practice and rote learning are studying.	Homework in pattern practice is important and is expected.

some Asian attitudes toward education and their educational implications. The relative importance of each of the attitudes differs from culture to culture.

As shown in Table 3-1, there are incongruities between Asian students' learning styles and American teachers' teaching styles. These differences can lead to teachers' misconceptions of students and students' confusion over the "proper" way of schooling, particularly with the naturalistic, whole-language approach to treatment, especially of preschool-aged and early elementary school–aged children. Again, the relative importance of each of the concepts varies with cultural group and among individuals within the group. Educators need to be sensitive to cultural tendencies of various APA groups. These tendencies, however, should not be viewed as static cultural rules. Generalizations must be avoided and predictions should not be made based on a superficial survey of the culture.

Cultural Characteristics of Asian and Pacific Peoples

All APA groups and the individuals in those groups present some common background as immigrants or descendants of immigrants. Each may have a very different story to tell. Such diverse personal and group experiences must be taken into consideration when working with individuals.

Clearly, intra- and intergroup differences exist among the Asian and Pacific Islander immigrant and refugee groups. Refugees are generally not prepared for emigration and leave their country of origin suddenly. Immigrants go through long periods of application and petition and are generally prepared for emigration. As stated earlier, caution should be taken to avoid overgeneralization of this information in relation to a particular client or family, because the APA clients and their families represent diverse social, cultural, and linguistic backgrounds.

The Chinese

Immigration History
The Chinese first immigrated to the United States in the 1800s. Records document the arrival of Chinese in the United States in 1785. Chinese immigrants, who came in greater numbers beginning in 1848, worked as miners and farmers and provided the major labor force for building the railroads. During the Sino-Japanese war, there was little immigration. Since the end of World War II, Chinese have been immigrating to the United States mainly from Taiwan and Hong Kong to study, join their families, or for business purposes. In recent years, more Chinese from the People's Republic of China have entered the United States. Immigrants from the People's Republic of China constituted one of the largest groups of immigrants in the 1990s. Today, the Chinese are the largest group of persons from Asia in the United States.

Religion and Values
There are 56 ethnic groups in China. They practice a variety of religions, including Buddhism, Taoism, Catholicism and other forms of Christianity, and Islam. They also believe in ancestral worship and Confucianism. One of the most important ideals of the Chinese culture is the pursuit and maintenance of harmony. Value is placed on outward calmness and on control of undesirable emotions such as anger, jealousy, hostility, aggression, and self-pity. Open expression of emotion and confrontation is viewed as undesirable. The three least desirable characteristics in Buddhism are greed, anger, and ignorance.

The Family
Chinese culture places a heavy emphasis on respect for elders and the strength of the family as a unit. Each member of the family has a role that is clearly defined through an intricate kinship system. Traditionally, the father was responsible for all decisions, with the mother having direct responsibility for caring of the elderly and the oldest son or daughter having responsibility for the care of his or her younger siblings. Parents taught their children to behave according to strict rules. In recent decades, the changing role of women and China's zero-population-growth policy has had significant impact on the roles of women and children.

Education

The Chinese traditionally believe that education is extremely important. Chinese Americans work hard to remove any linguistic and cultural barriers to obtaining a good education. Most traditional Chinese families expect their children to do well in school. Teachers are highly respected. If a child is successful in school, the entire family receives credit. Parents do not praise their children readily, even when they excel, because excellence is generally expected. If a child does poorly in school or needs special attention, the parents often feel ashamed, perceiving the difficulties as a sign of their own failure. Many Chinese American parents take their children to a Chinese language school on weekends and expect them to learn Chinese and maintain the culture.

Chinese students who have immigrated recently from Taiwan have had quite different educational experiences from students who immigrated from the People's Republic of China. Chinese students who have gone to school in the People's Republic of China, however, do reasonably well in U.S. schools, because they have had a competitive education similar to that in the United States. The terms *model minority* and *silent minority* have been used to describe the success of Chinese students. Their communicative disorders may be overlooked because they are quiet and often invisible.

Language

More than 80 languages and hundreds of dialects are spoken in China. The Chinese dialects are extremely complex. Some are closely related, whereas others are mutually unintelligible, even though their words are graphically represented by the same characters (Cheng, 1991). Of the Chinese population, 94% are reported to speak Han (a Sino-Tibetan language) and its dialects Mandarin, Wu, Yue (Cantonese), Xiang, Gan, Kejia, and Min. More than two-thirds speak the Mandarin dialect of Han. The two main dialects spoken by the Chinese in the United States are Mandarin (i.e., the national language of Taiwan and of the People's Republic of China) and Cantonese.

The languages spoken by the peoples of China are classified into five broad language groupings: (1) Sino-Tibetan, (2) Altaic, (3) Malayo-Polynesian, (4) Austroasiatic, and (5) Indo-European. Chinese has a logographic written system, which means that words are represented graphically by logographs or ideographs, with a single logograph or a combination of logographs, or both, representing a meaningful unit (Li & Thompson, 1981). Clinicians need to know the actual language or dialect spoken by their clients and patients to find appropriate interpreters.

Chinese is also a tonal language. Each character is phonetically represented by a single syllable, with each syllable having a tone mark. In Mandarin Chinese, there are four tones (and a neutral tone): The first tone has a high level, the second tone is rising, the third tone is falling-rising, and the fourth tone is falling. The same spoken syllable has different meanings, depending on the tone and various characters that the syllable represents. Each Han dialect has its own tonal system with differing numbers of tones. Deaf and hearing-impaired individuals find tones an added challenge in their acquisition of oral language, because tones are phonemic and carry meaning (Ching, 1990). Alaryngeal speakers also are challenged by the lack of ability to produce the different tones. Individuals with motor speech and voice disorders also often encounter difficulties in controlling the various tones. A syllable in Mandarin and Cantonese consists of segmental and suprasegmental features (Chi, 1999). Segmental features include an initial consonant (optional) and a final sound. Suprasegmental features include the distinct tones that are an intrinsic part of the phonologic makeup of a Chinese syllable. It may also be difficult for Chinese speakers to learn English intonation patterns, such as those signaling the difference between questions and statements.

There are several major differences between the phonetic systems of Chinese and English. Chinese characters are each composed of a single syllable. The rules for syllabification and syllabic stress in English can present difficulty for a Mandarin or Cantonese speaker. The speakers may sound telegraphic and may truncate words.

Because there are only two final consonants in Mandarin, /n/ and /ŋ/, and only seven final consonants in Cantonese, /m/, /n/, /ŋ/, /p/, /t/, /k/, and glottal stop /ʔ/, Chinese speakers often omit final consonants when speaking English. There are no consonant clusters in Mandarin or Cantonese, making the double and triple consonant clusters such as /spl/ and /str/ difficult for Chinese speakers, sometimes resulting in consonant deletion. Chinese learners of English may use Chinese sounds when speaking English if the sounds are phonetically similar in the two languages, such as /s/ and /ʃ/. The differing vowel systems can also cause some confusion. Cantonese speakers, for example, may substitute /e/ for /ɛ/ and /æ/, /i/ for /I/, /ou/ for /ɔ/ (e.g., "boat" for *bought*), or /u/ for /ʌ/ (e.g., "roof" for *rough*).

Unlike English, Chinese is noninflectional and does not use plural markers, tense markers, copulas, the verb *has*, the auxiliary *do*, articles, or conjunctions. In addition, the rules for the use of prepositions, pronouns, negatives, and other morphologic and syntactic forms vary—for example, "me no like it" instead of "I don't like it"—causing considerable difficulty for Chinese speakers when they are learning English. The semantic differences between English and Chinese words further compound the difficulty Chinese speakers have in learning English.

The pragmatic rules of the Chinese language such as turn-taking, greeting, social distance, proximity, and politeness vary a great deal from those of the English language. Because Chinese speakers generally do not interrupt a speaker to ask questions, students may appear to be passive or nonparticipatory. A socially appropriate Chinese greeting is "Have you eaten?," to which the accepted response is "Yes," which is similar to the English greeting "How are you?" and the answer "Fine." Social distance is determined by such attributes as age, class, and marital status. Chinese may not express emotion in public, and hugging, kissing, and touching are not frequently observed. A giggle can be used as a sign of embarrassment. The Chinese are taught to be humble and when praised are generally embarrassed. When someone says, "Thank you," the correct response is generally, "No need to thank me" rather than the English "You are welcome."

The Koreans

Immigration History

Koreans have one of the oldest surviving civilizations on earth and have maintained a significant number of their cultural traditions. For many centuries, the Koreans refused to compromise with other nations and remained closed to foreign ideas. As a result, they became a "hermit" nation (Kim, 1978). Since World War II, South Korea and North Korea have been clearly divided politically. In 2000, the two governments finally began talking. President Kim of South Korea won a Nobel Prize for Peace in 2000.

Korean immigration to the United States began in the early twentieth century, when Korean laborers went to Hawaii to work in the pineapple and sugarcane plantations and later went to the mainland. Before World War II, however, the Korean community in the United States was not visible because of its small population. Approximately 800,000 Koreans were living in the United States in 1990 (U.S. Bureau of the Census, 2000). More Koreans have emigrated in the last two decades.

Religion

Korean immigrants are primarily Christian. Many Christian churches in Korean communities conduct services in the Korean language. These churches also provide social and emotional support, informational help, and to serve as acculturation agents (Kim, 1981).

The Family

As with other Asian cultures, Koreans value the extended family, which typically includes three generations (Kim, 1978). Traditionally, the father is the head of the family and represents the family honor. He is responsible for the welfare of the family and is typically the sole provider. The father or other men in the Korean family do not typically help with household chores (Kim, 1984). The Korean mother, who centers her work on the home, usually represents the family in dealing with the school. The elderly family members previously received a great deal of respect from younger family members.

Parent-child conflicts based on language and cultural differences have increased between immigrant children and parents. Due to economic pressures, the size of the Korean family has decreased in the United States. Children have begun to question the traditional role of the father and to challenge his authority.

Education

Since 1945, the educational system in South Korea has been patterned after the American educational system of elementary school, junior high, senior high, followed by 2 years of junior college or 4 years at a university (Kim, 1978). Teachers have a great deal of authority. Korean classrooms are orderly. Korean children are socialized into an environment in which going to the best schools is highly valued. They are accustomed to working extremely hard to obtain high scores on college entrance examinations to get into the best colleges. They are directed from the very beginning into specific fields such as business, science, medicine, or engineering and are not typically encouraged to go into fine arts and human services. There is little room for other alternatives or for students who are not capable of high achievement.

Language

The Korean language belongs to the Altaic family. Koreans in North and South Korea speak the same language. There are some variations among the various regional dialects, but they are mutually intelligible. Until 1443, the Koreans used the Chinese written system. After that time, the Hangul system was developed. The Korean written language has 19 consonants and eight vowels. The sound of a letter is pronounced differently depending on its location in a word.

The phonetic systems of English and Korean are quite different and cause difficulty for Koreans learning to speak English. Fricatives and affricates do not occur in the final position of words, and final stops are often nasalized when they occur before a nasal sound (e.g., "banman" instead of "batman"). Because there are no labiodental, interdental, or palatal fricatives in Korean, speakers may make the following substitutions: b/v, p/v, s/sh, s/z, t/ch, and dz/th. Korean does not have vowel distinction so that the following vowels are problematic: /i/, /I/, /u/, /ʌ/, and /au/. Because [r] and [l] belong to the same phonetic category, they may be used interchangeably (e.g., r/l and l/r) (Chu, 1999).

Because there is no word stress in Korean, Korean speakers can sound monotonous and have difficulty with interrogative intonation, which is typically found in English question forms. In addition, there are several syntactic and morphologic differences between English and Korean that lead to difficulty for Koreans in learning English. Korean has no gender agreement, no articles, no verb inflections for tense and number, and no relative pronouns.

Korean communication behavior has been influenced by the Chinese. Important factors are harmony, filial piety, social order, fairness, reverence for elders, and the maintenance of human relationships. The choice of words and grammar denote the relationship between the communicators and the importance of that relationship (Chu, 1990). Nonverbal communication is very important, because taciturnity reduces the amount of verbal interchange. Silence is a much more important part of communication for the Korean speaker than for the English speaker (Chu, 1990). Korean has four different levels of speech (higher honorific, simple honorific). Korean children acquire the basic rules of honorifics by the time they enter elementary school (Chu, 1999).

The Japanese

Immigration History

Because land in their native island country was limited, large numbers of Japanese began to immigrate to the United States (first to Hawaii and then to California) between 1891 and 1907. Once in the United States, the Japanese worked at the lowest paying jobs in agriculture, mining, fishing, railroad building, and small businesses (Cheng, 1991). Since that time, the Japanese have spent considerable energies to educate themselves and to improve their standard of living. Japanese Americans have assimilated well and participate in social, business, civic, political, and religious groups outside Japanese American communities. They continue to integrate into predominantly white residential neighborhoods. Japanese Americans are the third largest Asian group in the United States.

Religion

Shintoism, a form of Buddhism, is the dominant religion in Japan today, although Christianity has been adopted by a large proportion of its population. In the United States, many Japanese Americans are Christians. The Japanese are the largest ethnic group in Hawaii, and many are practicing Christians.

The Family

The Japanese Americans are primarily U.S.-born, second-, third-, fourth-, and fifth-generation Japanese Americans. The terms *ni-sei* (second generation) and *san-sei* (third generation) are commonly used to refer to the number of generations the family has been in the United States. Japanese families generally value obedience, dependence on the family, formality in interpersonal relationships, and restraint in the expression of emotions. As in other Asian families, Japanese family members have well-defined roles and positions of power. Japanese children are expected to maintain emotional bonds with and dependence on their parents and only secondarily develop self-reliance (Ima & Labovitz, 1990). Japanese parents, wanting children to be receptive to adult expectations, continually refer to duty and obligation and invoke fear of ridicule and shame to control their children's lives.

Education

The teaching profession is one of the most highly regarded professions to the Japanese. To the Japanese, education is of prime importance. The Japanese student is expected to be attentive, work cooperatively, and be willing to accept the teacher's word as significant (Ima & Labovitz, 1990). In the United States, Japanese American students are often sent to after-school classes or to private tutors to ensure academic success. This contributes significantly to the pressures placed on children to be successful.

Language

Japanese is part of the Altaic language family. The Japanese writing system, which was adopted from the Chinese system, uses characters in writing called *Kanji*. The Japanese modified the Chinese symbols for phonetic purposes, organizing a syllabary called *Kana* in which each symbol represents one syllable (Cheng, 1991). Japanese is polysyllabic and has an elaborate inflectional system. Japanese is not tonal, with every syllable being given equal stress.

Japanese has five vowels (/a/, /i/, /u/, /e/, and /o/) and 18 consonants (/k/, /s/, /t/, /n/, /h/, /m/, /y/, /r/, /w/, /g/, /d/, /b/, /z/, /p/, /tʃ/, /ʃ/, and /j/). Vowels vary in duration, as they do in English. Only the /n/ phoneme occurs as a final consonant. Double consonants such as /kk/ and /pp/ may occur. Difficulties encountered by Japanese people learning English are substitutions of r/l, s/θ, z/ð, j/voiced, /th/, and b/v; the addition of vowels to words ending in consonants (deske/desk, miluku/milk); and approximations of phonemes (/f/ phoneme is pronounced between /f/ and /h/, resulting in /food/hood/. Japanese syllable structure consonant-vowel may result in a vowel insertion after the final consonant or between consonants in clusters such as /spaleshes/ for /splashes/. In Japanese, the sound is actually a vowelless bilateral fricative [/ɸ/] made by holding the lips together loosely and blowing air through them. As for the Japanese, /r/ sound lies somewhere in between the English /l/ and /r/. The closest approximation to the voiceless /θ/ is [t] in English. The [d] comes closest to the voiced /ð/ in English. The Japanese /b/ comes closest to the English /v/, and the Japanese /j/ comes closest to the English /z/ as in *azure* (Whitenack & Kikunaga, 1999).

Several grammatical features of Japanese interfere with learning English. Personal pronouns are often omitted, because they are inferred from the context. No distinction is made between the singular and plural, so that, for example, *hon* means book and books, with the meaning inferred from context. Because *yes* and *no* questions are marked by a final particle, question markers (e.g., *what* and *where*) are not needed at the initial position of a sentence. In a study of narrative and pragmatics among the Japanese, Minami and McCabe (1991) found that Japanese children speak succinctly about collections of experiences rather than elaborating on any one experience in particular. Furthermore, they found that Japanese mothers request proportionally fewer descriptions from their children, pay more verbal attention to boys than to girls, give fewer evaluations, and show more verbal attention than parents in North America. In the Japanese culture, the concept of rapport and empathy (*omoiyari*) says that the children are expected to anticipate what will be asked of them and to do it without being asked directly.

There are distinct cultural differences between the Japanese and Americans in classroom interaction. For example, group behavior and cooperation, important cultural concepts in Japanese society, are taught and learned in preschool. Peak (1991) professes that going to school in Japan is primarily training in group life or *Shudan seikatsu*. Lewis (1995) asserts that Japanese students do not just work *in* groups, they work *as* groups. Teachers create groups and group activities to help children enhance one another's strengths and overcome one another's weaknesses. Japanese children in the United States may still be expected to behave this way because of parental influence.

The Southeast Asians

Southeast Asia is comprised of Vietnam, Thailand, Laos, Cambodia (Kampuchea), and Burma. These countries have similar foods and are similar in geography and climate but differ in culture and religion. Because the Burmese and Thai are few in number in the United States, these groups are not discussed in this chapter.

Immigration History

Before 1975, there were few Southeast Asians in the United States. After 1975, however, more than 1 million Southeast Asians fled their countries because of communist takeover of their governments.

The first wave of Southeast Asian immigrants (refugees), who arrived in the United States in 1975, were Vietnamese who had worked for or been affiliated with the U.S. government during the Vietnam war. They were well educated and had some previous exposure to Western ideology and culture.

The second wave of Southeast Asian refugees arrived between 1979 and 1982. This group included Vietnamese, Cambodians, Laotians, Hmong, and ethnic Chinese who emigrated to Southeast Asia having escaped after considerable hardship. The second wave of immigrants were less well educated, less likely to have had contact with Western culture, less likely to know English, mainly rural, and likely to have spent a long period of time in refugee camps before immigrating.

The third wave of refugees came in 1982. The main purpose of this program was to allow Amerasians, the elderly, and unaccompanied minors to immigrate to the United States. Some of these refugees were preliterate or illiterate.

Many of the refugees took advantage of numerous programs established to assist in their resettlement. For them, life is stable and prosperous, with the children being able to finish school and obtain gainful employment. Other refugees did not adjust well, have not learned English, are underemployed, and feel a sense of loss and isolation. The problems of isolation are particularly serious for women who, because of staying at home to care for the children, have not had opportunities to learn English or adapt to their new surroundings (Ima & Keogh, 1995). There is now a significant number of elderly persons who require home health care and rehabilitation, and there are no trained bilingual SLPs to help them.

The Vietnamese

The Vietnamese practice a variety of religions. The majority practices Buddhism, but Taoism, Christianity, and Confucianism are also followed. The teachings from these religions form the foundation of all traditions, customs, and manners.

The Vietnamese celebrate many holidays. The greatest national holiday is the Tet festival, or Lunar New Year, which lasts several days. It is a time for family reunions, spring festivals, paying homage to ancestors, correcting faults, pardoning others, and paying debts. During the Tet festival, all birthdays are celebrated, because everyone becomes a year older on the last day of the twelfth lunar month. The Vietnamese also celebrate the death days of their parents and grandparents.

The Family

In the Vietnamese culture, the family is paternally oriented and is the chief source of social identity for the individual. The family members live and work together and look first to one another in times of crisis. The family usually consists of multiple generations that live under one roof and includes the husband and wife, their unmarried children, the husband's parents, and their sons' wives and children. Both parents share in disciplining the children. Discipline is usually of a soft, verbal type, with no corporal punishment and no extensive limits on behavior. Often, the responsibility for the children is given to older siblings.

Vietnamese names usually consist of three parts, which occur in the following order: family or clan name, middle name, and given name. A common middle name for men is *Van* and *Thi* for women. Common family names include *Nguyen, Tran,* and *Le* (Chhim, Luangpraseut, & Te, 1987). There are only approximately 300 family names; therefore, using the family name by itself has little meaning. The given name holds the most meaning. Individuals are normally addressed, for example, as "Mr." plus the given name. A married woman retains her own family name but can be referred to as "Mrs." plus the husband's given name. It is important to keep the correct order, as reversing it means addressing a different person. Also, when writing someone's name, the writer should include diacritical markings, which help to distinguish similar-looking names. For example, My Luong Tran is really Tran My Luong. *Tran* is the last name and *My Luong* is the first name.

Language

Vietnamese is a monosyllabic tonal language. Diacritical marks are used to signify the tone of each word. Proficient and educated speakers speak two forms of Vietnamese: the high (formal) form and the vernacular (informal) form (Chuong, 1990).

The following differences exist between English and Vietnamese phonetic systems (Te, 1987):

- Vietnamese words are typically monosyllabic.
- Vietnamese has only a limited number of final consonants, including /p/, /t/, /k/, /m/, /n/, and /ŋ/.

Vietnamese includes many words derived from other languages, such as English, French, Malay, and Chinese. Vietnamese speakers may mispro-

nounce certain English phonemes by substituting a similar Vietnamese phoneme. In Vietnamese, language pronouns are used to maintain proper social
distance and interpersonal relationships and show the intensity of respect or
disrespect (Chuong, 1990).

The Hmong
Immigration History

Originally from China, the Hmong (also spelled Miao, Mung,
Muong, H'mong, Hmoob, and Hmuoung) moved to the mountainous area of
Southeast Asia, primarily Laos, centuries ago. After the fall of South Vietnam in 1975, approximately 100,000 Hmong fled to escape retaliation for
assisting the South Vietnamese in the struggle against the Communists.
Most of them had never been outside their mountain homeland before evac-
uation. The majority of the Vietnamese were illiterate. Before their uproot-
ing, they had not been exposed to the conveniences (and stresses) of the
"modern world."

Most Hmong congregated in the so-called Indochinese communities,
the *de facto* Southeast Asian ghettos in Los Angeles, Fresno, Sacramento,
and cities of the midwest, especially Minneapolis. The immense social and
psychological upheaval the older Hmong had experienced left them physically and financially dependent on their children, physically and psychologically isolated, lacking in self-esteem, and with few of the skills that are
necessary for life in American mainstream society. The elderly Hmong in
the United States continue to practice folk medicine and perform indigenous religious rituals.

Education

The Hmong view of education is different from that of other
Asian refugee groups, in that they have not had a long tradition of literacy and
schooling. Oral tradition is much more important to the Hmong people. History is passed down from generation to generation by storytelling and rituals.

Language

The linguistic characteristics of the Hmong language create
difficulties for Hmong people attempting to learn English. The Hmong language, which is a Sino-Tibetan language, has two dialects: White (*Hmoob
Dawb*) and Green (*Hmoob Ntsuab*). Hmong has 56 initial consonants,
seven tones, and one final consonant /ŋ/ and 16 vowel phonemes. There
are four series of stopped consonants, voiced and voiceless fricatives,
nasals, liquids, and a single voiced glide. Several consonant sounds, such as
/p/, /r/, and /t/, have aspirated and unaspirated forms. The sound /r/, which

is a stop rather than a liquid, is produced in the midpalatal area and may sound like /t/ when aspirated or /d/ when unaspirated. Consonant clusters, which occur only in the initial position of words, include nasals plus stops (e.g., /np/ and /nt/) and nasals plus stops plus /l/ (e.g., /npl/).

Tones and vowels are more important for understanding than the many initial consonants. The sounds of Hmong are represented in the Roman alphabet. Tones are indicated by final letters but are never produced as final consonants in Hmong.

Phonologically, Hmong is a tonal language. Although linguists classify it as a monosyllabic language family, it contains sizable numbers of disyllabic and polysyllabic words. A typical Hmong word consists of a consonant, vowel, and tone marker (e.g., "kuv," *k* is a consonant; *u*, the vowel; and *v*, the tone marker).

Pronunciation problems are the result of the direct transference from Hmong consonantal sounds that correspond directly with English, mainly due to the correct places and the manners of articulation.

The Hmong orthography was phonemically based on the Romanized popular alphabets. Thus, its consonantal phonemes consist of single, double, triple, and quadruple consonantal clusters. Although there are more consonants in Hmong than in English, Hmong students may have problems with phonemic awareness and the pronunciation of certain sounds in English. Hmong speakers may experience difficulty with final consonants, particularly final consonant clusters. On the other hand, pronouncing polysyllabic words with correct primary and secondary stress is fairly easy, once the syllables are thought of as individual words with tones. A Hmong speaker may place too much importance on the vowel sound in unaccented syllables, not understanding that in English these vowels are often schwa sounds.

Unlike English, Hmong is a noninflectional language. Although many Hmongs have oral English fluency, they may still experience difficulty with tenses, using infinitives and gerunds, stringing several verbs together, and using adjectives after nouns.

The Cambodians
Immigration History
Cambodia, also known as Kampuchea, is located in mainland Southeast Asia. France colonized the region in the mid-1800s; in 1863, Cambodia became a French protectorate. In 1953, however, Cambodia gained independence, and the country was proclaimed the Khmer Republic in 1970. When Cambodia fell into the hands of the communist Khmer Rouge in 1975, there was a complete devastation of the economic, social, and educational systems.

Many of the 7 million Cambodians tried to escape the communist take-over. Those caught trying to escape faced horrible brutalities, including torture, robbery, and rape. The families that successfully escaped were settled in refugee camps. A majority of the families who arrived in the United States were headed by single parents (usually mothers), many of whom had mental health problems from the years of brutality and devastation during and after the war.

Because of hardships experienced during the war and in the refugee camps, elderly Cambodians in the United States may display considerable distrust.

Religion

Approximately 85% of the population in Cambodia adheres to Buddhism, the official religion. The temple was the place of worship and was traditionally located in the center of each rural community. Since the communist takeover, all religious activities in Cambodia have been suppressed (Chhim et al., 1987).

Education

After Cambodia gained independence from France in 1953, interest in education grew tremendously to serve the needs of the people. A reform in education called the "Khmerization of Education" began in 1967 after the Khmer language was substituted for French as the language of instruction (Ouk, Huffman, & Lewis, 1988). When the Khmer Rouge took total control of Cambodia in 1975, schools were destroyed, and educated people were executed. Because education was not available after the communist takeover, Cambodians born after this time have most likely had no formal education. Khmer children in the United States today have to rely almost entirely on the school for learning, because many of their parents have had little or no education.

Language

Khmer is a language of the Austroasiatic family, which consists of more than 100 languages scattered from Eastern India to the South China Sea. Approximately 90% of Cambodians speak Khmer, although many other languages such as Thai, Lao, and Cham are also spoken (Ouk et al., 1988). Khmer is a homogeneous language with very little dialectal variation from one region to the next. Several dialects can still be identified.

Standard Khmer is the form of the national language taught in schools and used for mass communication. Various groups of people must be addressed differently in Cambodia. Therefore, four different forms of Khmer exist: the language of the ordinary people, formal language, language of the clergy, and royal language.

Khmer words are usually monosyllabic or disyllabic, with stress always on the second syllable. The few polysyllabic words are compound words or derived from other languages. Khmer is a nontonal language. Many lexical terms are derived from the French, particularly technical terms such as *aeroplane, café,* and *poste* (stamp).

There are 50 vowels and diphthong sounds in Cambodian or Khmer. Many consonant sounds are shared between Khmer and English, but some English consonant sounds do not occur in Khmer. Others that are shared may not be exactly alike. There are 85 initial consonant clusters in Khmer but no final clusters. Most, but not all, are very different from those in English (e.g., *Mtyul* and *Sdap*). Khmer stops /p/, /t/, /k/, /ʔ/, and /d/ are aspirated and nonaspirated. There are only two fricatives.

Khmer speakers learning English often substitute /k/ for /g/, /v/ for /w/, /f/ for /b/, /tʃ/ for /s/, /s/ for /θ/, and /t/ for /θ/. The /r/ is approximated as a trill *r*. Many final consonants such as /r/, /d/, /g/, /s/, /b/, and /z/ are omitted. The /b/ and /d/ are implosive, and there are possible vowel distortions of /ɛ/, /i/, /u/, and /æ/.

The Khmer often have difficulty with forms of the verb *to be*, including copula and auxiliary verbs and progressive and future tense markers. In addition, they may experience difficulty with placement of negative markers.

The Laotians
Immigration History
As part of French Indochina, Laos was under French rule between 1893 and 1954. Soon after the fall of South Vietnam and the Vietcong invasion in 1973, many Laotians, fearing for their lives, escaped and resettled in the United States. Laotians have encountered many challenges in adjusting to the U.S. culture, because they were rural agrarians and were illiterate in their native language. In addition, they encountered difficulty in obtaining training and employment in the United States. Over the last two decades, many have learned some English and found gainful employment in factories and low-paying jobs.

Religion
The Laotian refugees brought many customs and beliefs with them to the United States. Most Laotians are Theravada Buddhists. Most Laotian men are required to spend 2 or 3 weeks as monks before they marry. Many believe in the practice of folk medicine and the ritual of Baci. In the belief that every human being has 32 souls, many Laotians ask a sorcerer to perform the ritual of Baci to call back the soul outside of one's body of a person who is sick to bring about that person's recovery (Lewis & Luangpraseut, 1989).

Education

Many Laotian refugees lacked basic literacy skills when they first immigrated to the United States, so they found it difficult to learn English. The main focus of Laotian education is the Pagoda, which teaches how to read the sacred Buddhist texts. It takes great effort for Laotian parents to convince their children to continue their education beyond high school. Students work for prestige or community recognition, but education in itself is not seen as a requirement.

Laotian students generally do not say "I don't know," believing it is a sign of disrespect to the teacher. Similarly, they rarely say "no," because they think that saying "no" will hurt the teacher's feelings.

Language

In the Laotian language, most words are monosyllabic, although there are some compound and polysyllabic words borrowed from Indian languages. In their system, there are more symbols than sounds. Laotian is tonal like Chinese and Vietnamese. There are six tones (Chhim et al., 1987). Laotians learning English may find phonetic interference with distortions (e.g., /c + Sh/ for /tʃ/), substitutions (e.g., s/sh and s/ch), and omission of final consonants.

Laotian culture plays an important role in the lexicon. Contrasting sets of lexical items are used in conversations with people of different social status. For example, seven different words may be used by a Laotian to refer to himself or herself, depending on the partner in the conversation. Consequently, Laotian speakers must determine the listener's social rank before having a conversation. If the rank is unclear, Laotians are uneasy about responding (Lewis & Luangpraseut, 1989).

Six different tones are used to denote syllables in Laotian. Individual words also have tonemes. Laotians sound monotonous because there is no stress in the language. Laotian words usually end in a vowel. Indicating stress and adding final consonants are therefore difficult for Laotian speakers learning English.

The basic word order of Laotian is similar to that of English (i.e., subject + verb + object), although the subject can be omitted; however, there are many syntactic and morphologic differences that interfere when a Laotian is learning English. Adjectives follow nouns, plurality and possession are expressed with different combinations of words rather than morphologic markers, and there are no tense markers. In addition, there are no articles, the verb form does not change when there is a change in subject (e.g., "I go," "you go," "he go"), and there is no verb *to be* for sentences with predicate adjectives (e.g., "food good," "dress beautiful"). Interrogatives are marked by placing *bo* at the end of the sentence.

The Indians

Immigration History

India is one of the most populous countries in the world, with a population of nearly 1 billion. It is the largest country on the Indian subcontinent, which includes India, Bangladesh, Nepal, Pakistan, Sri Lanka, and Bhutan. In the 1980s and 1990s, more Indians came to the United States than all of the years before combined. According to the 2000 Census, there are 847,562 immigrants from India in the United States (U.S. Bureau of the Census, 2000). Persons from India are the fourth largest Asian group in the United States.

Religion

India is the birthplace of many religions including Hinduism, Jainism, Buddhism, and Sikhism Most Indians believe in a God, but there may be a few atheists. All Hindus believe in the doctrine of karma or predestination. The caste system is another unique feature of Hindu life. The Brahmins have the highest place as the priestly clan, Kshatriyas are the warrior class, Vaisyas are the cultivators and merchants, and Sudras are the menials only in some remote parts of India. Post-independence reform abolished the caste system legally, but, in practice, it still lingers. Most Indians in the United States came from the Brahmin group. As such, they represent a people of considerable wealth who place a very high value on education and professional careers, particularly those in science and medicine.

The Family

Families in India are typically very large and include extended families. All members, including three or four generations, often live under the same roof or in close proximity to one another. In the United States, family structure is changing, and nuclear families are quite prevalent. In contrast, immigrant Indian families in the United States are smaller in size. Although the traditional caste system is no longer promoted, individuals from different castes still do not maintain contact. Intercaste marriages are becoming quite common. The "untouchables" are still considered the lowest in the social stratum only in some rural areas and among the uneducated. Marriage is a necessity for Hindus on religious grounds. Among the Hindus, a male child is more desirable, because eventually he will become the head of the household.

Education

The educational system in India is based on the British system. English is taught in the schools. The educated are bilingual or multilingual. The illiteracy rate is high in India, owing to the large number of people living in extreme poverty (Shekar & Hegde, 1995). Immigrants to the United States, however, have achieved high academic success and are, in general, well educated. Most are college educated and are fluent English speakers. Indian immigrants have the highest educational attainment of all ethnic groups in the United States (U.S. Department Commerce, 1993a, 1993b). They tend to hold technical, managerial, professional, and sales positions. They also have higher income than the general U.S. population (Shekar & Hegde, 1995).

Languages

Linguists have listed 845 dialects and 225 distinct languages in India. The constitution of India recognizes 21 major languages, including Sanskrit and English. Hindi, the national language, is spoken or understood by 40% of the population.

Most of the immigrants from south Asia to the United States speak a language of the Indic or Dravidian family and many speak English very well.

According to Shekar and Hegde (1995), Hindi and Kannada share a similar vowel system. Each has five short vowels /i/, /e/, /u/, /o/, and /a/ and their long counterparts. Vowel length is phonemic in Hindi and Kannada. Hindi also has nasalized vowels.

Hindi and Kannada have five tense vowels /ɑ/, /e/, /i/, /o/, and /u/ and their lax counterparts. The following Hindi and Kannada consonants are not found in English: (1) voiced bilabials and velar aspirated stops, (2) dental and retroflex consonants, (3) voiced and voiceless palatal affricates, and (4) palatal nasal. In English, /v/ is a labiodental fricative, whereas in Hindi the /v/ phoneme is a bilabial fricative. The English /w/ is an allophonic variation of the Hindi phoneme /v/. Hindi and Kannada speakers often substitute /f/ with a voiceless bilabial fricative, /ɸ/; /v/ with a labiodental approximate, /ʋ/; or /θ, ð/ with dental stops /t/ and /d/ (Wells, 1982). Indian speakers often substitute the alveolar series /t, d, l, r, n, s, z/ with their counterparts retroflex found in Indian languages. Bansal (1978, 1990) pointed out the distinct stress and intonation patterns of Indian English, which can negatively affect intelligibility.

The Filipinos

Immigration History

Before 1521, the Philippines was a sovereign state that traded with China and many other Eastern and Middle Eastern nations. In 1521, the Philippines was taken over and ruled by the Spanish until 1898, when, after the Spanish-American War, it became a protectorate of the United States. It was granted independence after World War II. Due to its history of trade and repeated colonization, the Filipino culture is a mosaic, with influence from Spanish, American, Chinese, Malay, Indian, and other cultures.

Filipino immigration to the United States began after the onset of American rule because of an unstable political climate, poverty, the search for better economic and educational opportunities, and reunion with family members. The Filipinos came to the United States in three major waves.

The first wave, which began in 1903, consisted of a highly select group of young men seeking a college education. They gained a reputation of being serious scholars (*pensionado*) (Takaki, 1989). These students returned to the Philippines after completion of their education and encouraged other young men and women to seek education in the United States (Melendy, 1977). Between 1910 and 1938, almost 14,000 Filipinos were educated in the United States (California State Department of Education, 1986).

In the second wave of immigration, between 1906 and the 1930s, Filipinos settled in Hawaii, seeking agricultural employment in pineapple and sugarcane plantations. Many Filipinos eventually moved to the mainland of the United States and were employed in agricultural jobs on the West Coast. The third wave of Filipino immigration, which began in 1965, included many well-educated families with school-age children, many of whom were seeking to unite with their family. Between 1980 and 1990, the Filipino population in the United States increased by 81.6% to 1.5 million people. In the 1990s 70.5% of the U.S. Filipino population was living in the west, with nearly 800,000 living in California, Washington, Arizona, and Texas and 170,000 living in Hawaii. Other regions with heavy populations of Filipinos include 10.2% in the northeast states, including New York, New Jersey, Pennsylvania, Maryland, and Virginia; 8.1% in the midwest including Michigan, Illinois, and Ohio; and 11.3% in parts of the south, including Florida, Georgia, and the Carolinas (U.S. Bureau of the Census, 2000). Today, the Filipinos are the second largest Asian group in the United States, just behind the Chinese.

The Family

The Filipino people practice a bilateral system of family responsibility, by which they are obligated to both sides of the family. The extended family is common. The Filipino culture places importance on specific roles and responsibilities that are hierarchically defined. The specific roles remain in effect even after children reach adulthood. The child is not viewed as an individual but rather as an extension of many generations of the family. Families tend to be large with frequent contact of immediate and extended members.

Education

Public education is compulsory through the elementary level in the Philippines, although this is not enforced by the authorities. The Filipino people are status conscious and view education as a key measure of status and the key to success. As a result, parents are eager for their children to do well in school and to perfect their English language skills (Monzon, 1984).

Languages

Authorities disagree on the exact number of Filipino languages. It is estimated that there are 75 mother tongues. All of the languages are from the Malayo-Polynesian group. The major languages are Tagalog (the national language), Ilocano, and Visayan. However, Tagalog, or Filipino, is the national language of the Philippines is the native language of approximately 25% of Filipinos, and is the first or second language of more than half of all Filipinos. *Many persons from the Philippines speak English, as it is the language of most education and business.*

Tagalog is a polysyllabic language with its own dialectal variations. It uses many Spanish and English words (Rafael, 1995). The sound system has 27 phonemes. There are sounds that are different from those in English and sounds that do not exist in English. Most words consist of roots and affixes. The combination of the root and its affix or affixes determines the meaning of the word. The usual word order in a sentence in Tagalog is the reverse of that in English (i.e., predicate plus subject, as in "slept the dog").

The Tagalog lexical, syntactic, morphologic, and phonologic features of language also can interfere with learning English. The Tagalog verb system does not make true time distinctions but characterizes something as begun or not begun and, if begun, as completed or not completed. Also, verbs are not inflected for number but are the same form for singular and plural. Furthermore, Tagalog does not indicate gender in third-person singular pronouns.

The phonetic and syntactic differences between English and Tagalog cause many frustrations for the native Filipino learning English. In the following excerpt, this frustration is expressed by a tenth grade Filipino boy who immigrated to the United States at age 14 (Olsen, 1988):

> There is lots of teasing me when I don't pronounce right. Whenever I open my mouth I wonder, I shake and worry, will they laugh? They think if we speak Tagalog that we are saying something bad about them, and sometimes they fight us for speaking our language. I am afraid to speak English, I am afraid to try. And I find myself with fear about speaking Tagalog.

Tagalog has 27 phonemes: 16 consonants, including the significant glottal stop; five vowel sounds; and six diphthongs. Although many of these phonemes are similar to those used in English, nine English phonemes do not occur in Tagalog: /v/, /z/, /t/, /d/, /dz/, /f/, /ʃ/, /ʧ/, and /z/. The Philippine speaker substitutes /p/, /b/, /s/, and /t/ for /f/, /v/, /z/, and /d/, respectively, because these sounds closely resemble sounds produced in Tagalog. Differences in vowel boundaries lead Philippine speakers to have difficulty distinguishing, for example, between "lift" and "left."

In Filipino languages, plurality is marked by the word *onga* placed before the pluralized nominal (e.g., "onga bata" meaning *children*) or by another word carrying the concept of plurality (e.g., "dala wang bata" meaning *two children*). The Filipino speaker learning English has difficulty with the marking of plurality with the morpheme *-s*, particularly when it is redundant to the context (e.g., many friends).

In a recent experimental study (Acenas, 2000) comparing Tagalog-English bilinguals to age- and education-matched monolingual controls, Tagalog-English bilinguals showed a higher rate of retrieval failures when naming pictures of low frequency objects (e.g., cymbals). These findings were obtained even when the analysis was limited to bilinguals who reported that English was their dominant language, and even though Tagalog was not used during the testing session (thereby perhaps causing interference between the two languages). These results are not unique to Tagalog-English bilinguals and have also been observed in Hebrew-English and Spanish-English bilinguals (Gollan, Acenas, & Smith, 2000; Gollan & Silverberg, in press). They imply that, to properly assess confrontation naming skills in bilinguals, such as Tagalog-English bilinguals, it will be necessary to develop tests that cater to bilinguals' levels of experience with words.

There are several communication rules that are important to providing clinical service to persons of Filipino descent. Filipinos are comfortable in one-on-one conversations that begin with small talk. In greeting, Filipinos enjoy a strong and longer handshake. Placing the freehand on top of the hand being shaken and patting or placing the free hand on the shoulder of the person being greeted is a common practice. It can be expected that Filipinos will be a few minutes late in keeping appointments. Early arrival indicates overeagerness and is usually avoided. Filipinos use nonverbal communication to express ideas, especially if they do not believe the listener understands what they are saying. For example, they may point with tightly closed lips rather than the finger, or they may use a clenched fist with the thumb hidden and palm turned upward to indicate consent.

The Pacific Islanders

The Pacific Islands are grouped into three clusters: Polynesia, Melanesia, and Micronesia. Most numerous among the Islanders are the Hawaiians, Samoans, and Chamorros, in that order. The Pacific Islanders have different views and ways of life based on their experiences. The Hawaiian, Tongan, Samoan, Fijian, and other groups may share commonalities. The abundance of food, the mild temperature, the collective nature of their traditions, and the ritualized behavior of a group make it less important for an individual to strive and compete to become the best.

The Pacific Islanders treasure and value collective behavior (i.e., the reliance of existence on the group rather than on the individual). In the school environment, children read, chant, and practice in unison. The American tradition of individualism and focus on individual achievement violates the Pacific Islanders' principles of collective work and community-oriented achievement and education.

Religion and Folk Beliefs

Many religions are practiced in the Pacific Islands. As a result of contact with people from the United States, Pacific Islanders practice various forms of Christianity, including Catholicism, Mormonism, and Protestantism. In addition, many have combined Western religions with indigenous folk beliefs. Suruhana and Surahano (practitioners of folk medicine) are often consulted for treatment in a case of illness.

The Family

Families in the Pacific Islands are usually extended and can include three generations living in the same house. Islanders' families place heavy emphasis on authority and expect children to comply with the wishes of elders and authority figures. The primacy of parents corresponds to the apparent lack of concern over the individual and the focus on the well-being of the family.

Education

Formal education was not part of Pacific Islander history until the Europeans came in the 1900s. Much of their educational tradition is based on oral learning. Learning style is usually passive, with rote memorization being preferred (Cheng, 1989). Teachers are respected, and children go to great lengths to please their teachers. Studies of Hawaiian, Tahitian, and Samoan children have suggested that they are likely to be unaccustomed to interacting with adults on a one-on-one basis, because they are often in situations in which direct communication is with other children and not adults. In addition, absenteeism is common, reflecting not only the more relaxed style of the Islanders but also a different emphasis on academic expectancies, such as being on time and completing projects.

As a result, when Pacific Islander children come to school in the United States, they are struck by the differences between the two cultures. The culture of the U.S.-based schools emphasizes the individual, individual excellence, and creativity. This contradicts the Pacific Islanders' learning style, and it basically undermines their sense of well-being (the *aloha spirit*), as their identity is tied to the group and is not individualistic. As a group, the Pacific Islanders perform at much lower levels in school than their Hispanic and African American counterparts (Ima & Labovitz, 1990).

Languages

Among the 5 million inhabitants of the Pacific Islands, more than 1,200 indigenous languages are spoken. The five *lingua francas* used by the Pacific Islanders are French, English, Pidgin, Spanish, and Bahasa Indonesian. Languages are heavily influenced by multicultural sources.

The People of the Hawaiian Islands

The Hawaiian Islands are the closest of the Pacific Islands to the U.S. mainland. They were discovered and settled by the Polynesians in approximately 300–750 AD and explored by Captain James Cook in the late 1700s. Hawaiians are American citizens, because Hawaii became the fiftieth state to join the union in 1959, beginning an age of tourism and development on the islands.

The Hawaiian Islands are multiethnic and multicultural. Much like the American Indian, the Hawaiian has become a minority group in its own land. Although in the last few years there has been a rebirth of traditional cultural values, only 6% of the residents of the islands are pure-blooded Hawaiians. The Hawaiians are a mixture of persons of many races and ethnic groups who mix and interact, yet maintain their own unique cultural values. The majority of residents are white, followed closely by Japanese, Chinese, and Filipino. Filipinos make up 16% of the Hawaiian population. Approximately 10% of the population is Korean, Samoan, and a mixed group of many other ethnic groups. There are more than 1.1 million residents on the Hawaiian Islands, including 115,000 persons in the U.S. military. Most residents live on Oahu, Waikiki, and Honolulu, with others living on Maui, Kauai, Molokai, and Lanai.

At least 22 languages are spoken by children enrolled in the Honolulu public schools, representing the major languages from Southeast Asia and the Pacific Islands. The most important values are expressed by *aloha*, meaning generosity, graciousness, spirituality, friendliness, and hospitality. The extended family, or *ohana*, is highly valued (Kanahele, 1986).

There are few Hawaiians who are able to speak native Hawaiian. The State of Hawaii outlawed the Hawaiian language and made English the only language spoken in the schools. Over the past decade, privately funded schools and programs have begun to revive the language in the hope that it would survive. The Hawaiian language is polysyllabic and alphabetical. It has the smallest alphabet in the world, with five long vowels (a, e, i, o, and u) and eight consonants (h, k, l, m, n, p, w, and ?). There are two ways to pronounce /w/. It may be pronounced as /w/, as in English; however, in the first syllable, it is often pronounced as /v/. The basic phonologic rules are that the stress is placed on the second to last syllable, consonant clusters do not exist, the final phoneme is always a vowel, and the glottal stop is phonemic.

Pidgin (meaning the language of business), Hawaiian Creole English, is an important part of the communication system among Pacific Islanders, including Hawaiians. Although looked down on by some, it is the mode of communication that was first established by plantation workers who came from many different backgrounds as a way to understand each other.

The Samoans

In the beginning of the nineteenth century, Samoa was visited by missionaries and traders from Germany, Great Britain, and the United States. In 1899, Western Samoa became a German colony. The United States acquired American Samoa for its naval station. After the defeat of Germany in World War I, Western Samoa was given to New Zealand under a League of Nations mandate. In 1962, Western Samoa became an independent nation. American Samoa continues to be a possession of the United States.

In the 1950s, large groups of Samoans left for Hawaii and the U.S. mainland. There are approximately 60,000 Samoans living in the United States (including Hawaii) and only 30,000 remaining in American Samoa. Among the many reasons Samoans gave for leaving their homeland are a search for a better life, access to health care, better education, and an escape from the traditional authoritarian system (Cheng, 1989).

The People of Guam

A territory of the United States, Guam has a population of approximately 116,000 (U.S. Bureau of the Census, 1995). Chamorros make up the largest ethnic group in Guam, representing approximately 42% of the total population.

Guam is an island society of diverse ethnic elements that draws its strength from Asian, American, and indigenous Chamorro sources. The Chamorro people control the political structure of the government of Guam. As many as 40% of all Chamorros now reside outside of Guam and the Northern Marianas (U.S. Bureau of the Census, 1995). Forty-nine thousand people from Guam lived in the United States in 1990 (U.S. Bureau of the Census, 1995).

Chamorro, the official language of Guam, has six vowels and at least 11 vowel allophones. There are 18 consonants and one semiconsonant, /w/. Words are divided into classes, and each class has separate rules it follows.

Chamorro speakers are likely to have difficulty learning English because of the characteristics of their native language.

The diversity that exists among Pacific Islanders and persons from other Asian groups is challenging and interesting. The above section provides a glimpse of this diversity. For speech-language pathologists and audiologists, the diversity among people in the Pacific Islands offers the beginning of a long journey to the quest of cross-cultural communicative competence. The following section offers guiding principles on assessment and intervention of APA populations.

Assessment and Intervention

Assessment Strategies

Chapter 13 focuses on assessment. This section offers brief principles and guidelines specific for the APA population.

APAs learning English as a second language with communication disorders face tremendous challenges in meeting the demands of school and assimilating into the American mainstream. To provide quality clinical service to children and adults with possible speech-language and hearing disorders, linguistically and culturally appropriate assessment is necessary. The purpose of assessment is to identify strengths and weaknesses of the individual so that appropriate clinical intervention can be provided, if necessary. As in all assessment, it is necessary to distinguish between language differences and disorders. This is particularly challenging in the assessment of communication in children who may still be in the process of developing language. It is also challenging because of the many cultures, languages, and dialects of the APA people, the amount of exposure to English, and the difficulty in identifying clinicians competent to make an assessment in the first language of the client.

APA children and adults who are in need of speech, language, and hearing services often are underserved due to a lack of trained bilingual professionals and understanding of the life history of the clients. The number of speech-language pathologists and audiologists in the United States who speak Vietnamese, Laotian, Khmer, Chamorro, Tagalog, Hmong, or Korean is minuscule. Only a few speech-language pathologists speak some of the other more widely used Asian languages, such as Mandarin and Japanese. Consequently, speech-language disorders in APA children and adults are sometimes not identified, and language differences are identified incorrectly as language disorders. According to the Individuals with Disabilities Education Act, assessment of the abilities of children with limited English proficiency should be conducted in their native language. This may necessitate seeking the assistance of interpreters. (For additional information on the use of interpreters in assessment, see Chapter 13.)

Clients have diverse linguistic, paralinguistic, stylistic, and discourse backgrounds and experiences. It is important that clinicians determine the degree to which the communication behaviors observed are due to cultural and linguistic differences, rather than to a disorder. As indicated earlier, Asian and Pacific Islanders have many different values and beliefs. An awareness of the particular cultural and linguistic values of the particular population to which the individual client belongs is an essential tool for the SLP. The clinician must not assume the characteristics of the client's language and culture. It is essential that the clinician regard each individual client as an individual with unique cultural and linguistic characteristics and a unique degree of assimilation and acculturation. Because of the uniqueness and heterogeneity of APA clients, the traditional mode of assessment may not be appropriate.

Traditional Approach to Assessment

Traditional assessment approaches that use standardized formal tests designed to measure discrete areas of language are not able to effectively account for cultural and linguistic diversities. When incongruities between the native culture and the mainstream American culture exist, clients, particularly children, tend to experience confusion. The translation of standardized tests into other languages to accommodate the needs of culturally and linguistically diverse students is inappropriate. There are many words that cannot be translated from one language into another language without losing meaning. Also, words or concepts that may be considered common in English may not be common in the language of the APA being tested. According to Cheng (1991), these may include names of household objects, clothing, sports, musical instruments, professions, historically related events and holidays, as well as games, values, and stories. Thus, formal assessment instruments, translated tests, and their interpretive scores are inappropriate for this population.

Recommended Assessment Procedures

The following guidelines for assessment are often referred to as the *RIOT procedure* (Cheng, 1995b). They are adapted here for APA populations:

1. **Review.** Review all pertinent documents and background information. Many Asian countries do not keep cumulative school records. When available, the records may not be in English. The academic subjects on the records may not match those of the traditional American curriculum. Oral reports are sometimes unreliable, yet they may be the only way to find the necessary information. Parents may be reluctant to discuss social and family background. An interpreter may be needed to obtain this information because of the lack of

English language proficiency of the parents or guardians. Medical records may also be difficult to obtain. Pregnancy and delivery records might not have been kept, especially if the birth was a home birth or in a refugee camp. The client may be reluctant to share personal information. Medical care may have been provided by a family member or other person who would not have kept records. Records, if available, may not be provided in English. Interpreters may need to be used to get background information about pregnancy and birth history.

  2. Interview. Interview teachers, peers, family members, and other informants to collect data regarding the client and the home environment. The family can provide valuable information about the communicative competence of the client at home and in the community, as well as historical and comparative data on the client's language skills. The clinician needs information regarding the client's proficiency in the home language. A description of the home environment and any cultural differences must also be discovered. The language used in the home, proficiency of family members in different languages, patterns of language usage, and ways the family spends time together are some areas for investigation. It is important to determine the family concerns and priorities. Teachers and other professionals can provide information about the child's communication behavior in relation to classmates, attempts to communicate, and to revise and clarify communication failure. Interview questions are available from multiple sources (Cheng, 1990, 1991; Langdon & Saenz, 1996). Questions should focus on obtaining information on how the client functions in his or her natural environment in relation to age peers who have had the same or similar exposure to language or to English. Questions about comparing behavior with playmates or a play group might reveal useful data.

  3. Observe. Observe the client over time in multiple contexts with multiple communication partners. Observe interactions at school, inside and outside the classroom, and at home. This cognitive-ecological-functional model takes into account the fact that clients often behave differently in different settings. Clinicians determine how the client interacts with others, reacts to different situations and individuals, and adapts to social communication barriers. Direct observation of social behavior with multiple participants allows the clinician the opportunity to observe the ways the client communicates. Observe family dynamics with consideration to the family role. Observe the proficiency of the parents in the native language and English. What language do the parents and family members use in addressing the client? Do they use the same level of language in addressing the client as they do to his or her age peers?

  4. Test. Test the client using informal dynamic assessment procedures in English and the home language. Use the portfolio approach by keeping records of the client's performance over time. Interact with the client, being sensitive to his or her need to create meaning based on what is perceived as important,

the client's frame of reference, and his or her experiences. Describe the client during genuine communication in a naturalistic environment with low anxiety and high motivation. Assessment procedures should be culturally and pragmatically appropriate.

Collect narrative samples using wordless books, pictures, or other stimuli. Asking the client to describe experiences, retell stories, predict future events, and solve problems provides rich data for analysis. Literature from the client's background or narratives can be used to assess skill in accounting (description of a present event), recounting (description of a past event), and event casting (description of a future event) (Heath, 1983). Stories translated into English may not be easily adapted to make them culturally appropriate. The clinician should then determine whether there are difficulties in communication due to possible cultural and social mismatches between the two languages or to a true disorder.

Special Challenges in Intervention

What clinicians learn from the assessment should be integrated into their intervention strategies. Intervention should be constructed based on what is most productive for promoting communication and should incorporate the client's personal and cultural experiences. Salient and relevant features of the client's culture should be highlighted to enhance and empower the client. Care should be taken not to consider differences in communication style as indicators of a communication disorder.

The following verbal and nonverbal communication behaviors can easily be misunderstood by clinicians in working with APA clients:

Delay or hesitation in response
Frequent topic shifts and difficulty with topic maintenance
Differences in the meaning of facial expressions, such as a frown signaling concentration rather than displeasure
Short responses
Use of a soft-spoken voice
Lack of participation and lack of volunteering information
Different nonverbal messages, including eye contact, such as avoiding eye contact with adults and body language, such as avoiding being hugged or kissed
Embarrassment over praise
Different greeting rituals, which may appear impolite, such as looking down when the clinician approaches
Use of Asian language–influenced English, such as the deletion of plural and past tense (Cheng, 1999).

APA clients may be fluent in English but use the discourse rules from their home culture, such as speaking softly to persons in authority, looking down or away, and avoiding close physical contact.

Surface analysis of linguistic and pragmatic functions is not sufficient to determine the communicative competence of children and might even misguide clinicians in their decision-making process. The home culture and discourse rules of the clients need to be explored by the clinicians, and discourse rules must be explained explicitly and modeled repeatedly before APA clients can make sense of the socialization process (Cheng, 1989, 1996). Cultural rules are not static but fluid. Children as well as adults learn to adjust to different languages and cultures by code switching and making necessary accommodation. It is difficult for adults to make the switches, because their native culture is deeply ingrained.

Working with the Family

Sociologic and psychological difficulties may arise in the conflict of culture, language, and ideology between new generation Asians, their parents, and the American educational system. These difficulties can include the background of traditions, religions, and histories of the APA population; problems of acculturation; the understanding of societal rules; contrasting influences from home and the classroom or society; confusion regarding one's sense of identity relating to culture, society, and family; the definition of disability; and the implications of special education services.

Intervention activities and materials can be selected based on the client's family and cultural background using activities that are culturally and socially relevant. Alternative strategies should be offered when clients or caregivers are reluctant to accept the treatment program recommended by the clinician. Inviting the family to participate in special classes or speech and language sessions is a useful way to provide the needed information. Seeking assistance from community leaders and social-service providers may also be necessary to assure that services will be provided in a culturally appropriate manner and to convince the clients of the importance of therapy or recommended programs. The clients or caregivers may also be asked to talk with other persons in the community who have experiences with treatment programs. Other individuals can be effective in sharing their personal stories about their experiences with therapy. The clinician should be patient with the clients by letting them think through a problem and waiting for them to make the decision to participate in the treatment program. Several additional resources are provided in Appendix 9-1 and Chapter 13 to assist the clinician in providing culturally appropriate services.

Working with Other Professionals

Clinicians need support from other professionals in their attempts to examine the cultural dimensions of interaction between themselves and their clients. While trying to comprehend cultural differences, clinicians must also guard against stereotyping the clients.

Intervention

Activities that provide interesting content and natural opportunities for social interaction can provide a rich environment for language learning to occur (Goodman, 1986). The principles of experiential learning can be applied to speech-language intervention with the APA client with the understanding that the approach is contrary to the teaching and learning styles of some cultural groups in which more direct instruction is the norm.

Johnston, Weinrich, and Johnson (1984) provided therapy guidelines useful for pragmatic activities, some of which can be adapted for APA clients. For example, the conversation module includes talking on the telephone and asking for directions.

The following are specific guiding principles for all clinicians and other professionals to enrich language learning in real-life contexts for APA clients (Cheng, 1994):

1. Use language in multiple social contexts. Clients should be encouraged to participate in high-interest activities that are familiar to them. For example, Japanese clients could be encouraged to tell a native folk story. Chinese clients could be asked to demonstrate how to use chopsticks or to relate an event or story important to the culture.

2. Facilitate language learning in low-risk and low-anxiety contexts. The clinician should get to know the client as an individual and not rely on general knowledge usually attributed to a cultural group. He or she should learn and understand interests, likes, and dislikes of the client. The clinician should attempt to determine the areas of strength and interest of the client and use those areas to form the context of the clinical intervention.

3. Use language activities that are experiential and relevant. When a clinician learns more about the clients and their experiences, the clients can be asked to share stories about experiences that are not only relevant but also meaningful to the client. Such activities can be a source of learning and bonding for everyone.

4. Encourage language interactions in comprehensible contexts, starting from the least demanding and proceeding to more cognitively challenging tasks. Art, music, and experiential activities with lower reliance on

verbal language should be used before activities that require high verbal ability or high cultural knowledge, such as reading text on difficult topics. Contexts relevant to the client's interest and occupation serve as a support for learning new language skills.

5. Respect differences between home language discourse rules and discourse rules or expectation in English (Cheng, 1994). Clinicians need to make the effort to explain explicitly what is expected in discourse in the new language. Games and activities that are common and understood by American children may be unfamiliar to clients who have recently arrived in the country. The concepts of winning a game may also be new. Concepts in games such as Monopoly may be unfamiliar to clients unfamiliar with the American system of real estate and finance.

6. Seek natural support systems and allow clients to have self-selected cooperative groups. Clients should be allowed to select their own groups, seeking out peers with whom they are comfortable. Such an atmosphere provides the support they need to socialize.

7. Provide culturally familiar activities and unfamiliar activities. Most Asian newcomers do not know much about the Cub Scouts, the YMCAs, YWCAs, the PTA, Boys and Girls Clubs, and the numerous programs that the schools and community offer to the students and their families. They should be guided to participate in some of these programs. The schools, on the other hand, can invite family or community members to come into the schools and provide information on ethnic cultural activities from the various ethnic groups, thus providing the family and client the opportunity to show their peers the activities that they are familiar with and value. This exchange is mutually empowering and provides the school-home-child connection.

8. Use a "talk story" approach. Au and Jordan (1981) propose establishing contact with students first by chatting with them without any set agenda, capitalizing on the preexisting cognitive and linguistic experiences of the children. The approach allows the students to "talk story" (a major speech event in Hawaiian culture).

Special Clinical Considerations: Accent, Stress, Voice, and Tones

Accent identifies a person as a member or nonmember of a particular linguistic community (Ainsfeld, Bogo, & Lambert, 1962). Everyone speaks with an accent, ranging from a New York accent to a Southern accent to a Cantonese accent. For tonal languages, tones are phonemic, and each syllable is assigned a specific tone. In English, intonation patterns are suprasegmental, and a variation of tones does not result in a completely different meaning. Individuals with tonal languages may apply their tonal patterns in their delivery of English, which makes their speech patterns distinct; hence, there are many versions of the English language, including French-influenced English, Hindi-influenced English, Tagalog-influenced English, Singaporean English, Australian English, British English, American English, and so on. Many of the distinct patterns and accents are not easy to change and can interfere with communication. Voice patterns also differ from culture to culture. A deep, soft voice indicates authority in Japan, but the same voice pattern may be viewed as a disorder in the United States. The aesthetics of voice also differ from culture to culture. For example, Chinese opera singers can use falsetto for performance, which sounds very pleasant to the audience; however, to the Western ear, Chinese opera may sound piercing and unpleasant. An easy way to understand this is to compare Chinese opera or Japanese opera with Western opera. An appreciation of the linguistic diversity of APA will facilitate better communication between service providers and their APA clients. (For information on reducing accent in intervention, see Chapter 13.)

Conclusion

Providing speech-language and hearing services to individuals from Asia and Pacific Island countries is challenging. Pre-assessment information on the language, culture, and personal life history of the individual lays a solid foundation to further explore the client's strengths and weaknesses. Assessment procedures need to be guided by the general principles of being fair to the culture. Results of assessment should take into consideration the cultural and pragmatic variables of the individual. Intervention can be extremely rewarding when culturally relevant and appropriate approaches are used. The goals of intervention must include the enhancement of appropriate language and communication behaviors, home language, and literacy. Clinicians need to be creative and sensitive in their intervention to provide comfortable, productive, and enriching services for all clients.

References

Acenas, L. (2000). *Tip-of-the-tongue states in Tagalog English bilinguals: A senior honors thesis.* University of California, San Diego.

Ainsfeld, M., Bogo, N., & Lambert, W. (1962). Evaluational reactions to accented English speech. *Journal of Abnormal Psychology, 65,* 223–231.

Au, K., & Jordan, K. (1981). Teaching reading to Hawaiian children: Finding a culturally appropriate solution. In H. Trueba, G. P. Guthrie, & K. Au

(Eds.), *Culture and the bilingual classroom* (pp. 139–152). Rowley, MA: Newbury.

Baker, C., & Pryor Jones, S. P. (1998). *Encyclopedia of bilingualism and bilingual education.* Clevendon: Multilingual Matters.

Bansal, R. K. (1978). The phonology of Indian English. In R. Mohan (Ed.), *Indian writing in English* (pp. 101–114). Bombay, India: Orient Longman.

Bansal, R. K. (1990). The pronunciation of English in India. In S. Ramsaran (Ed.), *Studies in the pronunciation of English: A commemorative volume in honor of A.C. Gimson.* London: Routledge.

Butler, K., & Cheng, L. L. (Eds.). (1996). *Beyond bilingualism: Language acquisition and disorder—A global perspective. Topics in Language Disorders* 16(4), 1–6.

California State Department of Education. (1986). *A handbook for teaching Filipino-speaking students.* Sacramento, CA: California State Department of Education.

Cheng, L. L. (1989). Service delivery to Asian/Pacific LEP children: A cross-cultural framework. *Topics in Language Disorders, 9*(3), 1–14.

Cheng, L. L. (1990). The identification of communicative disorders in Asian-Pacific students. *Journal of Child Communicative Disorders, 13,* 113–119.

Cheng, L. L. (1991). *Assessing Asian language performance: Guidelines for evaluating LEP students* (2nd ed.). Oceanside, CA: Academic Communication Associates.

Cheng, L. L. (1993). Deafness: An Asian/Pacific Island perspective. In K. M. Christensen & G. L. Delgado (Eds.), *Multicultural issues in deafness* (pp. 113–126). White Plains, NY: Longman.

Cheng, L. L. (1994). Difficult discourse: An untold Asian story. In D. N. Ripich & N. A. Creaghead (Eds.), *School discourse problems* (2nd ed.) (pp. 155–170). San Diego: Singular.

Cheng, L. L. (1995a). *Integrating language and learning for inclusion: An Asian-Pacific focus.* San Diego: Singular.

Cheng, L. L. (1995b, July). *The bilingual language-delayed child: Diagnosis and intervention with the older school-age bilingual child.* Paper presented at the Israeli Speech and Hearing Association International Symposium on Bilingualism, Haifa, Israel.

Cheng, L. L. (1996). Beyond bilingualism: A quest for communicative competence. *Topics in Language Disorders, 16*(4), 9–21.

Cheng, L. L. (1998). Beyond multiculturalism: Cultural translators make it happen. In V. O. Pang & L. L. Cheng (Eds.), *Struggling to be heard* (pp. 105–122). Albany, NY: SUNY Press.

Cheng, L. (1999). Sociocultural adjustment of Chinese-American students. In C. C. Park & M. Chi (Eds.), *Asian-American education.* London: Bergin & Garvey.

Chhim, S., Luangpraseut, K., & Te, H. D. (1987). *Introduction to Cambodian culture*. San Diego: San Diego State University Multifunctional Service Center.

Chi, M. (1999). Linguistic perspective on the education of Chinese-American students. In C. C. Park & M. Chi (Eds.), *Asian-American education*. London: Bergin & Garvey.

Ching, T. (1990). Tones for profoundly deaf tone-language speakers. *Chinese University of Hong Kong Papers in Linguistics, 2*, 1–22.

Chu, H. (1990, September). *The role of the Korean language on the bilingual programs in the United States*. Paper presented at the Asian Language Conference, Hacienda Heights, CA.

Chu, H. (1999). Linguistic Perspective on the education of Korean-American students. In C. C. Park & M. Chi (Eds.), *Asian-American education*. London: Bergin & Garvey.

Chuong, C. (1990, September). *The speech island: A Vietnamese perspective*. Paper presented at the Asian Language Conference, Hacienda Heights, CA.

Fadiman, A. (1997). *When the spirit catches you and you fall down*. New York: The Noonday Press.

Gollan, T. H., Acenas, L., & Smith, E. (2000). *Tip-of-the-tongue incidence in Spanish-English and Tagalog-English bilinguals*. San Diego: University of California.

Gollan, T. H., & Silverberg, N. (in press). Tip-of-the-tongue states in Spanish-English Bilinguals. San Diego: University of California.

Gollnick, D. M., & Chinn, P. C. (1990). *Multicultural education in a pluralistic society*. New York: Merrill-Macmillan.

Goodman, K. (1986). *What's the whole in whole language?* Portsmouth, NH: Heinemann.

Hammer, C. S., & Weiss, A. L. (2000). African-American mothers' views of their infants' language development and language learning environment. *American Journal of Speech-Language Pathology, 9*(2), 126–140.

Heath, S. B. (1983). *Ways with words*. New York: Cambridge.

Heibert, E. H. (Ed.). (1991). *Literacy for a diverse society: Perspective, practices and policies*. New York: Teachers College, Columbia University.

Ima, K., & Labovitz, E. M. (1990, March). *Changing ethnic/racial student composition and test performances: Taking account of increasing student diversity*. Paper presented at the annual meeting of the Pacific Sociological Association, Santa Ana, CA.

Ima, K., & Keogh, P-E. (1995). "The crying father" and "my father doesn't love me": Selected observations and reflections on Southeast Asians and special education. In L. L. Cheng (Ed.), *Integrating language and learning for inclusion: An Asian-Pacific focus* (pp. 149–177). San Diego: Singular.

Jiobu, R. M. (1996). Recent Asian Pacific immigrants: The Asian Pacific background. In B. O. Hing & R. Lee (Eds.), *The state of Asian Pacific America: Reframing the immigration debate* (pp. 59–126). Los Angeles: UCLA Asian American Studies Center.

Johnston, E. B., Weinrich, B. D., & Johnson, A. R. (1984). *A sourcebook of pragmatic activities.* Tucson, AZ: Communication Skill Builders.

Kanahele, G. H. (1986). *Ku Kanaka: stand tall: A search for Hawaiian values.* Honolulu: University of Hawaii Press.

Kim, B. L. (1981). *The future of Korean-American children and youth: Marginality, biculturality, and the role of the American public school.* Urbana-Champaign, IL: University of Illinois School of Social Work.

Kim, E. C. (1984, April). *Korean Americans in the United States: Problems and alternatives.* Paper presented at the Annual Conference of Ethnic and Minority Studies, St. Louis.

Kim, R. H. (1978). *Understanding Korean people, language, and culture.* Sacramento, CA: California State Department of Education, Bilingual Education Resource Series.

Langdon, H. W., & Saenz, T. I. (1996). *Language assessment and intervention with multicultural students: A guide for speech-language-hearing professionals.* Oceanside, CA: Academic Communication Associates.

Lewis, C. C. (1995). *Education hearts and minds: Reflections on Japanese preschool and elementary education.* New York: Cambridge University Press.

Lewis, J., & Luangpraseut, K. (1989). *Handbook for teaching Lao-speaking students.* Folsom, CA: Folsom Cordova.

Li, C. N., & Thompson, S. A. (1981). *Mandarin Chinese: A functional reference grammar.* Berkeley, CA: University of California Press.

Ma, L. J. (1985). Cultural diversity. In A. K. Dutt (Ed.), *Southeast Asia: Realm of contrast.* Boulder, CO: Westview Press.

Melendy, H. B. (1977). *Asians in America: Filipinos, Koreans, and East Indians.* Boston: Twayne.

Meyerson, D. W. (1990). Cultural considerations in the treatment of Latinos with craniofacial malformations. *Cleft Palate Journal, 27,* 279–288.

Minami, M., & McCabe, A. (1991). Haiku as a discourse regulation device: A stanza analysis of Japanese children's personal narratives. *Language in Society, 20,* 577–599.

Monzon, R. I. (1984). *The effects of the family environment on the academic performance of Filipino-American college students.* Thesis, San Diego State University, San Diego.

Olsen, L. (1988). *Crossing the schoolhouse border: Immigrant students and the California public schools.* San Francisco: California Tomorrow.

Ouk, M., Huffman, F. E., & Lewis, J. (1988). *Handbook for teaching Khmer-speaking students.* Folsom, CA: Folsom Cordova Unified School District.

Peak, L. (1991). *Learning to go to school in Japan: The transition from home to preschool life.* Berkeley, CA: University of California Press.

Rafael, V. L. (1995). Taglish, or the phantom power of the lingua franca. *Public Culture, 8,* 101–126.

Shekar, C., & Hegde, M. N. (1995). India: Its people, culture, and languages. In L. L. Cheng (Ed.), *Integrating language and learning for inclusion* (pp. 125–148). San Diego: Singular.

Strauss, R. P. (1990). Cultural considerations in the treatment of Latinos with craniofacial malformations. *Cleft Palate Journal, 27,* 275–278.

Takaki, R. (1989). *Strangers from a different shore.* Boston: Little, Brown.

Te, H. D. (1987). *Introduction to Vietnamese culture.* San Diego, CA: Multifunctional Center, San Diego State University.

Trueba, H. T., Cheng, L., & Ima, K. (1993). *Myth of reality: Adaptive strategies of Asian American in California.* Bristol, PA: Falmer Press.

U.S. Bureau of the Census. (1995). *Statistical abstract of the United States:* (115th ed). Washington, DC: U.S. Bureau of the Census.

U.S. Bureau of the Census. (2000). *Statistical abstract of the United States: 2000* (120th ed.). Washington, DC: U.S. Bureau of the Census.

U.S. Department of Commerce. (1993a). *We, the American Asians.* Washington, DC: U.S. Department of Commerce.

U.S. Department of Commerce. (1993b). *We, the Asian and Pacific Islander Americans.* Washington, DC: U.S. Department of Commerce.

Van Kleeck, A. (1994). Potential bias in training parents as conversational partners with their children who have delays in language development. *American Journal of Speech-Language Pathology, 3*(1), 67–68.

Wells, J. C. (1982). *Accents of English 3: Beyond the British Isles.* Cambridge, UK: Cambridge University Press.

Westby, C. (1990). Ethnographic interviewing: Asking the right questions to the right people in the right way. *Journal of Childhood Communication Disorders, 13,* 101–111.

Whitenack, D., & Kikunaga, K. (1999). Teaching English to native Japanese students: From linguistics to pedagogy. In C. C. Park & M. Chi (Eds). *Asian-American education.* London: Bergin & Garvey.

Additional Resources

Chang, J. M., Lai, A., & Shimizu, W. (1995). LEP, LD, poor and missed learning opportunities: A case of inner city Chinese children. In L. Cheng (Ed.), *Integrating language and learning for inclusion* (pp. 265–290). San Diego: Singular Publishing Group.

Cheng, L., Chen, T., Tsubo, T., et al. (1997). Challenges of diversity: An Asian Pacific perspective. *Multicultures, 3,* 114–145.

Liu, E. (1998). *The accidental Asian: Notes of a native speaker.* New York: Random House.

Trueba, H. T., & Bartolome, L. I. (Eds.). (2000). *Immigrant voices.* New York: Rowman & Littlefield Publishers, Inc.

Kristof, N. D., & WuDunn, C. (1994). *China wakes: the struggle for the soul of a rising power.* New York: Times Books.

Mura, D. (1991). *Becoming Japanese.* New York: Doubleday.

Tan, A. (1996). Mother tongue. In G. Hongo (Ed.), *Under Western eye.* New York: Doubleday.

Young, R. (1998). Finding one's roots in uncertain lands: How the Asian Pacific American child copes. In V. O. Pang & L. Cheng (Eds.), *Struggling to be heard.* New York: SUNY.

Website Information

Websites were accurate and active at the time of publication.
http://www.sil.org/ethnologue/top100.html
http://www.krysstal.com/langfams.html
http://www.travlang.com/languages/index.html
http://www.sil.org/ethnologue/countries/Sout.html
http://www.zompist.com/lang8.html
http://www.gopacific.com

4

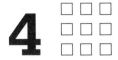

Middle Eastern and Arab American Cultures

Dolores E. Battle

The Middle East is a vast area of the world stretching from the lands surrounding the eastern edge of the Mediterranean Sea to the areas of Southwest India. Although the U.S. Census identifies several countries such as Iran and Iraq to be Asian, this text considers them as being in the Middle East. The distinction was made on the basis of the cultural roots of the countries and the roots of the languages spoken, rather than any political issues. The Asian cultures are discussed in Chapter 3.

People who practice Arab culture, speak Arabic natively, or have a solid kinship to the Arabic language and Islam can be defined as Arabs. Although *Arab* originally referred to the nomadic tribes of the Arabian Peninsula in southwestern Asia, the nomadic nature of Arab people has resulted in considerable ethnic diversity. Hence, the label "Arab" does not denote a single race of people.

Arab Americans and Arab people throughout the world are proud of their long and prodigious history. Over the centuries, they created great empires and established powerful centers of civilization. The Arab region is the center of the development of major contributions to the arts and sciences. In addition, it is the birthplace of three great religions of the world—Christianity, Judaism, and Islam. Moreover, the Middle East, the cradle of Arab civilization, has become one of the world's major melting pots of humanity.

At the heart of the Arab world and at the forefront of its accomplishments is the Arabic language. With the emergence and development of Islam, the fastest growing religion in the world, the Arabic language has increased in importance and significance. In recent times, Arabic language continues to maintain its noble status; however, complex social and cultural issues in the present-day Arab world directly impinge on the language and its users.

Geographic Diversity

The land of the Arab world lies in northern Africa and southwestern Asia. It ranges from Mauritania in the west to Oman in the east. The Arab countries from Egypt and Sudan eastward comprise the region of the world known as the Middle East. The Arab world throughout the ages has been an international crossroads. As a result, it has often come under foreign rule and influence. Vast deserts and mountainous terrain cover more than half of the Arab world, resulting in most Arabs living in selected areas. Owing to the shortage of water in the Arab world, most Arabs live in the Fertile Crescent valley of the Nile, Euphrates, and Tigris rivers or along the Mediterranean Sea.

Today's Arab world includes diverse countries from the Mediterranean area and northern Africa to southwestern Asia. The countries include the large cosmopolitan areas such as Cairo in Egypt, Jerusalem in Israel, Jeddah in Saudi Arabia, and Beirut in Lebanon. It includes the rich agricultural area of the Fertile Crescent, as well as the vast rural areas of the deserts in which the majority of Arabs continue to live. Countries of the Middle East include Egypt, Jordan, Syria, Lebanon, Iraq, Iran, Saudi Arabia, Sudan, Algeria, Morocco, Algeria, Turkey, and Tunisia. Other Arab nations include Kuwait, Mauritania, Oman, Palestine, Israel, Qatar, Somalia, Sudan, United Arab Emirates, and Yemen (Hsourani, 1991; Shipler, 1987).

The Middle East contains four main geographic regions that cut across national and political divisions. These are the northern tier, the Fertile Crescent, the largely desert south, and the western area. The northern tier, which encompasses Turkey, northern Iraq, and the northern and western sectors of Iran, consists mainly of mountains and semiarid plateaus. Much of the northern tier depends on irrigation and light rainfall to support agriculture. The major language groups in the northern tier include Arabic, Kurdish, Turkish, and Farsi (Isenberg, 1976). The primarily desert southern lands include the oil-rich United Arab Emirates, Oman, and the two Yemeni Republics (North and South). The Fertile Crescent consists of the Gulf States of Qatar, Saudi Arabia, and Jordan. The Fertile Crescent forms the southern border of the northern tier. It stretches northward through Israel and Lebanon and then arches across northern Syria to the valleys of the Euphrates and Tigris rivers in Iraq. The primary languages spoken in the Fertile Crescent and the southern sectors of the Middle East are Arabic, Hebrew, and dialects of Aramaic, Berber, and Nubian origin (Isenberg, 1976). Djibouti, Ethiopia, Sudan, and Egypt capsule the western areas of the Middle East. The languages of this vast area include French, Arabic, and Aramaic.

The Middle East is a predominately Arabic-speaking region that is populated primarily by Arabs. This notion requires clarification, however, because the term *Arab* itself is not strictly definable. In a purely semantic sense, no people can be classified as Arab, because the word connotes a mixed population with widely varying ethnologic and racial origins. Some people of Negro, Berber, and Semitic origins identify themselves as Arab (Wilson, 1996). Hence, *Arab* is best used within a cultural context (Lamb, 1987). Arab countries are those countries in which the primary language is Arabic and the primary religion is Islam. Consequently, the Middle East makes up the greatest portion of the Arab world, a world that reflects one of the most amazing achievements in history: the development and growth of Islam from an embryonic phenomenon into a vast sphere of influence and civilization.

According to Lamb (1987) and Mansfield (1992), approximately 200 million Arabs occupy the Arab world. The paradox of parallel modernization and political turmoil has influenced language, learning, and speech-language and hearing services in the Middle East. The hugely increased revenue flowing into the oil-producing Arab countries has facilitated the early phases of the development of speech-language and hearing services, while the turmoil of civil and regional wars has created populations of patients of all ages who need services to treat communication disorders.

Additionally, age-old traditions of consanguinity (blood relationships) contribute to a variety of communication problems among Arab speakers. Jaber, Nahmani, and Shohat (1997) studied the frequency of speech disorders in Israeli Arab children and its association with parental consanguinity. Twenty-five percent of 1,282 parents responding to a questionnaire indicated that their children had a speech and language disorder. After examination by a speech-language pathologist (SLP), rates of affected children of consanguineous and nonconsanguineous marriages were 31.0% and 22.4%, respectively ($p < .01$).

Arab Americans

Immigrants to the United States from the Arab nations came as early as the 1880s in search of opportunity and education. The early immigrants were from the countries of Ottoman-ruled Lebanon and Syria. More than 90% of the immigrants from the area at the time were Christian.

Although the area was predominantly Muslim, the Muslims were hesitant to come to the United States for fear that they would not be able to practice their religion. The early immigrants, who were called "Turks," "Armenians," and "Moors," settled in the urban areas of Chicago and New York. They were very industrious and made strides in the business community such that they were able to support their families in their new home, as well as their families in their home country. The early Arab Americans were fully assimilated when the second wave of Arab immigrants came to the United States.

The second major wave of Arab immigration began in the 1940s after World War II. They were primarily well-educated professional Muslims who, like their predecessors, sought the educational and financial opportunities in the United States. The new wave sparked a resurgence of ethnic pride among descendants of the early immigrants. Since the mid-1960s, the number of Arabs living outside of the Arab world has increased significantly. The United States, Germany, Brazil, Israel, England, France, Canada, and Sweden have among the largest populations of Arabs living outside of the Middle East.

Today there are 3–5 million Arab Americans in the United States (U.S. Bureau of the Census, 2001). Between 1981 and 1990, there were nearly 50,000 immigrants from Iran, 8,000 from Iraq, and 2,000 from Syria. This trend continued with nearly 35,000 from the countries between 1990 and 1994. However, there has been a significant decline of immigrants from the countries to the United States since the Gulf War in the mid-1990s, with a decline to fewer than 6,000 immigrants each year in 1995 and 1996 (U.S. Bureau of the Census, 2001).

Persons of Arab descent in the United States today are as diverse as the many countries of the origin of their descendants. They represent a variety of religions, values, and degrees of acculturation and assimilation. Because the major waves of immigration of persons from the Middle East occurred in the first half of the nineteenth century, 82% of Arab Americans are U.S. citizens, and 63% were born in the United States. As a cultural group, they are well educated, with 62% having at least some college (compared to 45% of the non-Arab U.S. population) and twice as many as in the non-Arab U.S. population having a master's degree or higher. More than 60% of Arab Americans hold white-collar or professional occupations, 12% are self-employed, and 20% are in retail trade businesses. Most reside in the urban areas of Detroit and Dearborn, Michigan; New York City; Washington, DC; Los Angeles; Chicago; Boston; Cleveland; and New Jersey (Immigration and Naturalization Service, 1998).

Although the Arab Americans are heterogeneous in origin and culture, they share in negative stereotypes and discrimination, particularly when there are political events involving the Arab nations, such as the Gulf War of the early 1990s (Suleiman, 2001). Although Arab Americans are less visible than other ethnic groups, the anti-Arab perception in the media makes them more visible in a negative way. There is considerable misunderstanding about the Middle Eastern people, particularly those of beliefs and practices of non-Christian religions. Holidays such as Ramadan (associated with Muslims) and Passover (associated with Judaism), modes of dress, prohibitions about food products, fasting, and other practices often result in misunderstanding and stereotypes that can have an impact on clinical practices. (For a more detailed discussion of religious practices see the Intervention section in Chapter 14.)

Arab American Families and Arab Lifestyles

Family life, religion, and harmony are important to nearly all Arab and Middle Eastern families. The family is the centerpiece of society in Arab states. It is the basic unit from which all other establishments revolve. Most Arab American families are large. It is not uncommon for several generations to live together as an extended family, with the oldest man being the head of each family; the families are patriarchal, being based around the father, his sons, their wives, and their children. Although separated from her natal family, ties between women and their blood relatives are continued. Women frequently consult their natal families if there are problems with the children or other problems. Clinicians need to respect the sanctity of the nuclear and extended family and the role of elders within the family (Schwartz, 1999). Inviting the family to participate in assessment and intervention can be useful in helping the family understand the needs of the individual.

In Muslim families, the women are responsible for instilling the proper cultural values in children through child-rearing practices.

The concept of honor is very important in the lives of Arabs and Middle Eastern society. Fear of scandal is a major consideration in their daily lives. Upholding the honor of the family is vital. Because Arabs are very sensitive to public criticism, clinicians should express concerns to Arab American families in a way that prevents the "loss of face" (Adeed & Smith, 1997; Jackson, 1995, 1997).

Women in Middle Eastern Culture

Islam stresses the concept of public morality, which is to be enforced collectively. It is believed that women are to be separated from men so that they are not overly sexually appealing. Young women must be modestly dressed, which has evolved into the tradition of veiling. In the past, women were seen as the weak link to the family's dignity. More modern trends, however, have led more women to work outside the home, particularly in the fields of medicine, education, and the social sciences. A woman's household duties with regard to the children are not reduced when she gains employment outside of the home.

Religion in Arab Life

Religion is very important to Arab and Arab American families. Although most are Muslim, many follow the Christian beliefs of their ancestors from the early wave of immigration. Some Muslim Arab American families send their children to private Muslim schools so they can receive education consistent with the religious beliefs of the family (Zehr, 1999). Some families opt to send their children to public schools. As the number of Arab American children in the public schools increases, many schools have adapted their programs and practices to accommodate the religious needs of the children. This includes adapting school menus to have alternatives to pork, which is not consumed by Muslims; allowing prayer at the noon hour; and adapting the program to allow for the fasting, required during Ramadan. Many school programs are reducing the emphasis on celebration of Christian holidays to relieve Muslim students from the stresses of participating in Christian and Judaic religious practices. Clinical materials and tests are being modified to remove items that may be specific to a particular Christian religion, such as items related to the celebration of Christmas. Clinicians should be sensitive to the religious beliefs of clients in selecting items for assessment and intervention.

Many Arabs continue to follow traditional ways, although modernization is rapidly changing their lifestyles. Historically, Arab cities, villages, and nomadic groups have remained interdependent. People in cities produce finished goods, villagers provide agricultural produce, and nomads supply animals that transport these products among the three kinds of communities. Owing to the uniformity of these lifestyles, Arabs are especially unique in their ability to maintain their cultural identity wherever they are located. Although most immigrants have their roots in the urban areas, there are some that are from a more traditional rural community with less exposure to more modern American-European traditions.

The majority of persons in the Middle East are farmers or laborers, although a great deal of the land space in the Middle East is unfit for agricultural use (Hitti, 1985). Because the oil wealth of the Middle East has benefited only a fraction of the Arab population, many inhabitants of the Arab world have speech, language, and hearing problems due to lack of medical, educational, and human resources services. These inhabitants are often born into communities that do not systematically provide these services. According to Isenberg (1976), the reality of limited natural resources in the vast majority of the Middle East explains why the Arab world must be considered among the underdeveloped sectors of the world. Limited resources, too few trained professionals, and lack of access negatively influence speech, language, and hearing integrity among large populations of Arab speakers. Persons seeking assistance for speech-language and hearing problems in the Middle East must send their child to other countries where services are available, such as Israel, Europe, or the United States. In some cases, clinicians are brought to the country to provide services, especially to those persons in oil-rich countries such as Saudi Arabia. Although there are attempts to provide more speech-language pathologists (SLPs) trained in the Middle East in the major cities such as Cairo, Jeddah, and Amman, the supply of clinicians is considerably below the demand for services. When the civil and regional political turmoil is considered, access to available services in the Middle East becomes even more restricted.

Ethnic Diversity among Arab American Speakers

The Arab world, owing to its ancient and current history, remains a diverse melting pot of humanity, largely due to Islamic pilgrimages. Because national languages and speech-language and hearing dynamics are influenced by histories of invasions, conquests, slavery, and, most important, the onset of Islam, the inhabitants of the Arab world are characterized by a multiplicity of racial groups, all struggling to coexist in a collision of cultures. The most useful method for classifying persons from the Middle East is according to the language they speak, religions they embrace, and traditions they honor (Mansfield, 1992). This categorization allows for four major national groups: the Turks, Iranians, Israelis, and Arabs. The extremely close relationships and overlapping of linguistic, cultural, racial, and sociologic factors of all these groups foster many of the chronic problems of Middle Eastern society.

Arab American Dialects

Two hundred million people speak Arabic or dialects of Arabic. The dialects are grouped into five geographic categories: (1) North African (Moroccan, Algerian, Tunisian, Libyan, and Mauritanian), (2) Egyptian/Sudanese, (3) Syrian or Levantine (Lebanese, Syrian, Jordanian, and

Palestinian), (4) Arabian Peninsular (Saudi, Yemeni, Adendi, Kuwaiti, Gulf, and Omani), and (5) Iraqi (Wilson, 1996). North African dialects were influenced by the Berbers and the language of the colonists from other North African countries. The Egyptian/Sudanese dialect is understood by most Arabs, because it is the dialect used in Egyptian movies, television, and radio that are seen and heard throughout the Arab world. Arabian Peninsular dialects spoken in Saudi Arabia, Yemen, Aden, Kuwait, Gulf, and Oman are considered the closest to Classical Arabic. They are the dialects closest to the language of the Koran (i.e., the holy book of Islam) and are considered by Arabs to be the most prestigious of the dialects. Egyptian, Syrian or Levantine, and Arabian Peninsular dialects are mutually comprehensible. North African, Iraqi, and Gulf dialects are difficult for others to understand (Almaney & Alwan, 1982; Wilson, 1996).

Written Arabic is different from spoken Arabic. Written Arabic, or Classical Arabic, is the language of the Koran. It is more complex, grammatically more difficult, and has a considerably larger lexicon than spoken Arabic (Wilson, 1996). To be truly literate in Classical Arabic requires many years of study. Even after 5 or 6 years of study, the average Arab may be functionally illiterate in Classical Arabic (Wilson, 1996). Because of its difficulty, good command of Classical Arabic is admired in the Arab culture. Because the dialects have no prestige, a person who does not know Classical Arabic may be thought not to know Arabic, even if he or she is able to speak the local dialect well (Ferguson, 1971).

Arabic Dialects and Language

Arabic Phonology

Wilson (1996) and Swan and Smith (1987) describe several features of Arabic phonology that influence the speech of Arabic speakers learning English. Because of the various dialects of Arabic, there is some variation in classifications or descriptions of the phonemes of Arabic. Arabic has eight vowels and 32 consonants. Short vowels have little significance in Arabic; they are often omitted or confused when Arabic speakers attempt to learn English. Frequent confusions include /I/ for /e/ (*bit* for *bet*), /eI/ for /E/ (*raid* for *red*), and /ou/ for /a/ (*hope* for *hop*).

The consonants /p/, /v/, /ŋ/, and /r/ do not have equivalents in Arabic. Several phonemes (/p/ and /b/, /f/ and /v/) are allophonic in Arabic. In addition, /ch/ and /sh/, /s/ and /z/, /d/ and /j/, and /g/ and /k/ are often confused. Most dialects of Arabic use /t/ and /d/ for /th/ unvoiced and voiced, respectively. In addition, /t/n/ is often produced as /n+ŋ/. Because in Arabic /r/ is a voiced flap, Arabic speakers often overproduce the post-vocalic /r/. Finally, many English two- and three-element consonant clusters do not occur in Arabic; therefore, Arabic speakers learning English often insert short vowels into the cluster (e.g., *sipring* for *spring*).

Among the other features of Arabic that influence production of English are exaggerated articulation with equal stress on all syllables, fewer clearly articulated vowels giving a staccato effect, and the use of glottal stops before initial vowels. In Arabic, spelling is phonetic. Arabic speakers, therefore, tend to produce English words phonetically, including all consonants, even those that are not pronounced in English (Wilson, 1996).

Arabic Syntax and Morphology

Arabic syntax and morphology are patterned and predictable (Wilson, 1996). The irregularities of English, therefore, pose particular difficulty for speakers of Arabic learning English. The verb is often placed before the subject noun. Negatives are formed by placing a particle before the verb. Adjectives follow their nouns. Because plurals are formed by internal vowel changes in Arabic, plural morphemes are frequently omitted when Arabic speakers are learning English. Arabic verb structure uses a simple present tense form for the English simple and present progressive tenses. There are no copula verbs, auxiliary "do," future tense, modal verbs, gerunds, or infinitive forms in Arabic. There are no indefinite articles.

Arabic Semantics

There is very little information on the development of semantics by Arab-speaking children published in English. Ferguson (1971) includes some information on early language development, including the use of child-directed or baby-talk talk in Syrian Arabic. Adults are reported to use baby-talk freely, with little concern that the use of baby-talk may inhibit the acquisition of adult language. Semantic fields in early language development include areas similar to those of children learning English (i.e., family names, food, body parts, and animals). Learning English vocabulary is particularly difficult for Arab speakers because there is little crossover between the languages. Some words that have been imported from Arabic include many words beginning with "al" (e.g., *algebra, alfalfa, alcove, alcohol, algorithm,* and *almanac*) and some foods (e.g., *coffee, sherbet, sesame, apricot, ginger, saffron, carob*), as well as *cotton, magazine, zenith,* and *tariff.* The following English words sound similar to vulgar words in Arabic and should be avoided, if possible: *zip, zipper, air, tease, kiss, cuss, nick, unique,* and *Biz* (Wilson, 1996).

Arabic Language and Religion

Arabs and Arab Americans place a high value on religion. Except for a small, aged generation of Jews and a small handful of Christians, religious minorities do not exist. Between 90% and 94% of the people are Muslims, and most speak or read Arabic. However, Arabs from Pakistan, India, and Iran speak Urdu, Hindi, and Farsi, respectively. Israelis and Palestinians speak Hebrew and Yiddish.

Throughout the history of the Middle East, religion has probably been the most important bond and source of conflict dividing the inhabitants (Davidson, 1991; Hitti, 1985). The majority religion of the Middle East is Islam; the largest minority religion is Christianity. Both religions have played an important role in shaping the Middle East. The Arabic language has had a tremendous influence on the shaping and development of the modern Middle East. This is largely due to the fact that the language of the Holy Koran is Arabic. Many links exist between Islam and Arabic. Arabic is the only official vessel for the transmission of Islam. Therefore, the purity and sanctity of Islam as a religion are strongly correlated with maintaining purity of linguistic integrity within the Arabic language. It is significant that Arabic is the medium of familial, societal, and national communication.

More than 95% of Arabic speakers in the Middle East and persons of Arabic origin are Muslim, and their standards for spoken and written Arabic are extremely high. Some are strict orthodox Muslims (Hitti, 1985), whereas others are more liberal. All regard their religion in a way that is difficult for the Western mind to grasp. The Arabic language is revered by Arabs as divine or holy, because the Prophet Mohammed revealed the Word of God in the Holy Koran in Arabic. (Clinical implications are presented in Chapter 14.)

Arabic Speakers and Culture

Arabic speakers typically use "national" versions of contemporary modern Arabic (CMA) in their everyday communication. Most Arabic speakers have formal and informal vernaculars that reflect social class, ethnographic background, and nationality. Typically, dialectal variations among native Arabic speakers reflect socioeconomic status, educational level, and nationality. French, English, and Turkish, as well as Spanish to a lesser extent, are language groups that have infiltrated CMA. The languages of northern India, Turkey, Iran, Portugal, and Spain are full of words of Arabic origin.

Socially, Arabic speakers use formal versions of CMA in business, academic, and religious settings. Typically, informal or colloquial Arabic is only used in informal communicative events that occur within family communication events. Because traditional Arab culture restricts interactions between nonrelated men and women, the use of informal Arabic is generally limited to family settings or intimate communication. Traditional Arab culture requires that "good" communicators use standard CMA (Lamb, 1987). Standard CMA refers to the hypothetical reference point for natural primary level (spoken) and standard secondary level (written) Arabic used by literate Arabic speakers. Standard CMA is derived from the Arabic of the Holy Koran and is spoken by the educated elite. In addition, native Arabic speakers are required to use formal or standard Arabic with their elders, authority figures, and religious leaders.

According to cultural mores, native Arabic speakers engage in lively interactive episodes of verbal communication that strongly adhere to highly stylized linguistic forms and rituals. Arab speakers across and within various national and language groups integrate Islamic and Arabic influences in all aspects of their communication. Younger communicators are expected to defer to their elders but are never excluded from participating in communication events. Typically, Arabic speakers engage in intense, interactive, communicative dialogues that allow several speakers to talk at one time.

Because Arab speakers strive to speak eloquently and to use their language creatively, a communication disorder may be perceived as having a greater social penalty for Arab speakers than it does for English speakers (Wilson, 1996).

Linguistic and Cultural Issues of Arab Americans in the Diaspora

Because the Arab world consists of a number of diverse countries, immigrants and political refugees that form the Arabic-speaking diaspora (United States, Canada, Europe, Sweden, and other countries), represent a myriad of dialectal and cultural variations. Thus, the Arab speakers that SLPs, audiologists, and educators may encounter in schools, hospitals, and other settings are likely to be diverse in linguistic and cultural backgrounds. Moreover, Arab speakers from Egyptian, Syrian, Palestinian, Lebanese, and Iraqi descent are likely to have higher levels of literacy in their native national language (i.e., Arabic or Farsi), as well as more English proficiency than other Arab speakers from less well-developed countries (Lamb, 1987). On the other hand, North and South Yemen, Sudan, Saudi Arabia, Kuwait, Bahrain, and Morocco have inhabitants with lower levels of literacy in Arabic and other languages (Lamb, 1987). However, they also have persons with high levels of literacy dependent on their ability to profit from the vast wealth of the oil-rich Saudi Arabia and United Arabic Emirates.

Wherever Arab speakers are found in the Arab Diaspora, the Arabic language is more than a medium of communication; it is an object of worship— an almost metaphysical phenomenon that bonds men and women to their God. Arabs, however, also view the mastery of other languages such as English and French to be important to economic prosperity. Therefore, Arab Americans and those in the Diaspora usually demand that their children be bilingual and that Arabic or their national language be the dominant language, regardless of where they live. Naturally, this position poses problems for some children who may have psycholinguistic deficits or differences that can negatively influence bilingualism. Therefore, careful, culturally and linguistically fair assessment and treatment services must be rendered based on comprehensive probes into the cultural and linguistic backgrounds of the clients. The family or appropriately informed family representatives must team with the SLP, audiologist, or educator and work with an Arab speaker to facilitate maximum and appropriate cultural input.

Educational and Clinical Implications

Because there are only approximately 100 Arab speech-language and hearing professionals worldwide (Wilson, 1993), those with communication disorders in the Arab world (i.e., the Middle East and other locations where significant numbers of Arabs live, such as Europe, Canada, and the United States) face a dearth of services. Collectively, these professionals include native Arabic, Hindi, Urdu, Farsi, and French speakers. Approximately 66% of Arab SLPs and audiologists reside in the Middle East, particularly in Israel, Jordan, and Saudi Arabia, whereas the other 33% live in the Arab Diaspora (Wilson, 1993). Consequently, only these Arab and other non-Arab SLPs, audiologists, and educators are available to work with Arab speakers who have communication and educational problems. This professional pool must meet the formidable challenge of not only providing the services but also of generating culturally and linguistically appropriate clinical and educational materials for a large number of Arab speakers who have communication disorders.

Linguistic, social, cultural, national, gender, and educational issues contribute to the constellation of variables that influence the management of the communication of native Arab speakers. These variables must be dealt with in a timely fashion to facilitate better speech-language, hearing, and educational services for Arab speakers. Therefore, considerable research, materials development, and SLP and audiologist personnel training are needed to improve the availability and quality of speech-language and hearing services to Arabs.

Implications for Service Delivery

A significant percentage of speech-language– and hearing-impaired individuals of Arab descent live in metropolitan areas worldwide. In the United States and the Arab Diaspora, families continue to engage in connubial practices based on strict tribal or family lineage. Consequently, it is thought that intermarriage is linked to a large number of the communication disorders found in Arab communities. Economic disparity, limited access to services, lack of trained native Arab SLP and audiologists, and limited educational support systems result in large numbers of underserved, communicatively impaired individuals in the Arab world. To increase the variety and range of SLP and audiologist services to those in the Arab world and the Arab Diaspora, the needs of the communicatively impaired must be examined from a worldwide perspective.

Arab Worldview and Communication Disorders

Limited knowledge about speech, language, and hearing often interferes with effective clinical service delivery in the Arab world and Arab Diaspora. *Worldview* refers to a set of belief systems and principles by which individuals understand and make sense of the world and their place in it. If clinicians are to effectively serve communicatively impaired Arabs, then fundamental differences between the belief systems of those of Arab descent and those of non-Arab culture must be acknowledged.

Mansfield (1992) observed that the Western world is characterized by reductionism and enriched by the expansiveness of modern technology. Conversely, the Arab worldview focuses on knowledge of the world and application of a lifestyle that is undergirded by the doctrines and influences of Islam. That is, Arab world sensibilities are driven by Islam, the Arabic language, family lineage, and a collective family-based culture. Another salient difference in worldview is reflected in Arab versus non-Arab values. For example, those of Arab descent typically value extended family, groupism, collectivism versus individualism, present time, holistic thinking, and religious roots (frequently Islamic-based doctrines). Each of these values must be viewed as a part of the Arab mosaic that has meaning only as a sum total. At the core of the Arab's worldview is the belief that all aspects of life are integrated or related to spirituality, even the secular aspects of everyday-life activities.

Because belief systems extend beyond systems of thinking to integrate traditional knowledge, professionals who engage in service delivery to Arabs must incorporate culturally appropriate tribal and traditional mores into the constructs of their treatment models. For example, traditional Arab stories, proverbs, songs, and literature should be incorporated into treatment materials regardless of the language of treatment. Useful and common sources of Arab literature known to most Arabs, Muslims, or non-Muslims are stories or conversations that report the actions or sayings of the Prophet Mohammed.

Clinical Intervention for Arab Americans and Middle Eastern Americans

Historically, Arabs in the Middle East and the Arab Diaspora have been expected to maintain their Arab culture regardless of where they reside. When those of Arab descent leave their cultural communities, they face particularly difficult cultural conflicts. In addition, levels of acculturation vary significantly among parents, children, and communities. SLPs must consider the unique cultural background of the client and the family to avoid the stress associated with cultural conflict. The communicatively impaired client of Arab descent without culturally appropriate services may experience coercive assimilation (Alireza, 1991) or, more simply, cultural collisions. Coercive assimilation unmanaged leads to issues of alienation and cultural identity confusion. Naturally, cultural alienation in the treatment process makes successful communicative management difficult. Acculturation stress and its subsequent alienation disturb cultural exchanges and the mediation of information exchange essential to good clinical management. When acculturation stress issues exist in the clinical process, a body of information is at risk. Acculturation-related stressors may be significant factors that interfere with successful management of the communicatively impaired Arab population.

The range of levels of cultural maintenance is extremely wide among communicatively impaired Arabs. The SLP or audiologist who treats the communicatively impaired Arab must recognize that some choice exists in current levels of acculturation for any Arab person or family. Variation in acculturation among those of Arab descent is typically influenced by lifestyle choices, geography, marriage patterns, and native-language retention, loss, or bilingualism. Cole (1989) reported acculturation variability as a spectrum of family systems, including the traditional, neotraditional, bicultural, and acculturated. Specifically, this variability is grounded in changes in modality behaviors, which include language, tribal lineage, folk practices, and religious-based mores.

Role of Parents

The extended family is very important in the Arab world; often, three generations may live together in one household (Sharifzadeh, 1998).

Because of the emphasis placed on strong Arab families in the Middle East and the Arab Diaspora, parent involvement in the clinical service program is critical. The relationships, role, and scope of Arab parents in the program must be clearly defined and continuous. Arab children are greatly cherished, and their education, growth, and personal development are of great importance to all segments of their nuclear and extended families. Typically, the parents and family members of communicatively impaired Arab patients go to great lengths to provide their family members with any necessary medical, educational, and rehabilitative services needed. Arab families may be uncomfortable using clinical services provided by non-Arabs, however. They may perceive social organizations as attempts to replace the traditional functions of the extended family (Wilson, 1996). They may be unwilling to talk about a disorder or disability, resulting in difficulty in obtaining an accurate or complete case history (Sharifzadeh, 1998; Wilson, 1996). If an Arab family member has a communication disorder, then the family would likely seek help; however, because the family perceives its role as that of caring for the disabled family members, it may not accept a long-term intervention program (Wilson, 1996).

Clinical intervention programs that involve clients or families of Arab descent must be sensitive to gender issues. Depending on fundamentalist religious beliefs, certain roles in the management of patients may only be assigned to men or women. For example, male clinicians may not be permitted to treat female clients without a male family member being present.

The more traditional family structure is patriarchal, with the man expecting to control all interactions between family and the clinician. The father or oldest male family member may make decisions regarding treatment, but the mother may be responsible for the child's development and for carrying out treatment suggestions (Wilson, 1996). Although Arab families expect their children to succeed in school, boys are expected to excel, whereas girls are only expected to receive a modest education (Wilson, 1996). Critical gender preferences must always be determined at the onset of the treatment process. Careful consideration of Arab cultural factors enhances the opportunities for successful cross-cultural communication management.

Cultural Variables in Assessment and Intervention

Because of the complexity and range of cultural differences among Arabs, clinicians must place the culture of Arabs from the Middle East and the Arab diaspora at the forefront of evaluation. The speech-language and hearing assessment of Arab speakers requires alternative, culturally relevant models that acknowledge the differences in narrative socialization and consider cultural factors that are fundamental to Arab culture (Guittierrez-Clellen & Quinn, 1993). For example, among Arab families, attachment and parent-child bonding are important. The families encourage interdependence among children and family members so that the mutual bonding necessary for adult life can occur. This may be in conflict with the frequent goal of independence in the intervention program often established in Western clinical programs (Wilson, 1996). Less physical contact between mother and child, later development of self-help skills, and later bedtimes to allow time to be with parents are typically in contrast with what is expected of American children (Wilson, 1996). In addition, language socialization practices may differ between American and Arab American children. Arab American children are discouraged from talking loudly and from talking during eating and meal times (Wilson, 1996). These have implications for expectations in the use of voice and expectation for discourse and conversation in intervention. Globally, the assessment of the speech, language, and hearing of Arab speakers must acknowledge all aspects of the speakers' language or languages within naturalistic environments (Damico, 1993).

Because clinicians have pursued information and cross-cultural research, systemic concerns must be addressed in language assessment and intervention. For instance, according to Wilson (1975), Butler (1989), and Damico (1991, 1993), the SLP who assesses the communication of the Arab Americans who speak Arabic must address critical factors such as normal second-language acquisition, dialectal influence, and cross-cultural interference. Thus, the successful assessment of the communication of Arab speakers poses some challenges for clinical services.

The core validity of virtually all existing tools and instruments is yet to be standardized for Arab speakers. Limited contemporary Arabic, Urdu, and other language tools and instruments exist. Of the instruments in existence, however, only a few have been standardized on Arabic speakers (Butler, 1989; Crago, 1990). Recently Wiig and El-Halees (2000) developed an objective and culturally and linguistically authentic Arabic language–screening test for children between 3 and 12 years. The development of the test was challenging because of the diversity among Arabic speakers, the diversity of Arab cultures, and the paucity of information on the speech and language development in Arabic-speaking children. The usefulness of the test is limited, because it was developed only for children in Jordan and Palestine. If it were used for children in other regions of the Middle East or other Arab-speaking communities, then scoring protocols and new standardizations would have to be developed.

The most useful techniques and tools available for the communicative assessment of Arab speakers are naturalistic descriptive instruments (i.e., language sampling, narrative probes, and behavioral assessments). Speech-language screening in Jordan, for example, uses nonsubjective measures to evaluate whether a child follows an expected course of language development. Among the methods used is to ask the child to recite a prayer commonly taught to 3-year-old children and to judge the production for intelligibility and articulatory performance (Wiig & El-Halees, 2000). Estimates of normal development are made against the normative data used for speakers of English.

Any SLP or audiologist model of service delivery for persons of Arabic descent must consider the components of Arab culture important to the client and family as a central component of the clinical process. The assessment and intervention process must validate Arab culture, individual human potential, and the cultural and linguistic references of the Arab speakers, including consideration of influences from the national community or country (e.g., Arabic, Urdu, English). The service delivery model must be comprehensive and address the ecologies of home, school, community, and any other cultural factors that might be relevant to the individual client. For example, some persons from the Middle East place a greater emphasis on memorization in education than Americans. The children may sing songs or recite poetry or nursery rhymes in a language they do not speak or understand. Because many Arab children are accustomed to rote learning and drill, they may not be responsive to indirect or facilitated language intervention in a naturalistic environment (Wilson, 1996).

Clinicians serving Arab Americans should respect traditional Arab attitudes toward clinical services and Arab communication style in all interactions. Group services should be considered, because they reflect the Arab value of collectivism. The group should be single gender. Clients may be reluctant to discuss personal information and personal feelings with unfamiliar persons. Respect for the privacy of the family should be considered in taking case history information. Certain information may not be provided until sufficient rapport has been established. The need for personal information and its relevance to the clinical situation should be explained. Because many Arab cultures maintain a close distance between communicators, Arab clients may be more comfortable sitting close to the clinician during interviews and other clinical interactions (Jackson, 1995).

The culturally appropriate service delivery model for SLP and audiologist management of Arab speakers must clearly validate Arab culture as a central component of the service delivery process. Wilson (1996) and Nydell (1997) have suggested several nonverbal and verbal cultural variables that should be observed and practiced when providing clinical services to those of Arab cultures. It is important to remember that the cultural variables important to a particular cultural group must be considered as individual to a client or family. The verbal and nonverbal variables cannot be applied across all groups without consideration of the specific preferences of the individual.

1. Sit with good posture to show respect. Do not lean against the wall or put your hands in your pockets.

2. Do not show the soles of your shoes when sitting with legs crossed. This is a sign of disrespect.

3. Arab men shake hands when greeting or parting. The handshake may appear to be prolonged according to Western practices. Some Arab men will not shake hands with a woman.

4. Greetings are long and formalized, with ritualized, predetermined expressions, and have a required response. Some formalized exchanges can last 5 or 10 minutes.

5. Formal dress is expected as an indication of professional respect. Women are not allowed to wear short skirts or pants in a formal situation.

6. Use of the left hand is considered rude. When handing objects, they should be placed directly in the right hand and not on a table or counter.

7. Some Arabs are frequently late for appointments or do not keep the appointment at all. Family needs may come before the need to keep to strict appointment times. However, among persons from Turkey, punctuality is important.

8. Arabs usually maintain a conversational distance of 2 feet between speaker and listener, in contrast to the usual American distance of 5 feet. Men frequently touch each other and use many gestures during conversation. Men do not usually touch women during conversations, especially women who are not close friends or family members.

9. During conversations, Arabs maintain steady eye contact with the listener.

10. A positive response ("yes") to a request may be an expression of goodwill, not an indication that the request will be carried out or agreement. Noncommittal answers usually mean "no."

The Arabic language is rich with forms of assertion, exaggeration, and rhetoric devices (e.g., metaphors, similes, and proverbs). Repeated words and overassertion are used in most routine exchanges for emphasis and to convince the listener that what is being said is actually meant. Emphasis and repetition should be used to stress meaning.

The ecologic approach, advocated by several researchers (Damico, 1993; Robinson & Cook, 1990; Wilson, F., 1975, 1990; Wilson, M., 1996), emphasizes the importance of placing culture to the frontline in the delivery of services to Arab American speakers. An ecologic assessment system takes into account client culture, ethnicity, socioeconomic status, attitudes, self-concept, and learning style. This is critical to service delivery and management of Arab speakers. SLPs who serve speakers of Arab descent must develop new skills, including the following:

1. Use descriptive situational assessment and intervention techniques within the context of interactions between the Arab speaker's culture and the culture of the SLP or audiologist.
2. Incorporate literature and information characteristic of the Arab speaker's background into clinical intervention.
3. Apply the Arab speaker's culture to the diagnostic and treatment process.
4. Be aware of historical and political factors that may influence the delivery of services.

Finally, the ecologic and dynamic assessment methodologies propagated by several researchers (Butler, 1989; Crago, 1990; Taylor & Payne, 1983; Wilson, F., 1975; Wilson, M., 1996) offer valuable approaches to the culturally fair assessment and intervention of Arab speakers. These methodologies include the following:

- Learn the history of immigration of the family and the client including their political associations. This is particularly important, given the volatile political climate in the Middle East.
- Identify roles and responsibility within the family and the support system. Determine who is responsible for the intervention program and who makes decisions within the family. Take care not to discount the role of the father in decision making, even if the direct contact is with the mother.
- Avoid touching without permission, especially areas around the head.
- Respect religious beliefs and practices by avoiding taboo topics such as pigs, pork products, and Christian holidays for Muslim clients.
- Avoid scheduling during the noon hour, which may be used for prayer, and on Fridays, the Muslim Sabbath.
- Respect concerns for services being provided by men to women or by younger clinicians to older clients.

Conclusion

Arabs in America are a composite of a changing society that is at once nostalgic about its past and eager to assume its role in the modern industrial world. It is a culture in which issues in male-female relations, dichotomies between urban-rural lifestyles and between traditional conservative tribal culture, and patriarchal authority contrast with the beneficiaries of the oil-rich land. The depiction of Arabs in America and the Arab Diaspora has changed in the past 40 years while being mixed with the impact of negative images in the media resulting from political conflicts in the region.

References

Adeed, P., & Smith, G. P. (1997). Arab Americans: Concepts and materials. In J. A. Banks (Ed.), *Teaching strategies for ethnic studies*. Needham Heights, MA: Allyn & Bacon.

Alireza, M. (1991). *At the drop of a veil*. Boston: Houghton Mifflin.

Almaney, A. J., & Alwan, A. J. (1982). *Communicating with Arabs*. Prospect Heights, IL: Waveland Press.

Butler, K. G. (1989). From the editor, language assessment and intervention with LEP children: Implications from an Asian/Pacific perspective. *Topics in Language Disorders, 9*(3), iv–v.

Cole, L. (1989). E pluribus pluribus: Multicultural imperatives for the 1990s and beyond. *ASHA, 31*(8), 65–70.

Crago, M. B. (1990). The development of communicative competence in Inuit children of Northern Quebec: Implications for speech-language pathology. *Journal of Childhood Communication Disorders, 13*(1), 54–71.

Damico, J. S. (1991). Descriptive assessment of communication ability in LEP students. In E. V. Hamayan & J. S. Damico (Eds.), *Limiting bias in the assessment of bilingual students* (pp. 157–218). Austin, TX: PRO-ED.

Damico, J. S. (1993). Clinical forum: Adolescent language. Language assessment in adolescents: Addressing critical issues. *Language, Speech and Hearing Services in Schools, 24*, 29–35.

Davidson, E. (1991). *Islam, Israel and the last days*. Eugene, OR: Harvest House.

Ferguson, C. A. (1971). *Language structure and language use*. Stanford, CA: Stanford University Press.

Guittierrez-Clellen, V. F., & Quinn, R. (1993). Assessing narratives of children from diverse cultural/linguistic groups. *Language, Speech and Hearing Services in Schools, 24*, 2–9.

Hitti, P. (1985). *The Arabs: A short history*. Chicago: The Gateway Edition, Regency Gateway.

Hsourani, A. (1991). *A history of Arab peoples*. Cambridge, MA: Belknap Press of Harvard University Press.

Immigration and Naturalization Service. (1998). *Annual report: Statistical yearbook*. Washington, DC: U.S. Government Printing Office.

Isenberg, I. (1976). *The Arab world*. New York: Wilson.

Jaber, L., Nahmani, A., & Shohat, M. (1997). Speech disorders in Israeli Arab children. *Israel Journal of Medical Science, 33*(10), 663–665.

Jackson, M. L. (1995). Counseling youth of Arab ancestry. In C. C. Lee (Ed.), *Counseling for diversity.* Needham Heights, MA: Allyn & Bacon.

Jackson, M. L. (1997). Counseling Arab Americans. In C. C. Lee (Ed.), *Multicultural issues in counseling* (2nd ed.) (pp. 333–352). Alexandria, VA: American Counseling Association.

Lamb, D. (1987). *The Arabs: Journeys beyond the mirage.* New York: Random.

Mansfield, P. (1992). *The Arabs.* New York: Penguin.

Nydell, M. K. (1997). *Understanding Arabs: A guide for westerners.* Yarmouth, ME: Intercultural Press.

Robinson, C. A., & Cook, V. J. (1990). Alternative assessment: Ecological and dynamic. *NASP Communique, 18*(5), 28–29.

Sharifzadeh, V. (1998). Families with Middle Eastern roots. In E. W. Lynch & M. J. Hansen (Eds.), *Developing cross-cultural competence: A guide for working with young children and their families.* Baltimore: Brookes Publishing Co.

Schwartz, W. (1999). Arab American students in public schools. *ERIC Digest* (Report No. 142). (ERIC Document Reproduction Service No. ED 429 144).

Shipler, D. K. (1987). *Arab and Jew: Wounded spirits in a promised land.* New York: Penguin.

Suleiman, M. (2001). Teaching about Arab Americans: What social studies teachers should know. (ERIC Document Reproduction Service No. ED 442 714).

Swan, M., & Smith, B. (Eds.). (1987). *Learner English: A teacher's guide to interference and other problems.* New York: Cambridge University Press.

Taylor, O. L., & Payne, K. (1983). Culturally valid testing: A proactive approach. *Topics in Language Disorders, 3*(3), 8–20.

U.S. Bureau of the Census (2001). *Statistical abstract of the United States* (120th ed.). Washington, DC: U.S. Department of Commerce.

Wiig, E. H., & El-Halees, Y. (2000). Developing a language screening test for Arabic-speaking children. *Folia Phoniatrica et Logopedica, 52*(6), 260–274.

Wilson, M. E. (1996). Arabic speakers: Language and culture, here and abroad. *Topics in Language Disorders, 16*(4), 65–80.

Wilson, W. F. (1975). *Dialect-fair evaluation of the syntax of kindergarten children.* Doctoral thesis, University of Illinois at Urbana-Champaign.

Wilson, W. F. (1990). *Prevalence of communication disorders: A comparative survey.* Paper presented at RCLMSS Seminar. Riyadh, Saudi Arabia: King Saudi University Press.

Wilson, W. F. (1993, November). *The role of speech-language pathology and audiology in the management of handicapped children in Saudi Ara-*

bia. Paper presented at the First International Conference of the Saudi Benevolent Association for Handicapped Children. Saudi Annals of Medicine, Riyadh, Saudi Arabia.

Zehr, M. A. (1999). Guardians of the faith. *Education Week, XVIII*(19), 26–31.

Additional Resources

Naff, A. (1983). Arabs in America. In S. Abraham & N. Abraham. *Arabs in the new world: Studies on Arab-American communities* (pp. 8–29). Detroit: Wayne State University Press.

Naff, A. (1998). *The Arab Americans.* New York: Chelsea House.

Nydell, M. K. (1997). *Understanding Arabs: A guide for westerners.* Yarmouth, ME: Intercultural Press.

Sharifzadeh, V. (1998). Families with Middle Eastern roots. In E. W. Lynch & M. J. Hansen (Eds.), *Developing cross-cultural competence: A guide for working with young children and their families.* Baltimore: Brookes Publishing Co.

5

Living in Harmony: Providing Services to Native American Children and Families

Carol Westby and Christine Begay Vining

In the popular media, Indians are generally depicted as relics of the past. "The tragedy of America's Indians—that is, the Indians that America loves, and loves to read about—is that they no longer exist, except in the pages of books" (Deloria in Elliott, 1991). As with any group of people, Indians have adapted and changed over time. To recognize the contributions of Indians in today's world, stereotypes associated with Indians of the past must be overcome.

Who Are Native Americans?

There is no consensus on whether members of this diverse group should be called *American Indians* or *Native Americans*. In this chapter, therefore, the two terms will be used interchangeably. Those called American Indians or Native Americans often prefer to identify themselves using terms specific to their native groups, such as *Nee-me-poo* (Nez Perce) and *Dineh* or *Diné* (Navajo). Each Native American group has always had a name for itself, which often translates to something like "The People." Official names have often been applied by outsiders, and, often, the Indians themselves now use these names. For example, the group known as *Sioux* is actually a number of related groups, including Ogala, Hunkpapa, and Yanktonia. The word *Sioux* comes from a French translation for a term applied to the group by their enemies, the Blackfoot, and means something like, "those who crawl in the grass like snakes." The Creek got their name from English settlers describing the location of their settlements next to creeks.

The American Indian population consists of Indians, Eskimos (Inuit), and Aleuts. Specifically, "Who is an Indian?," however, is a difficult question to answer, because no single federal or tribal definition is used to determine membership in this population. Three definition categories have been applied: biologic, mystical, and administrative. Biologic definitions are usually based on some minimum "blood quantum" or percentage of "Indian blood" (one-fourth, one-eighth, and so on). A congressional definition (Curtis Act of 1898) required that an individual have at least an Indian blood quantum of 25% to be considered an Indian for governmental recognition and services. This arbitrary governmental policy has resulted in divisiveness and dissension among Indians who have had to fight for limited funds and services. Many tribes have established their own blood quantum levels for a person to be classified as a tribal member. Among a few, the level is whatever can be proven; in some, it is one-half. Mystical definitions are spiritual or even fictional views of descent. Persons using a mystical view may claim to be Indians because they "feel like Indians." Administrative definitions often use biologic and mystical definitions to formulate governmental definitions of persons who are considered natives for some benefit or settlement purposes (Sutton, 2000). In the United States and Canada, Indians are viewed as distinct from the majority non-Indian population. In contrast, in Mexico, 75% of the population are of mixed Indian and non-Indian heritage (called mestizo), 20% full-blooded Indians, and 5% white; only those who speak native languages are considered Indios.

In the United States, there are approximately 700 native groups. Of that number, approximately 550, including some 223 village groups in Alaska, are formally recognized as sovereign nations, having government to government relationships with the United States. Another 150 native groups have applied for federal recognition. Reeves (1989) stated, "One of the major problems of American Indians at present is the fact that they are seen as 'one people with one need'" (p. 4). They are not a monolithic, generic group. The population is comprised of distinct tribal and native groups with vast differences regarding governance, customs, language, wealth, and religion. This diversity contributes to different worldviews and varied approaches to problem solving. Thus, "Indian people do not speak with one voice any more than America does" (Tijerina & Biemer, 1987–1988). Native Americans of one nation were, and are, as different from

Native Americans of another nation as the English are from the Spanish or the Swedes are from the Italians (Heinrich, 1991).

Native Americans do not fit the stereotype of "the vanishing American." Estimates of the Native population before the arrival of Columbus range from 8,000,000 to 18,000,000. After 1492, there was a population decline of approximately 95% that did not begin to reverse until the twentieth century. The contemporary Native American population is a young, rapidly growing group. A large proportion of the population is of childbearing age, which contributes to a birth rate 67% greater than for the U.S. general population (Indian Health Service, 1996). Today, the Native American population is approximately 2.4 million (U.S. Bureau of the Census, 1999).

Native Americans reside in every region of the United States in vastly different environments and geographic locations. Approximately three-fourths of the population is found in the West and rural areas. Relatively few are in New England or the Southeast. As of July 1998, the ten states with the largest Native American populations were California (309,000), Arizona (256,000), New Mexico (163,000), Washington (103,000), Alaska (100,000), North Carolina (98,000), Texas (96,000), New York (76,000), and Michigan (60,000). Although most of the Indian population resides off their reservations, approximately 48% of them live on or adjacent to Indian reservations (Bureau of Indian Affairs, 1991). Of 279 recognized reservations, only 18 had populations of 5,000 or more in 1990. The Navajo reservation (the size of West Virginia) is the largest in area and in population with 180,102 in 2000. The next largest reservation is Pine Ridge Sioux that had a population of 11,182 in 1990. Reservations vary in size from almost 16 million acres of land on the Navajo Reservation to less than 100 acres on smaller reservations. Some reservations are occupied primarily by tribal members, whereas others are inhabited by a high percentage of non-Indian landowners (Bureau of Indian Affairs, 1991). Over recent years, many Native Americans have shifted from reservation to urban residences. Thus, exposure to the dominant culture and the associated level of acculturation varies widely.

Levels of Acculturation

To understand the cultural diversity of Native American individuals, an examination of the concept of acculturation is imperative. *Acculturation* refers to learning the rules of another, nonnative culture. It differs from assimilation in that it is an additive, not subtractive, process and yields positive, not negative, psychosocial ramifications. For Native Americans, consideration of acculturation typically relates to the quality and quantity of cultural contact with the mainstream or white, middle-class culture. A continuum of acculturation exits within Native American communities, ranging from individuals who maintain a traditional lifestyle to those who operate primarily within and identify with the dominant culture. It is useful to consider acculturation to the mainstream culture on a spectrum and acknowledge that each Native American individual has some degree of acculturation. Red Horse (1988) proposed a spectrum of acculturation for Native Americans (traditional, bicultural, nontraditional/acculturated, and pan renaissance) involving behaviors of language, kin structure, religion, views of land, and health at various points of acculturation. Level of acculturation is related to a family's reservation or urban residence, with those living in urban areas tending to be more acculturated to the mainstream. Although urbanization clearly affects levels of acculturation, many urban Indian families maintain links to their reservations.

Traditional families adhere to culturally defined styles of living. Parents and grandparents speak the native language. Elders have respected roles because of their accumulated wisdom and have primary roles in child rearing. All family members are active in ritual ceremonies, and, depending on the tribal or village customs, they maintain bonds through clan relationships and activities such as ritual naming ceremonies.

Bicultural families have adopted much of the mainstream lifestyle. Parents often understand the native language but prefer to speak English. They do not teach the native language to their children or transmit traditional knowledge. Although they have acquired many characteristics of mainstream society, they are not totally socially integrated. They often prefer relationships with other American Indians and replicate traditional extended kin systems by incorporating non-kin friends into traditional roles. Their child-rearing practices are likely to reflect Indian values, although they may not be able to articulate these values explicitly (Miller & Schoenfield, 1975). They may attend powwows in urban areas or social dances in nearby reservations.

Acculturated families speak English and use mainstream cultural child-rearing practices. They have non-Indian religions and no linkages to land or kin. They may be aware of or uninterested in their Native American heritage. *Pan-renaissance* families are attempting to redefine and reconfirm previously lost cultural lifestyles. They and their parents may have become fully acculturated to mainstream values and behaviors, but they are now seeking to regain their lost heritage. They speak English and, when possible, attempt to learn the native language, reestablish clan connections, and participate in cultural activities.

It is important to realize that any one individual might show differing degrees of acculturation across different behaviors. That is, a person may retain traditional views about health and religion yet speak English and have no knowledge of his or her native language. The individual experience of acculturation will determine how each Native American person fits into native and non-native (mainstream) cultures. Each Native American individual will have his or her own values, beliefs, and worldview, depending on degree of acculturation.

Historically, Native Americans have been viewed by Euro-Americans as inferior, second-class citizens with a lesser culture. Recently, there has been a resurgence of Indian pride, and the perspective of most Americans has shifted to acceptance and admiration. As a result of rising political power, Indians are reasserting their sovereignty and regaining some control over sovereign rights to land, water, hunting and fishing, mineral resources, and religion. Northwest tribal groups have had fishing rights reaffirmed, and the Chippewa won a court decision granting them the right to hunt any resource within their territory without regard to state regulations. Tribal gaming is becoming a huge industry on many reservations. By 1999, at least 150 tribes had gaming facilities producing funds that allowed establishment of health and educational services, as well as, in some cases, the ability to buy back tribal lands (Sutton, 2000). There is an increasing presence of Native American views in music (e.g., the songs of Buffy St. Marie), literature (Harjo & Bird, 1997; Silko, 1992; Tapahonso, 1999), and science (Cajete, 2000).

Native Languages

Language Characteristics

Language scholars believe that before the arrival of Columbus, Native Americans spoke approximately 300 languages. Estimates of current language use vary, but there are indications that roughly one-half of these languages are now extinct (Krauss, 1998). Many of the remaining languages are considered near extinction, as they have few speakers and these speakers are all elders. Currently, there are 154 indigenous languages spoken in the United States. Table 5-1 shows the indigenous languages spoken by 100 or more persons. Of the 154, only approximately 20 are still spoken by people of all ages and are thus fully vital (Reyhner & Tennant, 1995). Some of these languages are spoken by only a few individuals; others such as Cherokee, Navajo, and Teton Sioux/Dakota are spoken by thousands (Estes, 1999). Projections suggest that by the year 2050, only 20 indigenous languages will remain (Crawford, 1999).

Acculturation and assimilation into the dominant society are contributing to use of English as a primary language in many Native American households. In some native groups, characteristics of the native language have been transferred to spoken English (Wolfram, 1991). This has occurred through a process in which native language characteristics are stabilized and then perpetuated in

Table 5-1   Indigenous Languages Spoken in the United States by More Than 100 Speakers

Speakers (No.)	Language	Location
148,530	Navajo	Arizona, Utah, New Mexico
35,000	Ojibwa, Western	Montana, Lake Superior, North Dakota
20,355	Dakota	Nebraska, Minnesota, North and South Dakota, Montana
12,693	Apache, Western	Arizona
11,905	Cherokee	Oklahoma, North Carolina
11,819	Papago-Pima	Arizona
10,000	Yupik, Central	Alaska
8,000	Ojibwa, Eastern	Michigan
6,413	Zuni	New Mexico
6,213	Muskogee	Oklahoma, Alabama, Florida
6,000	Lakota	Nebraska, Minnesota, North and South Dakota, Montana
5,264	Hopi	Arizona, Utah, New Mexico
4,580	Kerns, Eastern	New Mexico
4,280	Crow	Montana
4,000	Inuktitut, Northwest Alaska	Alaska
3,500	Inuktitut, North Alaska	Alaska
3,390	Kerns, Western	New Mexico
3,000	Yakima	Washington
2,284	Shoshone	Nevada, Idaho, Wyoming
2,100	Micmac	Boston, New York City
2,000	Paiute, Northern	Nevada, Oregon, California, Idaho
1,984	Ute-Southern Paiute	Colorado, Utah, Arizona, Nevada, California
1,800	Apache, Mescalero-Chiricahua	New Mexico
1,721	Cheyenne	Montana
1,631	Tiwa, Southern	New Mexico
1,301	Jemez	New Mexico
1,300	Tewa	New Mexico, Arizona
1,100	Yupik, Central Siberian	Alaska
1,092	Kiowa	Oklahoma
1,070	Cree, Western	Montana
1,062	Blackfoot	Montana
1,038	Arapahoe	Wyoming, Oklahoma
1,007	Havasupai-Walapia-Yavapai	Arizona
1,000	Chickasaw	Oklahoma
1,000	Hawaiian	Hawaii
927	Tiwa, Northern	New Mexico
887	Malecite-Passamaquoddy	Maine
854	Comanche	Oklahoma

Speakers (No.)	Language	Location
812	Apache, Jicarilla	New Mexico
800	Mesquakie	Iowa, Oklahoma, Kansas, Nebraska
775	Tlingit	Alaska
697	Nez Perce	Idaho
600	Koasati	Louisiana, Texas
539	Kikapoo	Kansas, Oklahoma, Texas
496	Mikasuki	Florida
406	Yaqui	Arizona
400	Yupik, Pacific Gulf	Alaska
365	Gwich'in	Alaska
343	Quechan	California
321	Cocopa	Arizona
300	Koyukon	Alaska
256	Alabama	Texas
250	Hocak, Winnebago	Nebraska
234	Mohave	Arizona
234	Shawnee	Oklahoma
200	Kalispel-Pend Doreille	Montana
200	Seneca	New York, Oklahoma
200	Tenino	Oregon
150	Assiniboine	Montana
141	Caddo	Oklahoma
138	Haida	Alaska
126	Karok	California
115	Tanana, Upper	Alaska
113	Tsimshian	Alaska
112	Okangan	Washington
107	Salish, Southern Puget Sound	Washington
102	Kutenai	Idaho, Montana
100	Hidatsa	North Dakota
100	Skagit	Washington
100	Walla Walla	Oregon

Source: Reprinted with permission from Estes, J. (1999). How many indigenous American languages are spoken in the United States? By how many speakers? *National Clearinghouse for Bilingual Education* [On-line]. Available: http://www.ncbe.gwu.edu/askncbe/faqs/20natlang.htm.

the variety of English used by members of the native group. As a consequence, distinctly indigenous ways of speaking English have been maintained (Bayles & Harris, 1982; Fletcher, 1983; Weeks, 1975; Wolfram, 1984).

There are as many forms of Indian English or Indian-influenced dialects as there are Indian languages. Leap (1993) identified some characteristics that appear in a number of Indian-influenced dialects as follows: (1) retention of the phonemic and phonologic characteristics of the tribal language, (2) retention of Indian language syntactic rules, (3) word formation and grammar markings from the tribal language may influence the English dialect, and (4) constructions found in other nonstandard variations of English are also found in Indian English (e.g., uninflected forms of *to be*). Silver and Miller (1997) have documented the basics of grammar in 160 native languages, along with discourse genres (language functions) and relationships between language and worldview. An understanding of the characteristics of the native language can enable speech-language pathologists (SLPs) to identify the ˙ characteristics of Indian-influenced English in particular Native groups.

In the Southwest, where Native languages continue to be spoken in many tribes, influences of the Native languages can be observed in the English language of adults and children. In Navajo, Apache, and the Pueblo languages, words generally begin with consonants and end with vowels. When speaking English, speakers of Navajo, Apache, and the Pueblo languages are likely to devoice final consonants or substitute a glottal, which is the most common consonant in the languages. If an English word begins with a vowel, then speakers may add an initial glottal. Voice onset time differs between these Native languages and English. These languages do not have the voice or voiceless distinction present in the plosives such as, /b/-/p/, /d/-/t/, and /g/-/k/. Instead, there are single plosives with voice onset times between /p/ and /b/, /t/ and /d/, and /k/ and /g/. As a result, children may have some difficulty distinguishing between these phonemes.

The Southwest Indian languages have a subject-object-verb sentence structure. Verbs are highly inflected. There are no gender pronouns or pronouns for "it." Pronominal prefixes on verbs code the relationships of subjects and objects to the verbs (possessor, agent, patient, benefactor) and person (first, second, third, fourth [passive]). Number is coded in the verb as one, two, and more than two. Location (coded by prepositions in English) is coded in the verb and is influenced by the characteristics of the objects (Fig. 5-1). Size comparisons are made on the basis of volume and plane in space (vertical or horizontal). Hence, there are no generic words for big and little. As a consequence, preschool children may be confused when confronted with tasks of classifying objects as big or little. One cannot use the same word to talk about a big snake and a big elephant.

Valiquette (1990) noted that in Keres (spoken in five Pueblo groups), infinitives are rare, and dependent clauses (which in English use connective words such as *when, while, until, because, before, after, although,* and *if*) are

**Figure 5-1 What does a Keres speaker say when told,
"Place this object(s) on the table. . ."?**

To know what to say, the Keres speaker must know how to categorize the objects. In English and other European languages, nouns influence verbs only in terms of number agreement—one or more-than-one (e.g., a boy runs; many boys run). In Keres, number is coded in the verb as one, two, and more-than-*two*. In English, location is coded by prepositions. In Keres, location is coded in the verb and is influenced by the characteristics of the subject. The Keres words in bold print would all be translated as "put on" or "place on." To know which verb form to use, persons must understand the Keres categorization system. Notice how the objects are grouped by their characteristics. Preschool Keres-speaking children know how to classify objects to use the appropriate verb form.

pishidiicha (enclosed container)	**picha (singular)**	**piguya (mass)**	**pit'cha (wide, flat shape of container)**
purse	pen	trashcan	basket
bag of popcorn	newsletter	chair	plate of cookies
sack of corn	cup	washing	basket of corn
groceries	ruler	machine	platter of chicken
carton of eggs	comb	TV	laundry
box of paper	scarf	apple	
	computer disk	10-gallon hat	
	spoon		
	coat		
	pencil		
	empty mug		
	magazine		
piwaisht'i (liquid in bowl)	**piisha (plural)**	**piy'aat'a (plural)**	**pisht'icha (liquid in it)**
bowl of posole	group of papers	three chairs	cup with water
	gloves		pot of coffee
			pitcher of milk

used but appear to be related to age privilege differences, not to age developmental differences. That is, as one matures and gains stature in the community, one uses dependent clauses with increasing frequency and a wider variety of purposes. Certain language forms are considered more formal and are associated with religious functions. Valiquette (1990) noted that a form of "and" is used as the connective in many dependent clauses in Keres. He suggested that this might be a result of Native Americans hearing the frequent use of "and" in English and Spanish and transferring it to their native language. It may, however, also be a reflection of how Native Americans perceive the temporal and causal relationships coded in dependent clauses (Hall, 1983). Time is not viewed as linear, and cause goes beyond physical principles (Cajete, 2000).

Even when there has been no contact with the Native language for many generations, the Native language may strongly influence the present English dialect. For example, Wolfram (2000) described and traced the roots of the Lumbee Indians in North Carolina. Although the Lumbee are not a recognized tribe, they are ethnically and culturally Native American. The Lumbee lost their language many generations ago. The Lumbee dialect shows the influence of early colonization by the English, Scottish, and Scottish-Irish, but Lumbee speech is distinctly different from the Anglo-American and African American English spoken in the area. Some vocabulary is unique to the Lumbee: *chauld* means embarrassed, a *juvember* is a slingshot, and *bog* is a helping of chicken and rice. The unique use of "bes" also sets the Lumbee dialect apart from others in the region: *Babies bes born like that; The train bes running.* SLPs must be alert to the varieties of Indian English and how they may affect children's performance on testing.

Language Policy

The U.S. government policy toward native language use has shifted radically over time. Previous assimilation and termination policies played a major role in the decrease of native language use. Many parents of children currently in school remember being punished if they were heard speaking their Native language. The recent shift to Native American self-determination, however, has been associated with native language revival efforts (Reyhner, 1992). The Native American Languages Act of 1990 recognized the importance of traditional native languages to the survival of Native American cultural identity and ensured that the U.S. government would act together with Native Americans in preserving and promoting the use of native languages. This act provided funds for language conservation and renewal. A number of tribes (e.g., Navajo, Tohono O'odham, Piqua, Yaqui, Northern Ute, Arapaho, and Red Lake Band of Chippewa) have adopted policies to promote the use of their ancestral tongues in schools and government functions, and others have developed model programs to teach languages that are being lost (e.g., Cree, Hawaiian, Arapaho, Inuktitut, and Choctaw [Crawford, 1998; Peacock & Day, 1999]). A number of programs begin in preschool mother and child programs. For example, in Wyoming, an Arapaho elder woman teaches parents traditional language used in caring for Arapaho children (Greymorning, 1999).

Native languages are integral to the cultural life and spiritual experience of Native communities. If the language were lost, then many of the cultural practices and rituals would no longer have meaning. It is through language that one is able to participate fully in cultural events. Without the native language, traditions such as hunts, songs, and dances would lose their significance, because embedded in the songs and stories are cultural values such as cooperation, kinship, respect (for self, mother earth, animals, and so on), and responsibility. The sense of place, belonging, identity, and values are expressed through language.

Questions are being posed by linguists and Native American communities regarding the merits and disadvantages of contemporary language maintenance efforts. Questions are asked such as "How do we make language a priority?" "What do we do, when do we do it, and how do we do it?" "Are there language maintenance strategies that have been proven successful with various native languages?" The implications and consequences of action versus inaction, attitudes toward language and its preservation, and resources available for language preservation and maintenance efforts are complex issues and impact progress across and within communities. What works for one language in one community may not be appropriate for another because of the circumstances under which the languages are disappearing.

Cultural Values

To interpret assessment data and provide appropriate and acceptable interventions for Native Americans, clinicians must have an understanding not only of a group's ways of knowing but also of the cultural values and beliefs that underlie these ways of knowing. A variety of approaches have been used to study cultural variations in values and beliefs among people (Cleary & Peacock, 1998; Hall, 1976; Hofstede, 1980; Kluckhohn & Strodtbeck, 1961; Triandis, 1995). Application of these approaches to mainstream and Native cultures reveals differences along several dimensions.

Individualism versus Collectivism

All societies must strike a balance between independence and interdependence between individuals and the group (Greenfield, 1994). Mainstream U.S. culture is strongly individualistic, whereas many Native American cultural groups are generally collective or oriented to the group. Individualistic cultures emphasize the goals of the individual, whereas collectivistic cultures emphasize goals of the group as having precedence over the individual's goals. In individualistic cultures, people are to look after themselves and their immediate family, whereas in collectivistic cultures people belong to in-groups or collectives that look after members of the group in exchange for loyalty (Triandis, 1995). Collectivistic cultures emphasize goals, needs, and views of the group over those of the individual. The collective orientation values the social norms of the group over individual pleasures, shared group beliefs rather than unique individual beliefs, and cooperation with group members rather than maximizing individual outcomes. The collectivist nature of the American Indian culture can influence assessment and intervention. Children in a collective culture are more likely to provide assistance to others, even in ways that mainstream teachers consider cheating. Individuals who are different are less likely to be singled out.

Although Indian communities function collectively and have responsibilities for one another, there is also a valuing of noninterference (Cleary & Peacock, 1998). One is not to interfere with the choices of others. Everyone is viewed as fulfilling a purpose, and, as a consequence, no one has the power to impose personal values on others. Autonomy is highly valued; children are expected to make their own decisions and operate semi-independently at an early age. They may be left alone to herd sheep or watch younger siblings at young ages. Children are allowed choices and freedom to experience the natural consequences of those choices. Despite the children's freedom to make choices, the impact of their choices on others is also emphasized (LaFromboise & Low, 1989). Children are allowed to make mistakes and learn from those mistakes without being scolded. Mainstream service providers have sometimes misinterpreted this parenting style of noninterference as an indication of neglectful or uninvolved parents.

Doing versus Being or Being-in-Becoming

Mainstream U.S. culture epitomizes the doing orientation in which there is "a demand for the kind of activity that results in accomplishments that are measurable by standards conceived to be external to the acting individual" (Kluckholn & Strodtbeck, 1961). Persons seek to be in control and in charge. In contrast, Native American cultures value a *being* and a *being-in-becoming*. The being orientation is concerned with who one is, not what one can or has accomplished. One is valued simply for being. One's worth is not decreased if one has a disability or as one ages and becomes less physically able. The focus on human activity in the being-in-becoming orientation is on striving for an integrated whole in the development of self. Therefore, there is no need to compete and prove one's self better than others. As a result, children do not need to strive to be better or to stand out from others.

Time Orientation

Orientation to human activity influences perceptions and use of time. In mainstream culture, because one must prove one's worth by getting much done, lists of activities are made, scheduled, and checked off when completed. Mainstream culture is driven by "clock time," whereas Native cultures are more attuned to "event time" (Harris, 1998). Hall (1976) refers to these two orientations toward time as *monochronic* and *polychronic*. Monochronic time emphasizes schedules, segmentation, and promptness. With the exception of birth and death, all important activities are scheduled. Polychronic time systems are characterized by several things happening at once. They stress involvement of people and completion of transactions rather than adherence to present schedules. No times are firm and changes in the time of important events occur right up to the last minute, creating frustration for those who value promptness and adherence to well-organized plans and schedules.

Scollon and Scollon (1981) reported that Athabaskan Indians believe it is inappropriate to speak of one's plans or to anticipate the future. Navajos believe that one should live a long life and not limit one's potential with a specific plan or timeline. If one sets a specific plan for future actions, then one may limit all other possibilities for living a long life (Mike, Bidtah, & Thomas, 1989). Although Native Americans may not be consciously aware of the reasons for not planning, they may have grown up in environments in which planning ahead was not done and time was not rigidly scheduled. Activities are done "when the time is right." Although one may be told that a dance or a chapter house meeting may begin at a particular time, this may only mean that the event will occur in the near future. The actual event may not begin for several hours. The idea of what constitutes "being late," then, differs between mainstream and Indian cultures. Children growing up in polychronic time systems are less likely to have experienced the pressure to perform quickly and, as a consequence, they may not perform well on timed tests.

American mainstream culture values time schedules and punctuality. Events flow linearly. Actions focus on the immediate present and the future. Activities are bound to the imposed rhythms of workdays, time clocks, overtime, saving time, and taking time out. Bruchac (1994) reflected that in mainstream culture, "The ticking of the clock is more important than the beat of the human heart" (p. 11). Mainstream service providers sometimes think that Native Americans have no sense of time because they may not honor imposed schedules (Hall, 1983). Native Americans, however, are quite conscious of time in its natural cyclical manner—days, months (moons), and years (seasons or winters). In fact, the Anazazi Indians, ancestors of the Southwest Pueblo Indians, were highly attuned to time. At Fajado Butte in

New Mexico, they arranged boulders and carvings in the rock mesa to mark the solstices and equinoxes of the sun and the 11-year cycle of the moon (Sofaer & Ihde, 1983). The "sun dagger" of Fajado Butte is considered the Stonehenge of the New World.

Cultural systems that place high value on traditions are said to have past orientations. The future orientation predominates where change is highly valued (e.g., mainstream U.S. culture). Acculturation to mainstream values results in Native Americans having some focus on the future, but at the same time, many continue to value and maintain the traditions of the past. As a consequence, elders are respected and hold power.

Relationship to Nature

The mainstream U.S. culture maintains a mastery-over-nature orientation. All natural forces can and should be overcome or be put to use by humans, or both. Human beings are viewed as superior to all life forms; consequently, mainstream Americans believe they have the right to manipulate nature and situations for their own comfort and convenience. As adults, they are responsible for mastering circumstances that arise. With this value system, mainstream families tend to think about the significance of a disability for the future. They may ask, "When will she learn to talk?," "Will therapy correct the problem?" or "When can he return to his teaching position?" They express concern regarding what persons cannot do, what they will be able to do, and when they are able to do it. Parents, spouses, or clients take responsibility for alleviating the disability. Persons with these mainstream values seek treatment for speech-language-hearing disabilities and are co-participants in their therapy.

Native Americans, in contrast, maintain a harmony-with-nature orientation that makes no distinction between or among human life, nature, or the supernatural. With their being-in-becoming and harmony-with-nature orientations, Native Americans tend to have a greater tolerance for variation, and they may feel less need to "fix things," focusing instead on learning how to accept and cope with their circumstances. Families may recognize that a family member is different but accept that difference as being who the person is. Because of such viewpoints and values, they may be less likely to seek out evaluation and treatment services. When they do become involved, it is important to include the extended family in decisions. According to Vining (2000), achieving and maintaining *hozho*, a state achieved through a balanced and harmonious life, is the essence of Navajo philosophy and teaching that sustains and guides the people. Navajo education focuses on preparing individuals to reach a state of *hozho*. All knowledge is viewed with respect to its ability to draw one closer to this spirit of harmony. Traditionally, individuals are taught the interrelationship and interdependence of all things and how they must harmonize with them to maintain balance and harmony.

Human Nature

Native Americans acknowledge that the world is made up of good and bad. They believe, however, that in the end, good people will triumph because they are good. This belief is reflected in the trickster tales from a number of Native groups. Coyote (Southwest), Raven (Northwest), and Iktomi (Plains trickster, also called Saynday, Na'pe/Old Man, or Wihio) fool, trick, cheat, and take advantage of good people, but, in the end, they usually lose (Sherman, 1996).

Communication Patterns

Conversation

Frequent miscommunication arises when Native American and mainstream persons interact, because their values and beliefs affect their styles of communication. Scollon and Scollon (1980, 1990) suggested that problems arise between non-Native speakers and Alaskan Athabaskan Native speakers in three areas: (1) the view speakers present of themselves, (2) organization of talk, and (3) contents of talk. Table 5-2 summarizes communication differences between non-Native and Native speakers that have been identified by a number of anthropologists and educators (Basso, 1990; Hall, 1959, 1976, 1983; Philips, 1983; Saville-Troike, 1989; Scollon & Scollon, 1980).

Non-Native persons get to know others by talking, and only when they know someone well do they think there is no need to talk. In contrast, many Native Americans prefer talking to those they know well; when they do not know someone well or in cases in which people have been separated for some time they prefer to watch and listen until they have gathered sufficient information about a person. Basso (1990) told the story of Apache parents waiting at the trading post for their children to arrive home from boarding school where they had been for several months. The children got off the bus and piled into their parents' trucks. Unlike mainstream families in which parents would question children about their activities over the past months, the Apache children and parents spoke minimally. When Basso (1990) questioned parents about this, they reported, "You just can't tell those children after they've been with White men for a long time. They get their minds turned around some-

Table 5-2 Cross-Cultural Perspectives of Speakers

Mainstream Perspective of Native American Speakers	Native American Perspective of Mainstream Speakers
Presentation of self	
Talk very little	Talk too much
Do not initiate	Always talk first
Avoid situations requiring talking	Talk to people they do not know
Only want to talk to close acquaintances	Think they can predict the future
Play down their abilities	Brag about themselves
Act as if they expect things to be given to them	Do not help people even when they can
Deny planning	Talk about what's going to happen later
Distribution of talk	
Avoid direct questions	Ask many questions
Never start a conversation	Always interrupt
Talk off topic	Talk only about their interests
Never say anything about themselves	Boast about themselves
Are slow to take a turn to talk	Do not give others a chance to talk
Contents of talk	
Are too direct and inexplicit	Too direct; are not careful when they talk about people or things
Leave without saying anything	Have to say "goodbye" even when they can see you are leaving

Source: Reprinted with permission from Scollon, R., & Scollon, S. B. (1980). *Interethnic communication*. Fairbanks, AK: Alaska Native Language Center.

times. . . . At school, some of them learn to want to be White men, so they come back and try to act that way. But we are still Apaches! So we don't know them anymore, and it is like we never knew them. It is hard to talk to them when they are like that."

When mainstream persons talk, the person in the dominant position (i.e., the teacher or clinician) asks questions and then listens to persons in the subordinate position to show what they know. Mainstream children learn and demonstrate what they know by performing. In contrast, Native children learn by watching; they do not perform until they have mastered the skill. When teachers ask Native children to display knowledge, the children may appear to become unruly. To the children, teachers appear incompetent because they are not doing most of the talking, yet they are acting superior (Scollon & Scollon, 1980).

In mainstream interactions, persons are expected to put their best foot forward. They are expected to speak well of themselves and have high hopes for the future. In contrast, in many Native cultures, it is not only inappropriate but also bad luck to speak highly of oneself, to highlight one's experiences, or to talk about plans for the future. As a consequence, parents may be hesitant to respond when asked about their child's strengths or specific needs.

Hall (1959, 1976, 1983) differentiated cultures on the basis of the communication style that predominates in the culture. A high-context communication or message is one in which "most of the information is either in the physical context or internalized in the person, while very little is in the coded, explicit, transmitted part of the message. A low-context communication is just the opposite, i.e., the mass of the information is vested in the explicit code" (Hall, 1976). Although no culture exits solely at either end of the low-high context continuum, the culture of mainstream United States is placed toward the low-context end of the continuum; Native American culture falls toward the high-context end of the continuum. When persons from high-context cultures communicate with persons from low-context cultures, they are likely to experience miscommunications. The indirect, nonspecific style of high-context Native American individuals appears vague to low-context mainstream individuals. The low-context individual is likely to suspect that the high-context individual is being intentionally evasive or uncooperative. The loud, explicit, direct style of low-context mainstream individuals appears impolite, rude, and disrespectful to high-context Natives.

Narrative Discourse

Native Americans learn much of their way of life through narratives (Cleary & Peacock, 1998; Sarris, 1993). Native American narratives differ in function, content, and structure from narratives in Euro-American cultures. By the time children are 9–10 years of age, however, schools expect children from all cultural backgrounds to comprehend and produce mainstream-style narratives (Hedberg & Westby, 1993). Native American narratives have a different purpose than many mainstream narratives. This difference in purpose was exemplified in an episode of the television show *Northern Exposure* in which a Native American medicine man attempted to understand a white person's stories. The Native American character reflected that Indian stories have a great healing power. They reflect on everyday life values and are told to influence people to change their life in some way. In contrast, the Native American character observed that many white persons' stories talked about mishaps, "put people down," and did not appear to have any value to change persons' lives. Basso (1990) noted the function of Native American stories to affect persons' lives. He discussed Apache historical tales that focus on persons who suffer misfortune as a consequence of actions that violate Apache standards for acceptable social behavior. Like arrows, these stories are shot at persons to warn them to change their ways. When using stories for assessment purposes, evaluators may need to establish a purpose for telling stories.

Mainstream stories usually have a linear, temporal structure, whereas Native American stories are known to have a nonlinear structure. Benally (personal communication, 1989), a Navajo educator, described the structure of Navajo narratives as being like Indian fry bread (a circular piece of dough fried in oil) with "an idea bubbling up here, another idea bubbling up over there." Lutz (1989) discussed the circle as a philosophic and structural concept in Native American narratives. The plots of Native American and mainstream Western stories are affected by these circular and linear orientations and by cultural values. In Western stories, a returning adventurer brings a happy ending with power, honor, respect, and material possessions for the individual. In Native American stories, the ensuing happiness and harmony that result from a person returning from a quest involve all persons within the circle (e.g., bringing rain clouds that affect the total environment rather than money for an individual). The cultural contrast in story plots is a contrast between a community, tribal, circular mode and an individualist, materialist, and linear mode (Lutz, 1989).

The structure of the first or native language can influence narrative organization and focus, even if the storyteller is telling the story in a second language. Lewis (1992) had Ute and Anglo children in first through sixth grades retell a favorite movie. She noted that non-Native students' narratives had story themes and linear sequences of beginnings, middles, and ends. In contrast, the Ute students' narratives were event focused, characterized by unconnected events and unexplained descriptions. The non-Native students presented the listener with some direction for the story; in contrast, the Native American students jumped directly into the story without providing the listeners the background information or reasons for the story. The nature of the Ute students' narratives anticipated a participatory speaker-listener engagement that is a guiding principle of Ute oral discourse (Leap, 1988). Ute storytellers assumed shared knowledge between the speaker and listener and believed that it was the listeners' responsibility to infer the meaning of the story or to question the storyteller. This expectation for listener participation in story comprehension can generate problems for students in classroom environments in which teachers expect predictable stories that stand alone.

A similar narrative discourse pattern was noted in beginning Navajo college students (Gregory, 1993). Gregory (1993) and other instructors who taught Basic English to secondary and beginning college students were able blindly to identify essays written by Navajo students. Gregory observed that the structure and language choice in the Navajo essays was determined by interaction of the topic and the audience. In contrast, their genre or purpose determined the structure of the non-Native essays. The Navajo students tried to make connections with the audience more so than the non-Native students. In oral language, Navajo students relied heavily on interaction to maintain clarity. They assumed that readers have the same responsibility with their written language. Navajo writers were more likely to address the audience directly (using *I, you,* and *we* in their writings) than the Anglo writers, and they expected the audience to assume responsibility for interpretation. This personalized approach to written discourse may present particular difficulties as students are expected to comprehend and produce increasingly decontextualized expository texts in science and social studies.

Health and Disabilities

Types of Disabilities

American Indians are among the poorest groups in the United States—32% have incomes below the poverty threshold. They attain fewer years of formal schooling than any other minority group. Dropout rates in urban high schools are particularly high, sometimes reaching 85%. Reservation and boarding schools, which educate almost 80% of Indian youth, have approximately a 50% drop out rate (Coladarci, 1983; Giles, 1985; St. Germaine, 1995). Almost 80% of Native American children receiving special education services are identified as learning disabled or speech-language impaired.

Native Americans have the highest rate of disabilities of all ethnic groups and the highest rate of infant mortality due to birth defects (Lynberg & Khoury, 2000). Cleft lip, palate, or both (Coddington & Hisnanick, 1996; Lowry, Thunem, & Silver, 1986; Edmonds et al., 1981); fetal alcohol syndrome or fetal alcohol effects (May, 1999; May, Hymbaugh, Aase, & Samet, 1984); and otitis media (OM) (Moore, 1999; Wiet, DeBlanc, Stewart, & Weider, 1980) are more prevalent among American Indians than other groups. OM is the most frequently identified disease of Indian children. OM includes not only fluctuating hearing loss but also severe complications resulting in hearing impairments of a more permanent nature (Moore, 1999). Racial, anatomic, and familial variables are associated with the incidence of OM (Todd & Bowerman, 1985). Inuit children are at particularly high risk for OM and its complications (Moore, 1999). After an extensive literature review, Stewart (1986) concluded that occurrence of OM in indigenous people was influenced by (1) ethnic (Asian) origin, (2) eustachian tube placement and insufficient middle ear aeration, and (3) relative inefficiency of the immune system. Because hearing loss and language impairment are often associated with OM, fetal alcohol syndrome, and cleft lip or palate, these conditions may account for the high rates of referral of Native children for speech-language and learning disabilities services. (See Chapters 11 and 12 for additional information on hearing loss.)

Diabetes and diabetes-related complications are also high in the Native population and are increasing. In some groups, 25% or more of the population are diabetic by age 40. Native American children are exhibiting increasing rates of diabetes. There has been a sixfold increase in diabetes in some groups of Native American children between 1976 and 1996 (Fagot-Campagna et al., 2000). Diabetes has multiple complications, including retinopathies resulting in vision loss, neuropathies and circulatory problems that can result in amputation, and strokes. Native Americans experience low rates of amputation but high rates of strokes.

Bowker (1993) stresses caution when interpreting the data on Native American low-educational achievement and a variety of poor health issues. Mainstream professionals should not conclude that the Native American culture fosters high school dropout rates, alcoholism, and poor health. Bowker notes that these behaviors are all highly correlated with poverty, and American Indians are the most poverty-stricken group in the nation.

Attitudes toward Disabilities

Words such as *disability, impairment, handicap,* and *rehabilitation* are not easily translated in Indian languages. Many Indian languages do not have words for *retarded* or *disabled;* instead, they may use words such as *incomplete* or *slow* (Locust, 1986). Cultures vary in the ways disabilities are explained. Some of this information may be available to mainstream professionals, but some is to be known only by tribal members. Many families live in the Native and mainstream culture, seeking services and explanations in both. Native Americans are to live harmoniously with Mother Earth and Father Sky, as well as to show respect for the circle of life that includes the environment, animals, plants, and humans. They believe that violation of beliefs and values may not only disrupt the natural order of life but also cause disharmony, which may manifest itself as ill health. Their holistic approach to health implies that all things in life are connected to one another and that people are connected in a spiritual and physical sense in this circle.

Views about the origin of disabilities are unique for each culture. Interviews with Navajo elders revealed that the origin of disabilities is related to violation of moral virtues by the First People (Vining & Allison, 2000). They believe that disabilities are becoming more prevalent, because people are no longer honoring traditional belief systems and teachings. In many Native cultures, expectant mothers and fathers need to be careful with what they may see, hear, feel, smell, and eat. In Navajo belief, supernatural projection on a baby within the womb results in the infant taking on characteristics of the entity being projected and may affect the child's physical, emotional, mental, and spiritual development. Although disabilities are often associated with violation of cultural beliefs and practices, the interviews with Navajo elders also revealed a positive perception of children with disabilities. They believed that people with disabilities are Images of the Holy People and, as such, should be considered sacred.

Although it can be useful for interventionists to know how a family explains a disability of a child or elder, the mainstream professional must exercise care in asking for this information. Many of these explanations are tied to religious beliefs and are not to be shared with the mainstream world.

Speech-Language Assessment

Native American children have often been inappropriately placed in special education; assessment and treatment approaches for children and adults often violate client and family values; and disabilities related to learning, speech-language, and social-emotional difficulties remain mis- or unidentified. Native American children are overrepresented in special education. More than 10% of Native American children in public schools (Pavel & Curtin, 1997) are placed in special education, and more than 18% of those in Bureau of Indian Affairs or tribal schools are in special education (Bureau of Indian Affairs, 2000). These students are most often identified as having a specific learning disability, a speech-language impairment, mental retardation, or emotional disturbance. The lack of culturally and linguistically appropriate materials and use of untrained interpreters complicate the assessment process.

Lack of Appropriate Materials

Material Content

The lack of culturally and linguistically appropriate materials for screening, evaluation, and intervention continues to be an issue that must first be addressed by Native American communities. With training and the availability of literature on the topic of culturally appropriate assessment and intervention with Native Americans, there is an increased awareness of appropriate materials and practices that respect cultural beliefs, and the use of inappropriate materials and practices that violate cultural beliefs and values appears to be declining. Professionals must be willing to listen and learn to respect the cultural beliefs of students and families from culturally and linguistically diverse backgrounds. For example, within the Navajo culture, certain animals such as the owl, snake, and bear are to be avoided. Clients should not be exposed to materials and experiences featuring these animals. Desalvo (1995) shared her experience of an incidence that resulted in a clash of cultures. When visiting the local zoo, a teacher called the children's attention to the grizzly bear, "Shash." The next day, many Navajo grandparents came to the school, upset because the bear had looked upon the children. The grandparents were concerned that the bear may have taken the children's minds. They would, therefore, be required to perform a ceremony that could cost more than $1,000 to restore each child to harmony.

This experience conveys the need to ensure that the materials and activities used with Native American students are culturally appropriate. Currently, materials and intervention activities for Native American students in special education—whether for evaluation or intervention—are intended for English-speaking students and primarily represent experiences in mainstream society. Materials that reflect tribal life, experiences that are culturally relevant, and materials intended for Native-speaking students should be used.

Standardized Tests and Test Translation

In an effort to evaluate bilingual, bicultural Native American children, service providers have attempted to translate various assessment tools. Parts of speech-language tests, for example, have been translated from English into several Native languages to evaluate students' vocabulary, syntactic, and semantic abilities. Assessors and translators need to be aware that vocabulary words are not necessarily equivalent. For example, there is not a single word in Navajo that can be translated for the word *construction*. The concept is translated as "there is a man hitting a board with a hammer." Clearly, the word *construction* has a more complex meaning than this translation implies. The phonologic and syntactic structures of Native languages are so markedly different from English that translation of articulation and syntactic tests is inappropriate and unrealistic (Allison & Vining, 1999).

Several speech-language assessment instruments have been locally normed on reservation Indians (Bayles & Harris, 1982; Miles, 1982; Uzdawinis, 1982). Currently, however, no research exists that specifically addresses the language development status of English-speaking Native American children or appropriate language assessment instruments for English-speaking Native American children. In recent years, research has been conducted with the Cherokee tribe in northeastern Oklahoma in an effort to identify language screening and assessment tools suitable for this population. Studies on nonreservation English-speaking Cherokee Indian children have indicated that standardized tests are of questionable use with this population (Long, 1998a). Long (1998a) reasoned that Indian children who live, socialize, and are educated among white individuals would evidence the same types of language skills as the white children. Nevertheless, Long and Christensen (1997) and Long (1998b) found a significant difference in the linguistic and social communication language skills between these two groups. When compared to 3- to 4-year-old white children, Cherokee Indian children had lower linguistic and social communication skills.

Alternative Assessment

Appropriate assessment of Native Americans requires the use of alternative forms of assessment. Teaming with other professionals to evaluate a student's academic, educational, and language abilities is beneficial, so that the functional relevancy of a client's communication disability can be documented. Informal procedures such as observations in the home or classroom or spouse, teacher, or parent report and informal tasks in the native language are necessary assessment procedures for English-speaking as well as Native American–speaking clients. Language samples in English and the native language, inventories and criterion-referenced testing, and work samples such as portfolios are excellent ways to evaluate cognitive and linguistic abilities and environmental influences that impact communication.

Dynamic assessment procedures involving test, teach, and retest methodology have been used with children from culturally and linguistically diverse backgrounds to differentiate students with language learning differences from those with language learning disorders (Lidz & Pena, 1996; Pena, 1996; Pena, Quinn, & Iglesias, 1992). Typically, these assessment tasks have focused on teaching noun labels. Label learning, however, may not be the most discriminating task for children from some backgrounds. Ukrainetz et al. (2000), working with Arapahoe and Shoshone Head Start children, initially attempted to use dynamic assessment procedures to measure their ability to learn labels for objects. This approach, however, did not differentiate between children developing language typically and those exhibiting language learning difficulties. Observation of the Head Start curriculum the children were exposed to revealed that they had been explicitly taught to label. Ukrainetz et al. (2000) then taught category identification (e.g., food, clothes, transportation, animals), because the Native American children were observed not to express categorical labels. This dynamic assessment strategy significantly differentiated children judged to be stronger or weaker language learners based on teacher report and examiner observation.

Intervention

Early Intervention

Requirements of Part C of the Individuals with Disabilities Education Act of 1997 require family involvement in the assessment and intervention process with infants and toddlers. Service providers need to understand Native American family values, beliefs, and views of the child's impairment and how they may want it treated. They must recognize family and kinship roles. The child's parents may not be the persons with the authority to make decisions regarding treatments for their child. Grandparents, aunts, uncles, and, sometimes, tribal elders must be involved in such decisions. For example, a mother of a young child had brought her son to Indian Health Services for a medical examination. The physician noted that the child had OM. He recommended that myringotomies be done that afternoon, in his mind, saving the mother a long trip back to the clinic at a later time. The nurse recognized the mother's discomfort. In talking with the mother, the nurse learned that the mother needed to have a traditional ceremony done for her son before he could have any type of surgery.

Families may wish to use traditional and Western medicine, and they may want explanations or an understanding of the disability in both cultures. A Native American mother of a toddler with Down syndrome commented that she had been told what caused her daughter's problem from the mainstream perspective, but she was not told how to understand it in her culture. She raised money and traveled some distance to consult with a medicine man and have an appropriate ceremony done. Early intervention staff working with a large Native population in the Southwest have reported assisting families in finding ways to raise money for traditional ceremonies that are not paid for by mainstream medical care.

Early intervention services are to be provided in natural environments. Some agencies and states have interpreted this to mean that services must be provided in the child's home. Although many parents appreciate this type of service, some American Indian parents who choose to use Native and mainstream practices have requested that therapy services be provided in hospital clinics or schools. Therapy services are viewed as Western or mainstream medicine and are to be carried out in mainstream sites.

Early intervention programs serving Native communities attempt to adjust activities to be compatible with Native practices of child rearing. *The*

Growing Path (Simons-Ailes & Valencia, 1983) describes traditional infant-parent behaviors such as wrapping, massage, shawl carrying, and cradleboards and explains how the activities help the child to develop. Olmstead (2001) and colleagues developed baby books in Yupik (an Alaskan Native language) with photographs of familiar people and things in the environment that are shared between caregivers and infants. A model parent-training program developed by the National Indian Child Welfare Association (1986) centers training on the use of traditional storytelling practices.

School-Age Children

The educational policies of the U.S. government and Bureau of Indian Affairs strove to alienate Native American children from their home cultures and to assimilate them into the mainstream culture (Kramer, 1991). Even through half of the twentieth century, Native American children were removed from their homes to be taught in boarding schools by government employees or missionaries. In these settings, their hair was cut, tribal clothing was replaced with uniforms, and they were punished for speaking their home languages and practicing their native religions.

Today, few Native American students attend boarding schools. The majority attend public or tribal schools on their reservations or in neighboring communities. Schools no longer actively attempt to destroy the culture of Native American students, but neither do they necessarily value the students' culture and attempt to sustain it. Native American students no longer need to run away from school; they simply drop out of school at rates of 50%, the highest of any ethnic group (McShane, 1983; St. Germaine, 1995; Yates, 1987). Current attitudes toward cultural and linguistic diversity urge teachers to assist students in living in two worlds by considering the learning styles of students and by including content familiar to these students while also teaching them the academic content of schools (Bennett, 1990; Chamot & O'Malley, 1994; Cummins, 1986; McLeod, 1994). Although such an approach is highly recommended, there are few guidelines as to how to accomplish it.

Some recent studies have suggested that children will achieve the best academic skills if they are taught in their first language through the early school years, at least until they achieve success in literacy in the language (Collier, 1989; Crawford, 1989; Hakuta, 1990). This has been done successfully in some Navajo, Alaskan Indian, and Inuit schools. A number of tribes, however, do not permit the use of the tribal language in schools. Schools represent the mainstream world, and the Native language belongs to the Native community and its culture; it is not something to be shared with everyone.

For the majority of Native groups, fluent speakers of the Native language are not available to teach it.

Cultural Influences in the Classroom

Many researchers have suggested the concept of cultural compatibility in teaching as a means of improving educational outcomes for minority students. The assumption is that education that is compatible with the cultural patterns of the students will be more effective (Au, 1980; Philips, 1983; Tharp & Gallimore, 1988). For many Native American students, the patterns of interaction and communication in the home environment are different from those in the school environment. Major differences between Native and mainstream cultures that have educational consequences are found in the following four areas:

1. *Social organization.* Mainstream North American classrooms use primarily whole-class organization with the teacher instructing or demonstrating to the whole group. Native American teachers are more likely to move from student to student and engage in lengthy individual teaching interactions (Leith & Slentz, 1984; Mohatt & Erickson, 1982). Native American students prefer to work in small same-gender groups, but schools encourage working in large mixed-gender groups (Tharp & Gallimore, 1988).

2. *Sociolinguistics.* Sociolinguistic variations among cultures encompass discourse style, wait time, and participant structures (Tharp, 1994). Mainstream discourse has a tight sequential organization on a particular topic. In contrast, Native American discourse style is loosely structured and moves fluidly from topic to topic. Native American students generally have longer wait times between conversational turns than mainstream teachers. Hence, teachers may not allow students sufficient time to answer questions (Saville-Troike, 1989; Scollon & Scollon, 1981). Mainstream teachers' questions require students to refer more to the written text, whereas Native American teachers' questions require students to refer more to their own general knowledge (White, Tharp, Jordan, & Vogt, 1989).

3. *Cognition.* Mainstream schools emphasize verbal learning and learning by trial and error; however, many Native American groups favor holistic visual learning and not attempting a task until one is sure how to perform the task well (Appleton, 1983; John, 1972; Longstreet, 1978; Suina & Smolkin, 1994).

4. *Motivation.* Mainstream North American schools value individual and independent attainment, whereas Native American groups generally stress interdependence and the well-being of the group as a whole (Greenfield, 1994). Schools generally motivate through public display of the individ-

ual—poor performance is reprimanded publicly and students receive rewards for being better than other students. In contrast, Native American students are trained to work to support the group and not to stand out as individuals. Efforts to control students' behavior, punishment, or contingent reward can violate cultural values (Mohatt & Erickson, 1982; Suinia & Smolkin, 1994; Tharp, 1994; Wolcott, 1987).

Even in situations in which schools are operated by tribes with Native American administrators and teachers, students' academic performance is often below mainstream standards (Peshkin, 1997). In an ethnographic study of an all–Native American school, Peshkin (1997) suggested that the Indian students believed that teaching and learning at school and in the community not only occur in separate places but also are separate processes as epitomized in a student's reflection: "With school, basically, all you have to do is try. You don't have to feel it in your heart" (p. 106).

Principles of Education for Diverse Cultures

Although the concept of culturally compatible teaching has merit, it is not easy to implement and does not adequately address the needs of culturally and linguistically diverse students to learn the skills and knowledge of mainstream academics. Instead, the concept of *instructionally congruent teaching* is advocated (Lee & Fradd, 1998). Such teaching integrates cultural understandings with the nature of academic disciplines in ways that encourage students' participation by building on prior experiences, while simultaneously promoting achievement that includes new ways of engaging in academic subjects. Tharp (1994) proposed four teaching and learning principles compatible with the concept of instructionally congruent teaching:

I. Develop competence in the language of instruction in all instructional activities of the school day.

II. Contextualize the teaching and curriculum in the experiences, skills, and values of the community. Schools teach through the use of abstract language, yet many communities do not teach in this way. Schools must assist students to understand how verbal descriptions and abstractions are drawn from the everyday world and how these abstractions can be applied to the everyday world (i.e., learning should be contextualized).

III. Use joint productive activity with peers and teachers (Sharon, 1984; Slavin, 1990).

IV. Teach by using *instructional conversations* (ICs) that involve dialogue between teachers and learners. ICs are discussion-based lessons geared toward creating rich opportunities for students' conceptual and linguistic development (Goldenberg, 1991). IC differs from the traditional "recitation script" in which the teacher repeatedly elicits and evaluates short responses.

According to Tharp (1994), these principles form a holistic view of education for diverse classrooms. IC approaches have been used to teach children from a variety of diverse cultures, including Native Hawaiian and Pueblo Indian children, in learning the mainstream narrative language style. The goal of education for Native children should be to facilitate their ability to live successfully in two worlds—the world of their community and the world of the public school—by mastering the discourse skills of both. Storytelling, which has a rich history in Indian communities, can provide a means of assisting children to live in two worlds.

Facilitating Narrative Discourse

Sarris (1993), a Coast Miwok and Pomo Indian author from northern California, claims that stories become an important device individuals use to interpret to each other their experiences with work, school, and their families. He describes a reading program for Pomo children designed to reduce the students' alienation from school by linking traditional Kashaya Pomo myths with the children's present-day experiences. Middle school students were given traditional mythic stories and told to illustrate them in a coloring book format that would serve as a reader for younger children. Working together with peers and conferring with parents, grandparents, and community members, the students created the *Pomo Supernaturals Coloring Book*, in which traditional characters were reframed into the students' present world experiences. For example, *coyote the trickster* became a low-rider or hoodlum. Sarris suggested that this approach to reading encouraged students to believe that they have equal power to the text they are reading and to the teacher who has given them the text.

Westby and Roman (1995) developed a narrative language arts curriculum for Pueblo Indian children in regular and special education using Tharp's (1994) principles of multicultural education to assist students in developing cognitive academic language proficiency (Chamot & O'Malley, 1994; Cummins, 1984). The program encouraged maintenance of traditional storytelling as well as giving students skills in comprehension and production of mainstream stories. The program involved the following elements:

1. *Contextualized lessons.* The SLP and teachers integrated familiar Native American stories and themes and stories of the Southwest with unfamiliar stories (mainstream stories and stories from other cultures). Students were encouraged to discuss personal experiences around the themes of the stories.

2. *Joint productive activities.* As a group, the students listened to stories read by the SLP or teacher, watched videos and interacted with computer CDs, discussed the stories and videos, and jointly constructed stories or completed related art or science activities.

3. *IC in lessons* (Goldenberg, 1991). This involved conversation with a thematic focus. Instructors activated students' background knowledge, provided direct teaching of concepts as needed, and promoted the use of complex language structures and justification of statements. They asked primarily open-ended questions that required students to predict, reason, and project into the thoughts and feelings of the story characters, and they were responsive to students' contributions.

The teachers selected themes for their teaching. The children were exposed to many stories related to these themes from their culture and from mainstream cultures. Native American storytellers told their stories in the school. Children were explicitly taught the structure of stories, and stories from different cultures were compared and contrasted.

As children produced their own stories, they often incorporated influences from the Native and mainstream cultures. For example, the children had read several versions of *The Three Little Pigs* (a traditional version [Galdone, 1970], *The Three Little Pigs and the Hawaiian Shark* [Laird, 1981], *The Three Little Javelinas* [a Southwest version; Lowell, 1992]). The students talked about how the environment affected the pigs, what they used to build their houses, and who their predator was. After doing a unit on rain forests, they were asked to write a version of the three little pigs in the rain forest. Before beginning their stories, they discussed what animals in the rain forest would take the place of the pigs and wolf. After the students decided that peccaries are piglike and their predator is a jaguar, they were asked to write their versions of *The Three Little Pigs.* The beginning and end of one child's story shows the influence of his Native culture and exposure to mainstream culture.

> The first boy peccary went north then the second peccary went south and then the third peccary went west, and the fourth went east. The first peccary saw a lady Kuna that had a bucket full of flowers. Then he said, "Can I have flowers to build a house for me?" The Kuna Indian said: "yes." Then the peccary went to build his house. After he finished his house he went to bed and slept and slept. When he got up he hear something. He look out the window, he saw a jaguar. Then he started to panic. Then he heard the jaguar say: "little peccary, little peccary let me come in. . . ."

Jaguar found them. The jaguar decided to ring the doorbell. They let him in even though they knew who he was. Right when he was about to attacked, the oldest peccary pulled out a paper in front of him. It was a restraining order against him. The jaguar was shocked. He started to cry and decided to leave but the peccaries decided to hug him good bye. After that they went on the trail for their long journey.

Although the title of the child's story was *The Three Little Peccaries*, his story had four peccaries going in the four cardinal directions, reflecting a common characteristic of Native stories of the Southwest. He ended his story with the jaguar being served a restraining order, which was probably a reflection of mainstream culture, not a part of traditional Pueblo culture.

There are many high-quality children's books addressing Native American narratives, history, ecology, and science, as well as current lifestyles. Care must be used in selecting materials, however, to avoid stereotypes, inaccurate representations, or incorrect and inappropriate content (Hirschfelder, Molin, & Wakim, 1999; Slapin & Seale, 1992). Appendix 5-1 presents guidelines for avoiding inappropriate Indian stereotypes in children's books. Tribal groups differ in terms of what is considered appropriate and inappropriate content. For example, many groups find the counting book *Ten Little Rabbits* (Grossman & Long, 1991) offensive, because it shows animals dressed in human clothing and participating in Native activities, whereas some find it acceptable and recommend it because it shows the variation among Native groups and accurately portrays differences in clothing and activities of the groups. In some tribes, it is inappropriate to use pictures or stories of certain animals such as snakes or owls; in other cases, stories about some animals can only be told or read at certain seasons of the year. For example, stories about coyotes, bears, snakes, and insects can only be told between the first and last frost, when the animals are in hibernation. To determine acceptability of materials, it is best to have liaisons from the Indian community review materials that will be used.

Beyond Stories

Success in mainstream education requires more than the ability to understand and produce stories. To succeed in the technological world of the twenty-first century, all students must also be scientifically literate (Westby & Valesquez, 2000). Cajete (1999), a Native American science educator, recommends using an ecological science approach in teaching Native children. He notes that "traditional Native American systems of educating were characterized by observation, participation, assimilation, and experiential learning rather than by the low-context formal instruction characteristic of European schooling" (Cajete, 1999). Use of indigenous science instruction allows for traditional styles of learning. Buffy Sainte-Marie's Cradleboard Teaching Project (King, 2000; http://www.cradleboard.org) has developed a series of science units (some of which are available on CD-ROMs) based on Native American (and Canadian First Nation) ways of life. For example, the physics of sound is taught by showing how Native American musical instruments make sound; friction is taught using examples such as grinding, tobogganing, and the game of ice snake.

Consider a weather unit taught in the upper elementary grades of a Pueblo school that weaves Native experiences with mainstream content. The teacher's goal was to have students develop an understanding of the water cycle and weather patterns. In the process, she exposed her students to an array of texts to acquaint them with the necessary vocabulary, concepts, syntactic structures (dependent clauses with temporal and causal connectives), and discourse styles from a variety of perspectives. The teacher read the book *Storm in the Night* (Stolz, 1988), which relates the experience of an African American child and his grandfather in a storm, and the poems *The Wind Picks Up* (Two Two, 1999) and *Clouds* (Holmes, 1999), from *When the Rain Sings* (National Museum of the Native American, 1999), a collection of poetry written by Native American children. The class then talked about their experiences with weather and storms. The teacher did a KWL activity, checking what the students knew about weather and storms, and what they wanted to know about weather and storms. (At the end of the unit, the students discussed what they had learned.) She asked the students what they thought caused storms. The students and teacher read the Cherokee myth, *How Thunder and Lightning Came to Be* (Harrel & Roth, 1995), and then read a scientific explanation of these events in *Wet, Wild, and Windy* (Llewellyn, 1997). Then, using activities from *How the Weather Works* (Allaby, 1995), the students conducted simulation experiments on the water cycle, lightning, and thunder. During the experiments, the teacher modeled procedural discourse (describing the steps of the activities) and encouraged students to describe the procedures they used. After the experiments, they reported their observations. Through interactive conversations, the teacher led the students into explaining their observations. She revised their responses, using a scientific language style (O'Connor & Michaels, 1996):

> Titania: and, well see, the lightning makes the air get real hot and so the air spreads out and that makes sound.
>
> Teacher: so, Titania, what you're saying is that lightning rapidly heats the air. The hot air expands quickly, making waves that we hear as sound.

The students compared the explanation for thunder and lightning given in the Cherokee story with what they had learned from their experiments and reading scientific texts. Next, the students read the story *Thunder Cake* (Polacco, 1990), which is about how a grandmother and her granddaughter prepared to bake a cake before an approaching storm arrives. They discussed how the characters in *Thunder Cake* used the lightning and thunder to judge the distance of the approaching storm and their feelings about the storm. After this story, they read and discussed *The Big Storm* (Hiscock, 1993), which is a factual account of a devastating storm that crossed the United States in 1982. The book provides explanations for the blizzards, hail, avalanches, and tornadoes that were spawned by the storm and pictures of the results. Students discussed predictions about the storm, related what they learned from the theoretical explanations of the water cycle and weather in *Wet, Wild, and Windy* (Llewellyn, 1997) and their simulation activities, and discussed results of the storm in terms of devastation of property and people's experiences and feelings. The teacher then raised the question of what would happen if something other than water, sleet, snow, or hail fell from the sky. The students read *Bartholomew and the Oobleck* (Dr. Seuss, 1949). They made oobleck (a mixture of cornstarch and water), explored its properties, predicted the consequences of oobleck falling in their own community, and designed solutions for cleaning up the oobleck. Each activity built on what came before. These science activities permitted Native children to make use of their observational skills to build language skills in reporting, predicting, and reasoning.

Cajete (1999) emphasized that Native American students are intimately involved with their families, culture, and community. Native American cultures are essentially spiritual, oral, nature centered, tradition based, and communal. Educators and SLPs must be aware of the students' cultural orientation and determine appropriate ways to incorporate these cultural orientations into the classroom. Cleary and Peacock (1998) offer the following suggestions for doing so:

- Get to know the norms and values of the community from which the students come.
- Be aware of the students' background knowledge and experiences.
- Discuss the students' learning style with them and help them to understand why they do what they do in learning situations.
- Be aware of any pacing of activities within a time framework that may be too rigid.
- Be aware of how questions are asked, and think about communication styles.

- Consider alternatives for those students who do not like to be singled out from the group.
- Provide plenty of time for students to observe and practice before performing.
- Be aware of personal space boundaries.
- Organize the classroom to meet the learning preference needs, and encourage cooperation and independent activity.
- Provide feedback that is immediate, consistent, and private when necessary; give praise often and for specific achievements.
- Be flexible and realize that educational goals or standards may be attained in a number of ways, so provide students with adequate choices for demonstrating their learning.

Native American culture and language have survived, to some extent, early Spanish and European contact and are thriving today in the midst of new pressures from within and without. Native American people continue to record their history and pass it on orally through stories, as they have done for centuries. The indigenous people of the Americas face an uncertain future, however, because of the tremendous outside influences and pressures that are eroding their languages and cultural way of life. Educators and SLPs serving these populations should seek to develop programs that will enable children and adults to live successfully in two worlds.

References

Allaby, M. (1995). *How the weather works*. Pleasantville, NY: Reader's Digest.

Allison, S. R., & Vining, C. B. (1999). Native American culture and language considerations in service delivery. In T. V. Fletcher & C. S. Bos (Eds.), *Helping individuals with disabilities and their families: Mexican and U.S. perspectives* (pp. 193–206). Tempe, AZ: Bilingual Review Press.

Appleton, N. (1983). *Cultural pluralism in education*. New York: Longman.

Au, K. H. (1980). On participation structures in reading lessons. *Anthropology and Education Quarterly, 9*, 91–115.

Basso, K. H. (1990). *Western Apache language and culture*. Tucson, AZ: University of Arizona Press.

Bayles, K. A., & Harris, G. (1982). Evaluating speech-language skills in Papago Indian children. *Journal of American Indian Education, 21*, 11–20.

Bennett, C. I. (1990). *Comprehensive multicultural education: Theory and practice* (2nd ed.). Boston: Allyn & Bacon.

Bowker, A. C. (1993). *Sisters in the blood: The education of women in Native America*. Bozeman, MT: Center for Bilingual/Multicultural Education.

Bruchac, J. (1994). The circle of stories. In M. A. Lindquist & M. Zanger (Eds.). *Buried roots and indestructible seeds: The survival of American Indian life in story, history, and spirit.* Madison, WI: University of Wisconsin Press.

Bureau of Indian Affairs (1991). *American Indians today: Answers to your questions.* Washington, DC: Bureau of Indian Affairs.

Bureau of Indian Affairs Division of School Program Support and Improvement (2000). *Special education eligibility document,* PL 105-17. Washington, DC: U.S. Department of Interior [On-line]. Available: http://www.oiep.bia.edu/eligibility_document.htm.

Cajete, G. A. (1999). *Igniting the sparkle: An indigenous science education model.* Skyland, NC: Kivaki Press.

Cajete, G. A. (2000). *Native science: Natural laws of interdependence.* Santa Fe, NM: Clear Light Publishers.

Chamot, A. U., & O'Malley, J. M. (1994). *The CALLA handbook.* Reading, MA: Addison-Wesley.

Cleary, L., & Peacock, T. (1998). *Collected wisdom.* Boston: Allyn & Bacon.

Coddington, D. A., & Hisnanick, J. J. (1996). Midline congenital anomalies: The estimated occurrence among American Indians and Alaska Native infants. *Clinical Genetics, 50*(2), 74–77.

Coladarci, T. (1983). High school dropout among Native American. *Journal of American Indian Education, 23,* 15–23.

Collier, V. P. (1989). How long: A synthesis of research on academic achievement in a second language. *TESOL Quarterly, 23*(3), 109–131.

Crawford, J. (1988). Endangered Native American languages: What is to be done, and why? In T. Ricento & B. Burnaby (Eds.), *Language and politics in the U.S. and Canada: Myths and realities.* Mahwah, NJ: Erlbaum.

Crawford, J. (1989). *Bilingual education: History, politics, theory and practice.* Trenton, NJ: Crane.

Crawford, J. (1999). *Bilingual education: History, politics, theory and practice* (4th ed.). Los Angeles: Bilingual Educational Services.

Cummins, J. (1984). *Bilingualism and special education.* San Diego: College-Hill.

Cummins, J. (1986). Empowering minority students: A framework for intervention. *Harvard Educational Review, 56,* 18–36.

Desalvo, A. (1995). Experience reported in *Los Ninos Preschool Press.* Albuquerque, NM: University of New Mexico Training and Technical Assistance Unit.

Dr. Seuss. (1949). *Bartholomew and the oobleck.* New York: Random House.

Elliott, J. (1991). America to the Indians: Say in the 19th century. In *Rethinking Columbus: A special issue of* Rethinking Schools (September), 23–30.

Edmonds, L. D., Layde, P. M., James, L. M., et al. (1981). Congenital malformation surveillance: Two American systems. *International Journal of Epidemiology, 10,* 247–252.

Estes, J. (1999). How many indigenous American languages are spoken in the United States? By how many speakers? *National Clearinghouse for Bilingual Education* [On-line]. Available: http://www.ncbe.gwu.edu/askncbe/faqs/20natlang.htm.

Fagot-Campagna, A., Pettitt, D. J., Engelgau, M. M., et al. (2000). Type 2 diabetes among North American children and adolescents: An epidemiologic review and a public perspective. *Journal of Pediatrics, 136*(5), 664–672.

Fletcher, J. (1983). What problems do American Indians have with English? *Journal of American Indian Education, 23*(1), 1–13.

Galdone, P. (1970). *The three little pigs.* New York: Clarion Books.

Giles, K. N. (1985). *Indian high school dropouts: A perspective.* Milwaukee, WI: Midwest National Origin Desegregation Assistance Center.

Goldenberg, C. (1991). *Instructional conversations and their classroom application.* Santa Cruz, CA: The National Center for Research on Cultural Diversity and Second Language Learning.

Greenfield, P. M. (1994). Independence and interdependence as developmental scripts: Implications for theory, research, and practice. In P. M. Greenfield & R. R. Cocking (Eds.), *Cross-cultural roots of minority child development* (pp. 1–37). Hillsdale, NJ: Erlbaum.

Gregory, G. A. (1993). *The texture of essays written by basic writers: Dine and Anglo.* Doctoral dissertation, University of New Mexico, Albuquerque.

Greymorning, S. (1999). Running the gauntlet of an indigenous language program. In J. Reyhner, G. Cantoni, R. N. St. Clair, & E. P. Yazzie (Eds.), *Revitalizing indigenous languages.* Flagstaff, AZ: Northern Arizona University. (ERIC Document Reproduction Service No. ED 428 924).

Grossman V., & Long, S. (1991). *Ten little rabbits.* San Francisco: Chronicle Books.

Hakuta, K. (1990). *Bilingualism and bilingual education: A research perspective. Focus No. 1.* Washington, DC: National Clearing House for Bilingual Education.

Hall, E. T. (1959). *The silent language.* New York: Doubleday.

Hall, E. T. (1976). *Beyond culture.* New York: Doubleday.

Hall, E. T. (1983). *The dance of life.* New York: Doubleday.

Harjo, J., & Bird, G. (1997). *Reinventing the enemy's language: Contemporary Native women's writings of North American.* New York: W. W. Norton.

Harrel, B. O., & Roth, S. L. (1995). *How thunder and lightning came to be: A Choctaw legend.* New York: Dial Books.

Harris, G. A. (1998). American Indian cultures: A lesson in diversity. In D. E. Battle (Ed.), *Communication disorders in multicultural populations.* Boston: Butterworth–Heinemann.

Hedberg, N., & Westby, C. E. (1993). *Analyzing storytelling skills: From theory to practice.* Tucson, AZ: Communication Skill Builders.

Heinrich, J. S. (1991). Native Americans: What not to teach. In *Rethinking Columbus: A special issue of* Rethinking Schools (September), 15.

Hirschfelder, A., Molin, P. F., & Wakim, Y. (1999). *American Indian stereotypes in the world of children.* Langham, MD: The Scarecrow Press.

Hiscock, B. (1993). *The big storm.* New York: Atheneum.

Hofstede, G. (1980). *Culture's consequences: International differences in work-related values.* Newbury Park, CA: Sage.

Holmes, K. (1999). Clouds. In L. Francis (Ed.), *When the Rain Sings.* New York: Simon & Schuster.

Indian Health Service (1996). *Trends in Indian health—1996.* Washington, DC: U.S. Department of Health and Human Services.

John, V. P. (1972). Styles of learning—styles of teaching: Reflections on the education of Navajo children. In C. Cazden, D. Hymes, & V. P. John (Eds.), *Functions of language in the classroom.* New York: Teachers College Press.

King, C. (2000). From cradleboard to motherboard. *Teaching Tolerance,* 10–13.

Kluckhohn, F., & Strodtbeck, F. (1961). *Variations in value orientations.* New York: Row, Pederson.

Kramer, B. J. (1991). Education and American Indians: The experience of the Ute Indian tribe. In M. A. Gibson & J. U. Ogbu (Eds.), *Minority status and schooling.* New York: Garland.

Krauss, M. (1998). The condition of Native North American languages: The need for realistic assessment and action. *International Journal of the Sociology of Language, 132,* 9–21.

LaFromboise, T. D., & Low, K. G. (1989). American Indian children and adolescents. In J. T. Gibbs., L. N. Huang, & Associates (Eds.) *Children of color: Psychological interventions with minority youth.* San Francisco: Jossey-Bass.

Laird, D. (1981). *The three little hawaiian pigs and the magic shark.* Honolulu: Barnaby Books.

Lee, O., & Fradd, S. H. (1998). Science for all, including students from non-English language backgrounds. *Educational Researcher, 27*(4), 12–21.

Leith, S., & Slentz, K. (1984). Successful teaching strategies in selected Manitoba schools. *Canadian Journal of Native Education, 12,* 24–30.

Leap, W. (1988). Assumptions and strategies in guiding mathematics problem solving by Ute students. In R. Cocking & J. Mestre (Eds.), *Linguistic and cultural influences on learning mathematics.* Hillsdale, NJ: Erlbaum.

Leap, W. (1993). *American Indian English.* Salt Lake City: University of Utah Press.

Lewis, J. M. (1992). The story telling strategies of Northern Ute elementary students. *Journal of Navajo Education, 9,* 24–32.

Lidz, C. S., & Pena, E. D. (1996). Dynamic assessment: The model, its relevance as a nonbiased approach and its application to Latino American children. *Language, Speech, and Hearing Services in Schools, 27*(4), 37–372.

Llewellyn, C. S. (1997). *Wild, wet, and windy.* Cambridge, MA: Candlewick Press.

Locust, C. (1986). *American Indian belief systems concerning health and wellness.* Tucson, AZ: Native American Research and Training Center, University of Arizona.

Long, E. E. (1998a). Native American children's performance on the Preschool Language Scale-3. *Journal of Children's Communication Development, 19*(2), 43–47.

Long, E. E. (1998b). Pragmatic language skills of English-speaking Native American children. Paper presented at the ASHA annual convention, November 1998, San Antonio.

Long, E. E., & Christensen, J. M. (1997). Indirect language assessment tool for English-speaking Cherokee Indian children. *Journal of American Indian Education, 38*(1), 1–14.

Longstreet, E. (1978). *Aspects of ethnicity.* New York: Teachers College Press.

Lowell, S. (1992). *The three little javelinas.* Flagstaff, AZ: Northland Publishing.

Lowry, R. B., Thunem, N. Y., & Silver, M. (1986). Congenital anomalies in American Indians of British Columbia. *Genetic Epidemiology, 3,* 455–467.

Lutz, H. (1989). The circle as philosophical and structural concept in Native American fiction today. In L. Coltell (Ed.), *Native American literatures.* Servizio Editoriale Universitario: Vicolo della Croce Rossa 5-56126, Pisa.

Lynberg, M. C., & Khoury, M. J. (2000). Reports on selected racial/ethnic groups special focus: Maternal and child health contribution of birth defects to infant mortality among racial/ethnic minority groups, United States, 1983 [On-line]. *MMWR Surveillance Summaries, 39*(SS-3), 1–6, 8–12. Available: http://www.cdc.gov/epo/mmwr/preview/mmwrhtml/00001671.htm.

May, P. A. (1999). The epidemiology of alcohol abuse among American Indians: The mythical and real properties. In D. Champagne (Ed.), *Contemporary Native American issues* (pp. 222–244). Walnut Creek, CA: Alta Mira Press.

May, P. A., Hymbaugh, K. J., Aase, J., & Samet, J. M. (1984). Epidemiology of fetal alcohol syndrome among American Indians of the southwest. *Social Biology Quarterly, 30,* 374–387.

McLeod, B. (Ed.) (1994). *Language and learning: Educating linguistically diverse students.* Albany, NY: State University of New York.

McShane, D. (1983). Explaining achievement patterns of American Indian children. *Peabody Journal of Education, 61,* 34–48.

Mike, E. H., Bidtah, L., & Thomas, V. (1989). *Cultural conflict.* Central Consolidated Schools, District 22, Title VII, Bilingual Education Program.

Miles, M. C. (1982). *Look, listen, and tell: A language screening instrument for Indian children.* Albuquerque, NM: Southwest Communication Resources, Inc.

Miller, M., & Schoenfield, T. (1975). *The Native Americans.* Austin, TX: National Education Lab.

Mohatt, G., & Erickson, F. (1982). Cultural organization of participation structures in two classrooms of Indian students. In G. Spindler (Ed.), *Doing the ethnography of schooling.* New York: Holt, Rinehart & Winston.

Moore, J. A. (1999). Comparison of risk of conductive hearing loss among three ethnic groups of Arctic audiology patients. *Journal of Speech, Language, and Hearing Research, 42*(6), 1311–1322.

National Indian Child Welfare Association (1986). *Positive Indian parenting: Honoring our children by honoring our traditions.* Portland, OR: National Indian Child Welfare Association.

National Museum of the American Indian (1999). *When the rain sings.* New York: Simon & Schuster.

O'Connor, M.C., & Michaels, S. (1996). Shifting participant frameworks: Orchestrating thinking practices in group discussion. In D. Hicks (Ed.), *Discourse, learning, and schooling.* New York: Cambridge University Press.

Olmstead, P. (2001). Yupik baby books born in Alaska. *The ASHA Leader, 6*(2), 2–20.

Pavel, D. M., & Curtin, T. R. (1997). *Characteristics of American Indian and Alaska Native education: Results from the 1990–1991 and 1993–1994 schools and staffing surveys* (Report No. NCES 97–451). Washington, DC: U.S. Department of Education. National Center for Education Statistics. (ERIC Document Reproduction Service No. ED 405 169).

Peacock, T. D., & Day, D. D. (1999). *Teaching American Indian and Alaska native languages in schools: What has been learned.* ERIC Clearinghouse on Rural Education and Small Schools [EDO-RC-99 10].

Pena, E. (1996). Dynamic assessment: The model and its language applications. In K. N. Cole, P. S. Dale, & D. J. Thal (Eds.), *Assessment of communication and language.* Baltimore: Brookes.

Pena, E. D., Quinn, R., & Iglesias, A. (1992). The application of dynamic methods to language assessment: A non-biased procedure. *The Journal of Special Education, 26*(3), 269–280.

Peshkin, A. (1997). *Places of memory: Whiteman's schools and Native American communities.* Mahwah, NJ: Erlbaum.

Philips, S. (1983). *The invisible culture: Communication in the classroom and on the Warm Springs Indian reservation.* New York: Longman.

Polacco, P. (1990). *Thunder cake.* New York: Putnam & Grosset.

Red Horse, J. (1988). Cultural evolution of American Indian families. In C. Jacobs & D. Bowles (Eds.), *Ethnicity and race: Critical concept in social work* (pp. 186–199). Silver Spring, MD: National Association of Social Workers.

Reeves, M. S. (1989, August 2). The high cost of endurance. *Education Week,* 2–4.

Reyhner, J. (1992). Policies toward American Indian languages: A historical sketch. In J. Crawford (Ed.), *Language loyalties: A source book on the official English controversy* (pp. 41–47). Chicago: University of Chicago Press.

Reyhner, J., & Tennant, E. (1995). Maintaining and renewing native languages. *The Bilingual Research Journal, 19*(2), 279–304.

Sarris, G. (1993). *Keeping slug woman alive: A holistic approach to American Indian texts.* Berkeley, CA: University of California Press.

Saville-Troike, M. (1989). *The ethnography of communication* (2nd ed.). New York: Basil Blackwell.

Scollon, R., & Scollon, S. B. (1980). *Interethnic communication.* Fairbanks, AK: Alaska Native Language Center.

Scollon, R., & Scollon, S. (1990). Cultural communication and intercultural contact. In Carbaugh, D. (Ed.), *Intercultural Communication* (pp. 259–286). Hillsdale, NJ: Lawrence Erlbaum Assoc., Inc.

Scollon, R., & Scollon, S. (1981). *Narrative, literacy and face in interethnic communication.* Norwood, NJ: Ablex.

Sharan, S. (1984). *Cooperative learning in the classroom: Research in desegregated schools.* Hillsdale, NJ: Erlbaum.

Sherman, J. (1996). *Trickster tales: Forty folk tales from around the world.* Little Rock, AR: August House Publishers.

Silko, L. (1992). *Almanac of the dead.* New York: Penguin Books.

Silver, S., & Miller, W. R. (1997). *American Indian languages: Cultural and social contexts.* Tucson, AZ: University of Arizona Press.

Simons-Ailes, S., & Valencia, E. (1983). *The growing path: Traditional infant activities for Indian children.* Albuquerque, NM: Southwest Communication Resources.

Slapin, B., & Seale, D. (1992). *Through Indian eyes: The native experience in books for children.* Philadelphia: New Society Publishers.

Slavin, R. E. (1990). *Cooperative learning: Theory, research, and practice.* Englewood Cliffs, NJ: Prentice-Hall.

Sofaer, A., & Ihde, A. (1983). *The sun dagger.* Bethesda, MD: Atlas Video.

Stewart, J. (1986). Hearing disorders among the indigenous peoples of North America and the Pacific Basin. In O. Taylor (Ed.), *Nature of communication disorders in culturally and linguistically diverse populations* (pp. 237–239). San Diego: College-Hill Press.

St. Germaine, R. (1995). *Drop-out rates among American Indian and Alaska Native students: Beyond cultural discontinuity.* ERIC Clearinghouse on Rural and Small Schools. (ERIC Document Reproduction Service No. ED 388 492).

Stolz, M. (1988). *Storm in the night.* New York: HarperCollins.

Suina, J., & Smolkin, L. (1994). From natal culture to school culture to dominant society culture: Supporting transitions for Pueblo Indian children. In P. M. Greenfield & R. R. Cocking (Eds.), *Cross-cultural roots of minority child development.* Hillsdale, NJ: Erlbaum.

Sutton, M. Q. (2000). *An introduction to Native North America.* Boston: Allyn & Bacon.

Tapahanso, L. (1999). *Songs of Shiprock fair.* Walnut, CA: Kiva Publishing.

Tharp, R. (1994). Research knowledge and policy issues in cultural diversity and education. In B. McLeod (Ed.), *Language and learning: Educating linguistically diverse students.* Albany, NY: State University of New York.

Tharp, R. G., & Gallimore, R. (1988). *Rousing minds to life.* Cambridge, MA: Cambridge University Press.

Tijerina, K. H., & Biemer, P. P. (1987–1988). The dance of Indian higher education: One step forward, two steps back. *Educational Record, 68*(4), 86–93.

Todd, N. W., & Bowerman, C. A. (1985). Otitis media in Canyon Day, Ariz., a 16-year follow-up in Apache Indians. *Archives of Otolaryngology, 111,* 606–608.

Triandis, H. C. (1995). *Individualism and collectivism.* Boulder, CO: Westview Press.

Two Two, R. (1999). The wind picks up. In L. Francis (Ed.) *When the Rain Sings.* New York: Simon & Schuster.

Ukrainetz, T., Harpell, S., Walsh, C., & Coyle, C. (2000). A preliminary investigation of dynamic assessment with Native American kindergartners. *Language, Speech, and Hearing Services in Schools, 31,* 142–154.

United States Bureau of the Census. (1999). *Statistical abstract of the United States* (119th ed.). Washington, DC: United States Department of Commerce.

Uzdawinis, D. C. (1982). *Let's talk: Screening instrument for Native American children.* Albuquerque, NM: All Indian Pueblo Council, Inc.

Valiquette, H. P. (1990). *A study for the lexicon of Laguna Keresan.* Albuquerque, NM: University of New Mexico.

Vining, C. B. (2000). *Navajo sociocultural perspective of developmental disability.* Albuquerque, NM: University of New Mexico Center for Development and Disability.

Vining, C. B., & Allison, S. R. (2000). *Navajo perceptions of developmental disabilities: Project Nanitin institute manual.* Albuquerque, NM: University of New Mexico.

Weeks, T. (1975). The speech of Indian Children: Paralinguistic and registral aspects of the Yakima Dialect. Paper presented at the Annual Meeting of the National Council of Teachers of English, San Diego.

Westby, C. E., & Roman, R. (1995). Finding the balance: Learning to live in two worlds. *Topics in Language Disorders, 15,* 68–88.

Westby, C. E., & Valesquez, D. (2000). Developing scientific literacy: A sociocultural approach. *RASE, 21,* 101–110.

White, S., Tharp, R. G., Jordan, C., & Vogt, L. (1989). Cultural patterns of cognition reflected in the questioning styles of Anglo and Navajo teachers. In D. M. Topping, D. C. Crowell, & V. N. Kobayashi (Eds.), *Thinking across cultures.* Hillsdale, NJ: Erlbaum.

Wiet, R. J., DeBlanc, G. B., Stewart, J., & Weider, D. J. (1980) Natural history of otitis media in the American native. *Annals of Otology, Rhinology, & Laryngology Supplement, 89*(3), 14–19.

Wolcott, H. F. (1987). The teacher as an enemy. In G. D. Spindler (Eds.), *Educational cultural process: Anthropological approaches* (2nd ed.). Prospect Heights, IL: Waveland Press.

Wolfram, W. (1984). Unmarked tense in American Indian English. *American Speech, 59*(1), 31–50.

Wolfram, W. (1991). *Dialects and American English.* Englewood Cliffs, NJ: Prentice-Hall.

Wolfram, W. (2000). *Indian by birth: The Lumbee dialect.* Raleigh, NC: North Carolina State University.

Yates, A. (1987). Current status and future directions of research on the American Indian child. *American Journal of Psychiatry, 44,* 1135–1142.

Additional Resources

Websites

Center for American Indian Research and Education: http://www.caire.org.

Index of Native American Resources on the Internet: http://www.hanksville.org/NAresources/.

Native Health Research Database: http://hsc.unm.edu/nhrd/index.html.
National Center for American Indian and Alaska Native Mental Health: http://www.uchsc.edu/sm/ncaianmhr.

Books

Cajete, G. (1999). *Igniting the sparkle: An indigenous science education model.* Skyland, NC: Kivaki Press.

Cleary, L. M., & Peacock, T. D. (1998). *Collected wisdom: American Indian education.* Boston: Allyn & Bacon.

Hirschfelder, A., Fairbanks, P., & Wakim, Y. (1999). *American Indian stereotypes in the world of children.* Lanham, MD: The Scarecrow Press.

Reyhner, J. (1992). *Teaching American Indian students.* Norman, OK: University of Oklahoma Press.

Slapin, B., & Seale, D. (1998). *Through Indian eyes: The Native experience in books for children.* Los Angeles: American Indian Studies Center.

Sutton, M.Q. (2000). *An introduction to Native North America.* Boston: Allyn & Bacon.

□ □ □
□ □ □
□ □ □

Appendix 5-1

Guidelines for Selecting Native American Books for Children

1. In ABC books, is "E" for "Eskimo" or "I" for "Indian"?
2. In counting books, are "Indians" counted?
3. Are children shown "playing Indian"?
4. Are animals dressed as "Indians"?
5. Do "Indians" have names like "Indian Two Feet" or "Little Chief"?

Inappropriate Presentations	*Appropriate Presentations*
• Native peoples are portrayed as savages or primitive people who are extinct. • Native cultures are oversimplified and generalized. Native people are all one color, one style. • The art is a mishmash of "generic Indian" designs (e.g., Plains facial features, Navajo dress). • There are insulting overtones to the language in the book. Racist adjectives are used to refer to Indian peoples. • There is manipulation of words like "victory," "conquest," or "massacre" to justify Euro-American conquest of the Native homelands. Native actions are presented as being responsible for their own "disappearance." The U.S. government is only "Trying to help." • The story encourages children to believe that Native peoples accepted defeats passively.	• Native peoples are shown as human beings, members of highly defined and complex societies. • Native cultures are presented as separate from each other, with each culture, language, religion, and dress unique. • Attention is paid to accurate, appropriate design and color; and clothes, dress, houses are drawn with careful attention to detail. • The language is respectful. • History is put in the proper perspective: the Native struggle for self-determination and sovereignty against the Euro-American drive for conquest. • The story shows the ways in which Native peoples actively resisted the invaders.

Inappropriate Presentations	Appropriate Presentations
• Native heroes are only the people who are believed to have aided Europeans in the conquest of their own people. • Native peoples are discussed in the past tense only, supporting the "vanished Indian" myth. The past is unconnected to the present.	• Native heroes are those who are admired because of what they have done for their own people. • The continuity of cultures is represented, with values, religions, and morals, as an outgrowth of the past and connected to the present.

Source: Adapted from information in Hirschfelder, A., Molin, P. F., & Wakim, Y. (1999). *American Indian stereotypes in the world of children.* Langham, MD: The Scarecrow Press; and Slain, B., & Seals, D. (1992). *Through Indian eyes: The native experience in books for children.* Philadelphia: New Society Publishers.

6

□ □ □
□ □ □
□ □ □

Latino Culture

Aquiles Iglesias

Over the last two decades, our service delivery system has focused on ensuring that service providers are sensitive to the needs of our ever-growing culturally and linguistically diverse population. Although a first step, the provision of appropriate services requires service providers to go beyond this level and shift from cultural sensitivity to cultural competence—a skill-based paradigm that focuses on equal access, equal usage patterns, and outcome-based quality indicators. To a large extent, service providers' present level of cultural competence with respect to cultural-linguistic minority populations has been limited, primarily to improving language access: the ability of the provider to speak with the patient in their primary language. Language is an important issue, but so is the sociocultural environment of our patients.

This chapter focuses on one segment of our population—Latinos—and is intended to provide an understanding of the sociocultural environment that has the potential of impacting our service delivery to this population. The provision of services that are responsive to Latinos requires an understanding of the demographic characteristics of the population, as well as their history, past experiences, cultural beliefs, and cultural norms. Furthermore, it requires an examination of how each of these variables, independently and collectively, guide us to what to do and how we do it to ensure quality of services. As culturally competent service providers, we must use these newly acquired skills and foster and promote a service delivery system that meets the patients in their own ground instead of forcing them to conform to a system developed for the mainstream segment of our population.

Before discussing the sociocultural context, it is important to discuss two terms often used interchangeably: *Hispanics* and *Latinos*. The term *Hispanic* was chosen by the U.S. government as a convenient, inoffensive label that applied to all people who trace their descent from Spanish-speaking countries. The term has no historical link to the people it describes and is considered by some to be a somewhat colonial term, reflecting Spain's conquest of the Americas and subjugation and annihilation of native people. In addition, the term does not reflect the native people of the Americas or the numerous diverse groups who voluntarily or involuntarily immigrated to Latin America. The less colonial term *Latino* is presently emerging, is used interchangeably with the term *Hispanic* in all U.S. publications beginning in 2003, and is used throughout this chapter.

In the last 30 years, Latinos have received a great deal of attention and have become part of the national consciousness for several reasons. One reason is the rapid increase in the size of the Latino population and projected growth as the largest cultural-linguistic minority group in the near future as a result of high levels of immigration coupled with a large representation of young people and high fertility rates. As America's fastest growing ethnic group (61% between 1970 and 1980 and 53% between 1980 and 1990), Latinos represent a major force in the U.S. economy, politics, and culture. However, it is their strong support for bilingualism and their large immigration that has raised the most attention.

Latinos are not a homogeneous group. They share a common past and a strong ethnic solidarity based on their support for cultural and linguistic maintenance. Nevertheless, beyond these areas of commonality, the subgroups differ significantly in many ways. Major historical, cultural, and demographic differences exist among the groups. As we examine the similarities and differences across groups, it is important to note that membership in a group or a subgroup does not determine behavior but makes certain types of behaviors more probable. Thus, the information provided should be seen as general trends in the Latino subpopulations and not reflective of any one of its members. After all, each family carries their unique genetic makeup and has their own history, past experiences, and beliefs.

Latinos in the United States

The Latino population in the United States, excluding the Commonwealth of Puerto Rico, is estimated to be 31.7 million or 11.7% of the total population. Adding the 3.8 million Latinos living in Puerto Rico would increase this number to 35.5 million. The substantiated undercounting of minority populations by the U.S. Bureau of the Census makes the real number much higher (Population Reference Bureau, 1999). Two-thirds of mainland Latinos (65.2%) are of Mexican descent, whereas individuals of Puerto Rican and Cuban descent accounted for 9.6% and 4.3%, respectively. Central, South

American, and "Other Hispanics" accounted for 20.6%. Latinos are highly concentrated in the Southwest, with five southwestern states (i.e., California, Arizona, New Mexico, Colorado, and Texas) being home to 61% of U.S. Latinos. More than half of the Latino population lives in the states of California and Texas. Outside of the Southwest, the largest concentration of Latinos resides in the states of New York and Florida, 9% and 7%, respectively. More than 80% of Mexican Americans live in the Southwest, 66% of Puerto Ricans are in the northeast, and two-thirds of Cubans live in Florida.

It is estimated that the size of the Latino population will represent one-fourth of the U.S. population, approximately 81 million Latinos, by the year 2050. During the last decade, the growth of the Latino population was shared by all states, including the District of Columbia. The largest numeric increase was experienced by the states of California (2.8 million), Texas (1.7 million), Florida (760,000), New York (447,000), Arizona (372,000), New Jersey (280,000), Nevada (180,000), Colorado (179,000), and Washington (162,000). The percentage of growth, however, reflects the trend of Latinos to move into areas with low Latino concentration. In the last decade, the highest percentage of growth of Latinos has been in the states of Arkansas (170%), Nevada (144%), North Carolina (129%), Georgia (119%), Nebraska (108%), and Tennessee (104%). This trend is also reflected at the county level, in which the largest numeric change occurred in communities with a large Latino population (Los Angeles, Miami-Dade, Houston, Phoenix, Chicago, San Diego, and San Antonio), but the highest percentage rate increase occurred in counties with a small population base in the states of Arkansas (Benton), Georgia (Forsyth, Paulding, Henry, and Coweta), and Illinois (Jefferson and Christian).

Migration and Settlement Patterns

Migration and settlement patterns of Latinos have been influenced by socioeconomic and political conditions in Latin American countries, as well as socioeconomic and political conditions within the United States. The socioeconomic and political conditions of their home countries provide us an understanding of the situations that precipitated the migration. They also provide information on potential areas in which these individuals might encounter difficulties in adjusting to new surroundings. For example, the psychology literature clearly suggests that many individuals who are uprooted owing to migration experience higher levels of stress; the degree of stress varies with the degree of conflict the immigrant has experienced (Harwood, 1994; Portes & Rumbaut, 1993). The reception that these individuals receive in the new host country will also affect their life trajecto-

ries and well-being. Issues such as legal context of entry, kinship and community support, and opportunities to interact with other subpopulations
will impact how they will perform in our society. Although closely inter-
twined, their success or failure will be determined more by the social, economic, political, and educational circumstances in this country rather than
those in their country of origin.

Although U.S. consciousness might be now heightened, the presence of
Latinos in what is now the mainland United States has a long history. By the
time St. Augustine—that is, the first permanent European settlement in the
North American continent—was established by Spaniards in 1565, a thriving
community had been developed in Puerto Rico for 57 years. Spaniards had
established colonies in the Carolinas, explored the Chesapeake Bay and areas
that were later to become California, Colorado, Georgia, Kansas, Louisiana,
Mississippi, New Mexico, Tennessee, and Texas. Not until 1607, 42 years
later, did the first permanent English colony in the New World appear in
Jamestown, Virginia. Eleven years before the Pilgrims landed on Plymouth
Rock, Latinos had settled Santa Fe, New Mexico. The Spaniards tended to settle in the southern portion of the North American continent, as well as in
Central and South America. The Northern region of North America (later to
become Canada) was originally occupied by the French. Groups from nations
who spoke different languages settled the land in between, with the British
becoming the dominant nationality and English the dominant language. By
1763, the British had expanded their control over most of Franco-America.
Strong Latino communities flourished in the West and Southwest before and
after they became part of the United States.

Many Latinos are long-established citizens who have lived in the United
States for generations. The vast majority is the product of one of the most
important immigration streams of the second half of the twentieth century.
Before 1950, most of the new immigrants came from Europe. In the 1950s, 20%
of new immigrants were from Latin America. Presently, 52% of immigrants are
from Spanish-speaking countries, with approximately 25% of the immigrants
arriving in the United States being from Mexico. Thirty-five percent of Latinos
were born outside of the continental United States, with approximately 50% of
the foreign-born Latinos coming into the United States in the last two decades.
Immigration accounted for two-fifths of the growth of Latinos in the 1990s. At
least half of the people who become immigrants each year are already living in
the United States under temporary visa or some other legal status or as undocumented aliens. The largest entry is of relatives of U.S. residents.

Although the size of the immigration is high, it is important to note that
the flow has always been there, although not necessarily in the numbers and
definitely not documented by Census data, which began to count Latinos as a

group in the 1970 Census (Mexicans counted in the 1930 Census; Spanish surname in 1950 and 1960; Mexican, Puerto Rican, Cuban, and Other Hispanic in 1970 and 1980; 30 Hispanic groups in 1990). Unless major restrictive immigration policies are implemented, it is predicted that the brisk rate of growth of the Latino population is likely to be sustained by immigration.

Immigration has been primarily owing to economic and political reasons. At times, some immigrants have been received with opened arms. In times of economic decline in this country, their reception has been less positive. Some of the immigration has been legal and some has not. Although individuals from all Latin American countries are represented in the United States, the sheer numbers of three groups—Mexicans, Puerto Ricans, and Cubans—deserve special consideration. This is not to say that the other groups are less important; in some communities, these subgroups constitute the largest Latino population.

Mexicans

Mexican migration to what is presently the United States must be viewed from an historical perspective, because Mexico's original northern frontier became part of the United States through war and purchase. The independence of Texas from Mexico in 1836, its subsequent admission to the Union in 1845, the Treaty of Guadalupe Hidalgo in 1848, and the Gadsden Purchase of 1854 provided the residents of these areas U.S. citizenship. The Mexican Revolution (1910–1921) encouraged thousands of Mexicans to emigrate across the border into the United States. From 1942 to 1962, a highly defined migration stream—the pattern of which has continued despite its termination—was created. The two countries established the Bracero program, which brought more than 4.5 million Mexican farm workers to the United States. During periods of economic prosperity and war, a welcoming environment has existed. However, during periods of economic downturn such as the Great Depression, the environment has been hostile, and incidences of massive repatriation have occurred.

Puerto Ricans

Puerto Rico became a possession of the United States in 1899 after the Spanish American War. The Jones Act of 1917 granted Puerto Ricans U.S. citizenship. It was not until 1947 that Puerto Ricans were able to elect their first Puerto Rican governor. In 1952, Puerto Ricans voted to create the Commonwealth of Puerto Rico, giving the island government control of internal matters. External matters such as commerce and foreign policy became the responsibility of the United States. Considerable disagreement still exists among Puerto Ricans as to whether they should pursue independence, maintain their commonwealth status, or seek U.S. statehood.

Puerto Ricans who migrate to the United States are not immigrants but U.S. citizens who move from one part of the country to another. Before 1940, Puerto Ricans did not immigrate to the mainland in large numbers, although there was a sizeable presence in New York City. However, after World War II, migration to the mainland has been constant, although this migration has been circular, with many Puerto Ricans returning to the island after spending time on the mainland. Most of the early migration was to the East Coast of the United States, where agricultural and manufacturing jobs were available. Increasing numbers of Puerto Ricans have settled in Illinois and California.

Cubans

Before 1959, the number of Cubans who migrated to the United States was relatively small, although a notable presence existed in New York City, New Orleans, Key West, and Ybor City. These last two cities in Florida were major centers for Cuba's independence from Spain in 1902. By 1959, approximately 40,000 Cubans lived in the United States. Since the Cuban Revolution in 1959, the pattern of immigration has reflected the availability of the means to leave Cuba. From 1959 to 1962, the first major wave of Cubans, approximately 200,000, immigrated to Florida using the regular commercial air traffic available. After a 2-year hiatus in which no flights were available directly to the U.S. mainland, flights were resumed until 1973, and a second wave of approximately 260,000 Cubans entered the country. After a 7-year period of slow immigration due to cancellation of flights between the two countries, a third major wave occurred as a result of the Mariel boat lift in which approximately 125,000 new refugees entered the country. Although Miami is the hub of the Cuban community in the United States, with approximately half of the Cuban population in the United States, well-established communities exist in Union City, New York City, and Los Angeles.

Other Latinos

In addition to Mexican Americans, Puerto Ricans, and Cuban Americans, the Latino population in the United States consists of Central and South Americans. Although collectively they represent 20% of the Latino population, the presence of individual subgroups is often overlooked because of the relative size of the population and their concentration in limited areas of the country. Approximately 43% of Central Americans are Salvadorans, 20% are Guatemalan, and 15% are Nicaraguans. Colombians are the largest group of South Americans (37%), followed by Ecuadorians (19%) and Peruvians (17%).

Before 1960, migration of Central and South Americans varied from decade to decade, reflecting U.S. demand for labor during World War I and subsequent legislative restrictions to immigration during the 1930s. The largest migrations of Central and South Americans have occurred since the 1970s, reflecting political or economic upheaval in the country of origin and ease of transportation. These migrations have been characterized by waves in which the richest and most highly educated segment of the population migrates first, followed by less educated and poorer waves of immigrants. In the case of Nicaraguans, the first wave consisted of those close to the Somoza government; the second wave was triggered when the Nicaraguan government was reorganized; and, finally, a third wave triggered by the fighting between Sandinistas and the U.S.-supported Contras. The Sandinista Revolution brought the largest wave of Nicaraguans to the United States during the 1980s, with immigrants concentrating in the city of Sweetwater, Florida (16 miles from Miami), and creating smaller communities in large urban centers such as Los Angeles and San Francisco. The Salvadoran experience is similar. The military coup of 1979 gave rise to a civil war in which thousands were killed and hundred of thousands were displaced. In the 1980s, an estimated 214,000 legal immigrants entered the United States, and an estimated 300,000–500,000 crossed the border illegally. The largest concentrations of Salvadorans are in the Pico-Union district of Los Angeles and the Adams Morgan and Mount Pleasant district of Washington, DC. U.S. military interventionist policies and shifting federal policies toward the conflicts in these two countries has resulted in great uncertainty as to the extent to which these new immigrants are refugees or immigrants seeking better economic opportunities.

The experiences individuals have as a result of their migration are unique, regardless of the condition that prompted their migration. Individuals have entered this country with different social, economic, and educational capital. The social and economic resources of the communities into which they have entered have also varied. For some, the migration has placed them in a path for success. For others, the circumstances have been less positive. As service providers, it is important that we are mindful of the struggles individuals have encountered and attempt to understand that an individual's life trajectory is greatly influenced by events in their lives. The extent to which an individual can overcome negative events or maximize positive ones will be greatly determined by the social, economic, and educational resources the individual possesses and the extent to which they are maximized and developed in their host communities.

Demographic Characteristics of the Population

To understand the Latino population, one must take into account, with caution, a series of interrelated demographic characteristics of the population; these characteristics should be considered simultaneously, because they influence and are influenced by each other. The data are, like many statistics, a static representation of the population average and do not reflect the fact that individuals may be in different life trajectories. The population mean on any particular measure only provides a general tendency of the population sampled and does not capture the general direction in which the population is changing or the rate at which this change will occur. Furthermore, neither the average nor the average movement direction can be assumed for any one member of the population. To illustrate this point, let us consider Figure 6-1, a sample population with a mean score of 1.7 on variable X. Individuals A and B are at the high end of variable X, whereas individuals C and D are at the lower end. The average of the total population does not reflect the values of A, B, C, or D. In some cases, it overestimates and in others it underestimates. As can be further seen in Figure 6-1, individuals B and C are in life trajectories, indicated by direction of arrows, which will result in higher numbers on variable X, whereas individuals A and D are in life trajectories that will result in no change. Let us hypothetically assume for a moment that variable X reflects the number of children born to individ-

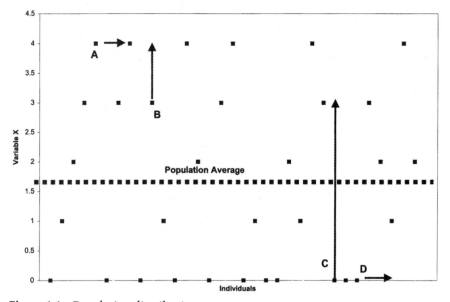

Figure 6-1 Population distribution.

uals in a particular group. The population average at this point in time does not quite reflect any of the four individuals and tells us nothing about what will happen once these individuals complete their life trajectory. If we only know the mean score of the population, then information as to what trajectories specific members of this population will take is also not available. The mean score of the population only tells us that on average at a particular point in time, the population is behaving in a particular way. It is with this perspective that we should view the demographic data presented.

Race

Latinos are an ethnic group, not a racial group. Latinos can be of any race. Most classify themselves as white, a minority classify themselves as black, and an increasing number identify their race as "other." From the social perspective of Latinos, race is not a significant issue. The large number of interracial marriages and the lack of marginalization of racial groups in the country of ancestry contribute to this view. This does not mean, however, that once these individuals come to the United States they are not marginalized by our society because of their race or that the race of other non-Latino populations with whom Latinos come in contact is not an issue.

As noted by Salas-Provance (1996), although there has been much discussion denouncing race as a biologic category (American Anthropological Association, 2001; Cavalli-Sforza, 1995), differentiation by race can be used to assist medical professionals in making differential diagnosis. However, the large racial heterogeneity of the Latino population presents a challenge when attempting to use prevalence data of any physical problem reported to be highly associated with race. For example, the prevalence of cleft uvula has been determined to be 1 in 80 for whites, 1 in 350 for blacks, and 1 in 14 for Native Americans (Jaffe & DeBlanc, 1972; Schaumann, Peagler, & Gorlin, 1970). Within the Latino population, it would be impossible to determine the genetic predisposition for any inherited disease or condition, given the admixture of individuals of different racial groups. Some other genetically based disorders such as sickle-cell disease might be missed, because they tend to be associated with other racial or ethnic groups; in reality, they are highly prevalent in some Latino subpopulations.

Fertility and Age Distribution

The large growth of the Latino population is partially attributed to its high fertility rate. Not only are more Latino women (*Latinas*) having

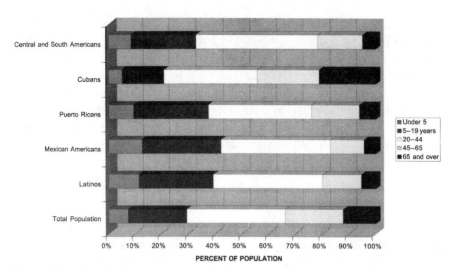

Figure 6-2   Population by age.

babies, but they are also having more babies than the general population. According to data from the National Center for Health Statistics (1999), the proportion of live births to Latinas has increased steadily from 14% in 1989 to more than 18% in 1997. In 1997, the total fertility rate of Latinas between the ages of 15 and 44 years was 102.8 per 1,000, as compared to 57.0 per 1,000 for non-Latino whites and 72.4 per 1,000 for non-Latino blacks.

Overall, the birth rate to teenage Latinas is 17% (National Center for Health Statistics, 1999). This rate varies across subgroups, with Puerto Ricans having the highest teenage birth rate (22.3 per 1,000) and Cubans having the lowest (7.4 per 1,000). These alarming statistics are significant, because teen childbearing has been associated with negative economic consequences for mother and child. Teen mothers are less likely to finish high school and to be employed. These consequences might reflect the economic conditions in which the mother lived before the birth of her child, rather than a consequence of her age.

One reason Latinos account for a disproportionate share of births is a function of the age distribution of the population. The Latino population is young, with nearly 70% being 35 years of age or younger. As can be seen in Figure 6-2, Latinos are overrepresented in the "under 5," "5 to 19," and "20 to 44" years categories and underrepresented in the older categories. The "graying" of America appears not to be occurring for the Latino segment of the population. As well attested in numerous school districts throughout the country, Latinos are increasingly becoming a large percent of the school-age population. Furthermore, the large numbers of Latinos in the childbearing years will likely increase the number of children in this age sector.

Language

More than 30 million Americans, 13.8% of the population, speak a language other than English, with more than half of these individuals speaking Spanish. Speaking Spanish is one of the major ties that binds the Latino population, and approximately three-fourths of the Latino population reportedly speaks it. The numbers of Latinos who speak Spanish, English, or both reflect the linguistic heterogeneity of the population. The vast majority of the Latino population considers themselves bilingual, and a small percentage is monolingual in English or Spanish. It is important to stress that the majority of Latinos are bilingual and self-report speaking English "very well." Only 21% of the Latino population report that they "do not speak English well" or "not at all." Variations across Latino subgroups exist, with Dominicans and Central Americans reporting the least amount of English proficiency. Among the three largest subgroups, Cubans are the group most likely to speak only Spanish and the least likely to speak only English.

The number of monolingual Spanish-speaking and English-Spanish bilinguals is not surprising, considering that 35% of the Latino population is foreign born and that the majority of foreign-born Latinos entered this country in the last three decades. Furthermore, the literature on language maintenance across generations (Hudson et al., 1995) suggests that the rate of language transmission from generation to generation is directly related to the extent to which the minority population is integrated into the mainstream culture. Native language loss (i.e., monolingualism in English for Latinos) could potentially be the cost of social and economic integration. The degree to which the historical pattern of language loss will occur in subsequent generations of Latinos is difficult to predict, given the constant influx of new Spanish-speaking immigrants, the strength of the Spanish media, and the strong tie between speaking Spanish and Latino identity.

The extent to which Latinos speak Spanish or English is not an isolated special interest fact but one that has educational and economic implications. It also has implications for our service delivery system. In California, for example, Latino enrollment is predicted to increase more than three times as fast as overall enrollment; the majority of Latino students come from non–English speaking backgrounds, and 80% of English learners are Spanish-speaking. The result will be a growing number of English learners in California's schools (California Department of Education, 2000). Consistent with the Regulations of the 1997 Amendments to Individuals with Disabilities Education Act of 1999 (IDEA, PL 105-17) (Individuals with Disabilities Education Act, 1999), tests and other evaluation materials used to assess a child must be selected and administered so as not to be discriminatory on a racial and cultural basis and are provided and administered in the child's native

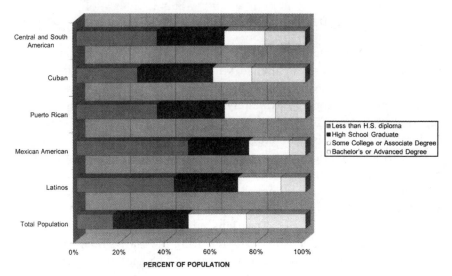

Figure 6-3 Educational attainment.

language, unless it is clearly not feasible to do so. As service providers, we must be mindful of any activity that would deny meaningful access and participation on the basis of language. Denial of access to any agencies' programs or activities could be considered as discrimination on the basis of national origin and a violation of Title VI of the Civil Rights Act of 1964.

Educational Attainment

The level of educational attainment of Latinos differs significantly from that of the total U.S. population (Figure 6-3). Although 15.9% of the total U.S. population has less than a high school diploma (11.6% for non-Latino whites), 43.0% of Latinos do not have a high school diploma. Latinos are also underrepresented at the "bachelor's or advanced degree" level, 10.6% for Latinos, 25.6% for the total population, and 28.1% for the non-Latino whites. Discrepancies can also be seen across Latino subgroups, with Mexicans being overrepresented in the "less than high school diploma" category. Although disturbing, these figures do not capture the educational disparity that presently exists among groups or the factors that contribute to the disparity. To capture the root of the disparity, we must look at the profile of children in our schools and identify factors that make many of the Latino children "at risk" for academic failure and limit their ability to proceed in the educational pipeline.

In 1990, there were approximately 55 million school-age children, of which 12% were Latinos. Although one-third of 3- and 4-year-olds were enrolled in pre-kindergarten, only one in five Latino children attended pre-kindergarten. Pre-kindergarten attendance was influenced by parental education, mother's age, family mobility, language, and income. The lower the parental education, the younger the mother, and the greater the family's mobility, the less probable that children would be enrolled. English-speaking ability of the parent in the household or the household's linguistic isolation also affected participation. Children whose family spoke "little or no" English were less likely to be enrolled in pre-kindergarten than those whose mother spoke English "very well" (National Center for Education Statistics, 1996b). The data on income and pre-kindergarten attendance shows that at all income levels, Latinos tended to underenroll their children in pre-kindergarten.

Enrollment rate data at all the elementary and high school levels further indicate that these same variables (i.e., parental education, mother's age, family mobility, language, and income) substantially impact the extent to which Latino children, especially teenagers, will participate and continue their education. When one compares enrollment across racial or ethnic groups, Latinos ages 14–19 years were less likely to be enrolled than any other group, reflecting the high dropout rate of Latinos. Teenagers in linguistically isolated households were less likely to be enrolled than teenagers in households in which English was spoken as a matter of course (National Center for Education Statistics, 1996a). This high dropout rate is significant, because teens who drop out of high school are three times as likely to live in poverty than those who complete high school (National Center for Education Statistics, 1996a). Latinos who attended school were likely to attend schools that were disproportionately poor, predominantly minority, underfunded, and underachieving (National Center for Education Statistics, 1996a). Thus, it is not surprising that 60% of Latino fourth graders read below the basic level (National Center for Education Statistics, 1999).

As noted previously, the above data should be viewed with caution. The data represent the conditions at one particular point in time and do not capture the positive trends that have been occurring over the last few decades; the rate of Latinos that complete high school and the rate of those who attend college have almost doubled (Freund, 1991). It is also important to remember that as new immigrants enter the system, averages of aggregate data may remain constant, but individuals who have been in the system for a while might be demonstrating positive trajectories.

Workforce, Earnings, and Poverty

The data on labor force participation indicate that Latinos participate in the labor force at a rate similar to that of non-Latino whites (67%

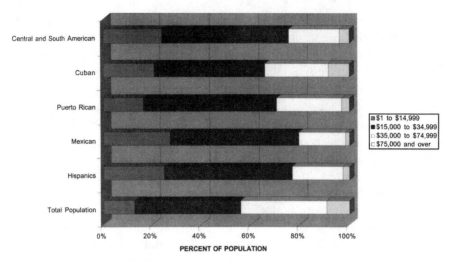

Figure 6-4   Earnings of full-time workers.

and 61%, respectively). However, the percent of unemployed individuals is significantly different across Latino subgroups. The unemployment rate of Latinos (6.7%) is almost twice that of non-Latino whites. It is also important to consider that Latinos are overrepresented in low-paying jobs (e.g., farming, laborers, manufacturing). Fifty-five percent of Latino men and 20.3% of Latinas are employed in low-paying jobs as compared to 40.9% and 9.9%, respectively, for non-Latino white men and women. Not surprising, the median family income of Latinos is 30% lower than for all Americans. Of all of the Latino groups, Dominicans had the lowest median income. As can be seen in Figure 6-4, Latinos were overrepresented in the lowest income brackets (76.5% make less than the average median income for the U.S. population). Furthermore, differences across the Latino groups are seen at the lower and upper end of the earning levels, with Mexican Americans having a disproportionate number of individuals in the "$1 to $14,999" level and Cubans having a relatively disproportionate number of individuals in the "$75,000 and over" level.

Based on 1999 income figures, Latinos were almost three times as likely as non-Latino whites to be living below the poverty level (22.8% as compared to 7.7%). The poverty rate ranged from 25.8% among Puerto Ricans to 17.3% among Cubans. Greatest discrepancies are seen across groups when one looks at poverty rates in children under the age of 18 years and the elderly. In 1999, 30.3% of Latino children lived below the poverty level, as compared to 9.4% for non-Latino white children. Noticeable differences exist across the various Latino groups, with 37.2% of Puerto Rican children living below the poverty level. Almost three times as many elderly Latinos (65 years of age and older) lived in poverty than non-Latino white elderly, 20.4% and 7.6%, respectively.

The issue of poverty cannot be ignored, because poverty has a confounding effect on many other variables such as health risk, access to health care, and academic achievement. At the same time, it is important to realize that increasing economic capital (e.g., increasing minimum wage) might decrease the gap in buying power of a group but does necessarily change many of the sociocultural conditions associated with poverty.

Health Indicators of the Latino Population

Although Latinos experience many of the same health problems as the rest of the population, striking disparities exist between the health status of Latinos and other racial and ethnic groups in the United States. Many Latinos face tremendous social, economic, and cultural barriers to achieving optimal health. The elimination of the disparity among major groups is one of the major goals of *Healthy People 2010* (U.S. Department of Health and Human Services, 2000). The disparities in health status are the result of an array of factors and exist not only across major racial and ethnic groups but also among the different Latino subgroups. Although genetic predisposition for specific conditions is a possible cause for some of the disparity, sociocultural factors appear to have a major impact and provide an explanation as to why Latinos consistently perform better in some indicators while typically doing worse in others. It is important to look at these sociocultural factors, because they are alterable and intervention can ameliorate the condition.

Healthy development begins in the prenatal period, with prenatal care providing the fetus a healthy environment. Prenatal care and smoking during pregnancy are two factors that can affect the health status of infants (Mathews, 1998). As a group, Latinas in the United States are less likely to seek early prenatal care than non-Latino white women, 73.7% and 87.9%, respectively. Among Latinas, Mexican American women reportedly had the lowest rate (72.1%) of first trimester care. The rate for Cuban women (90.4%) was higher than that of white non-Latinos, contributing to a higher overall percent for all Latinos. The rate of early prenatal care among Latinas increased during the 1990s, from 59.5% in 1989 to its present level of 73.7% (National Center for Health Statistics, 1997). Preventable birth defects, such as the documented elevated rates of neural tube defects among Latino infants, could be greatly reduced with greater prenatal care. The work of Byrd et al. (1996) suggests that when Latinas

perceive more benefit of prenatal care and when barriers such as long waiting times at the clinic, embarrassment of the physical examination due to
male physician, and lack of transportation were reduced, Latinas partici-
pated more in prenatal care. Smoking during pregnancy has been associated with adverse outcomes such as intrauterine growth retardation, low
birth weight, and infant mortality. Latinas are less likely to smoke (13.7%
as compared to 23.9% for white non-Latinas) and to smoke less on a daily
basis. Foreign-born Latinas have a much lower rate of smoking than U.S.-
born Latinas. Of the major racial and ethnic groups, Latinas have the lowest rate of smoking during pregnancy (4% as compared to 16% for white
non-Latinas). Although no data are available for individual subgroups of
pregnant Latinas, data on Latino subgroups indicate that cigarette smoking varies across subgroups, with approximately one-third (33.7%) of
Puerto Ricans reporting to be current cigarette smokers, compared to
23.6% of Cuban Americans and 25.4% of Mexican Americans (National
Institute of Health, 1995).

Low birth weight is a contributing factor to infant mortality and a risk
for poorer developmental outcome for survivors (Mathews, Curtin, & Mac-
Dorman, 2000). As a group, Latinos tend to fare better than non-Latino
whites. As indicated in Figure 6-5, the birth weight of Latino children is similar to that of the white non-Latino population and much lower than that of

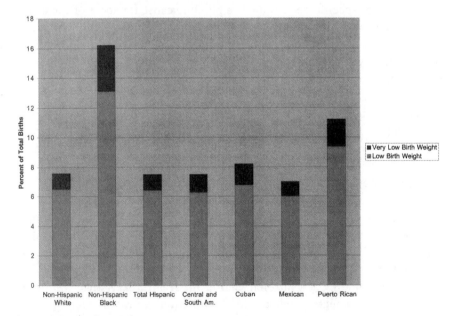

Figure 6-5 Birth weight.

non-Latino blacks. However, within the Latino groups, the Puerto Ricans have a higher percentage of children born in the "low birth weight" and "very low birth weight" categories. Infant mortality of Latinos (6.1 per 1,000) is slightly higher than that of the white non-Latino population (6.0 per 1,000). However, among Latinos, the infant mortality rate is highest for the Puerto Ricans (8.6 per 1,000) and lowest for the Cubans (5.1 per 1,000). In addition, infants born to U.S.-born Latinas were more likely to die before their first year than infants born to foreign-born Latinas. This discrepancy might suggest that as Latinas become more acculturated, they adopt U.S health behaviors that might have harmful health consequences (National Institute of Health, 1998; Palinkas et al., 1993) and birth outcomes might worsen (Mendoza et al., 1991; Scribner & Dwyer, 1989).

Although less documented, the Latino population is particularly vulnerable to environmental risk factors that impact their health. More Latinos live in areas that fail to meet the National Ambient Quality Standards; 80% of Latinos live in an area failing to meet one U.S. Environmental Protection Agency air quality standard, compared to 65% of black non-Latinos and 57% of white non-Latinos (Wernette & Nieves, 1992). Latino children under the age of 11 suffer from more active cases of asthma than do black non-Latinos and white non-Latinos; with asthma, rates are 11.2% for Puerto Ricans, 5.2% for Cuban Americans, 2.7% for Mexican Americans, 5.9% for black non-Latinos, and 3.3% for white non-Latinos. Latinos are more than twice as likely as non-Latino blacks or whites to live in areas with high levels of lead—18.5% of Latinos, 9.2% of black non-Latinos, and 6% of white non-Latinos. Farm workers are the largest group affected by pesticide poisonings, and Latinos comprise approximately 82% of the farm worker workforce.

Overall, Latinos experience many socioeconomic and demographic risk factors that should result in health outcomes to be substantially poorer. However, for some health indicators, they are doing better than other groups, and their health status should be the national benchmark. For example, Latinas have lower death rates from heart disease (64.7%) than do white non-Latinas, but they have the highest lifetime prevalence of depression (24%) of all women; nearly twice as many Latinas reported being depressed (11%) as African American women (6%) and white non-Latinas (5%). Latinas have the second highest mortality rate from acquired immunodeficiency syndrome (6.7 per 100,000). They are at least 2.5 times more likely to die from human immunodeficiency virus or acquired immunodeficiency syndrome than are white non-Latinas (National Institutes of Health, 1998). The renewed national focus on health disparities among underserved populations will provide us an opportunity to further explore the biologic, economic, and educational factors that interact to produce discrepancies among major racial and ethnic groups and among Latino groups, as well as the protective factors that buffer the effects of these factors.

Parity in Access and Use of the Health System

Access and use of adequate health services are crucial to providing a healthy environment for Latinos. Discrepancies in access and use have been attributed to factors such as socioeconomic status, insurance coverage, type and availability of health care services, culture, and language. As service providers, it is our responsibility to ensure that barriers that prevent equal access and use are eliminated and that initiatives to address financial and nonfinancial barriers are implemented. To accomplish this effort, we must understand the potential barriers and examine successful strategies that can be used to eliminate them.

Poverty, minority status, and absence of insurance exert independent effects on access and use of primary care (Newacheck, Hughes, & Stoddard, 1996). Patients who are poor, members of a minority group, or uninsured are more likely to lack consistent sources of care, nearly twice as likely to wait 60 minutes or more at their sites of care and use only approximately half as many physician services after adjusting for health status. Children living in very high poverty neighborhoods and those whose parent(s) have less than a high school education are the most likely group to be uninsured (17% and 19.7%, respectively) (Annie E. Casey Foundation, 2000; Newacheck, Hughes, & Stoddard, 1996).

A disproportionate number of Latinos (21%) are uninsured or rely on public, rather than private, health insurance. This is important, because the uninsured and those who rely on public health insurance are the ones most likely to lack a usual source of care, and having a consistent source of care is highly associated with a greater likelihood of seeing a physician. Over the last 20 years, rates of not having a usual source of care have increased significantly for all racial and ethnic groups, with Latinos having had the most marked increase in lacking a usual source of care (29.6% in 1996, compared with 19.7% in 1977) (Zuvekas & Weinick, 2000). Furthermore, uninsured children receive fewer aggregate annual physician visits than their insured counterparts, receive inadequate preventive services, and are inadequately immunized. In a time marked by profound changes in the organization and delivery of health care, we must ensure that our health system addresses the needs of the most vulnerable members of our society.

As members of the same society, we all have common experiences, beliefs, and values. As members of unique cultural-linguistic groups, we also have unique experiences, beliefs, and values that reflect our respective sub-cultures. The collective culture of our nation and that of the individual cultural-linguistic groups that make this nation can only be changed, or at least valued and respected, through contact with one another. The rise of Latino enclaves in which community members can function without the serious disadvantage of a language barrier and in which every product and service can be provided by the community has partially restricted the contact. So has the marginalization of these groups by our society. As a result of this lack of direct contact, many service providers' views and perceptions of Latinos are filtered not by their knowledge and experiences with the diverse population of Latinos but through their own ethnocentric experiences. Thus, views of appropriate health seeking behavior or prevention and management of illness might not be consistent between the service provider and the individual needing or seeking services.

Individuals of diverse ethnic backgrounds may have beliefs about health, disease, the meaning and cause of disability, and treatment that vary significantly from American practice. These beliefs may be influenced by length of time in the United States, age, and social economic status. Some individuals may incorporate folk medicine into their health care that may have an effect on their health or may interact with their course of treatment. Our challenge as service providers is to develop an awareness of the continuum of beliefs and practices represented in our pluralistic society and, without stereotyping, examine where in the continuum particular individuals are functioning (Iglesias & Quinn, 1997). We must do this without relying on reported ethnocultural characteristics of Latinos (Giger & Davidhizar, 1995; Keller & Stevens, 1997; Marin, 1989) that may or may not be accurate, because they ignore the variability and life trajectory of the Latino population in the United States.

A constellation of beliefs and values has been associated with Latino families. Some of these beliefs and values deal with the role and relationships among family members, whereas others deal with beliefs about health and illness, religion, and spirituality. The specific values and beliefs held by particular Latino families are dependent on their life trajectories. Some of these values and beliefs reflect Latino culture, some reflect social class, and others reflect degree of acculturation. Although it is sometimes difficult to disentangle the source of the individual characteristics, it is important to realize that during the early stages of migrations, immigrant families turn more intensely to the comfort and continuity of past practices. Thus, it is highly probable that new immigrants will reflect practices common to individuals in their country of origin, provided that these were practices in which they engaged before entering this country. Furthermore, these practices are less likely to be modified or eliminated when the individual or family have limited contact with members of ethnic groups other than their own. The children of these families, however, are more likely to be in direct contact with other ethnic groups. This differential contact results in intergenerational discrepancies in the rate of adaptation (Portes, 1997), although the intergenerational discrepancy might be less evident for particular subgroups that have strong contacts with the country of origin (Phinney, Ong, & Madden, 2000). Thus, children of immigrant families who come in contact with other ethnic groups are less likely to retain the values and beliefs about families and health that tend to be associated with the culture of origin. Family organizations vary across Latino groups. Traditionally, the basic social unit of Latinos has been considered to be the extended family—a large family network with flexible boundaries, sharing a belief in collectivism and mutual interdependence (Vega, 1990; Zayas, 1988). Poverty and social marginality of Latino subgroups has further promoted interdependence as an adaptive mechanism in an adverse and unfriendly environment (Sontag & Schacht, 1994). The extended family, which often includes non–blood-related members, such as *comadres* and *copadres* (literally, "godparents"), provide significant support and are often involved in the decision-making process. Greene and Monahan (1984) compared the use of formal and informal supports by Latino and white non-Latino elderly enrollees in a comprehensive case management system. Despite a tendency to exhibit higher levels of impairment, Latino elderly used significantly fewer agency services and significantly higher levels of informal support than did the white non-Latino elderly. Not surprisingly, it is this extended family that is often valued as the source of information rather than the intervention professional (Lareau, 2000). Because the extended family is an important support and, in some cases, the only source of support available to immigrant families living in the United States, absence of such a support system may place these families at greater risk for health complications. Failure by human service professionals to explore and use this natural resource in the development of intervention plan, program, and policies may result in an underuse of services.

As in every other modern society, the gender-role structure within Latino groups is being reexamined. The greater equality across genders calls into question the traditional static roles of *machismo* (male supremacy) and *marianismo* (women as dutiful individuals who will sacrifice their lives for their men and children). Higher education and higher economic independence of women have changed traditional female roles, as well as reduced the widespread cultural stereotype of the Latino man as the dominant, authoritative figure (Gutmann, 1996; Powell, Zambrana, & Silva-Palacios, 1995). As service providers, we must be cognizant of these changing roles and ensure that our interactions with individuals of various genders do not perpetuate stereotypes. At the same time, we must be aware of possible differences in gender roles and provide our services in a way that respects established roles and responsibilities.

Views on health and illness vary among Latinos (Maestas & Erickson, 1992). Some Latinos will rely on Western medical beliefs, some will rely on folk explanations, and some will rely on supernatural explanations. Most of the literature, however, portrays Latinos as maintaining a dual system of beliefs and practice in which Western medical and traditional folk-oriented and supernatural approaches share the stage (Applewhite, 1995). The extents to which non-Western medicine beliefs and practices occur appear to diminish with increased level of acculturation to Western theories of health and illness (García-Prieto, 1996). It is important that we become sensitive to the variety of beliefs about the etiology of particular disorders (e.g., *mal de ojo*, "evil eye"; *susto*, "fright"; *brujeri*, "witchcraft") (see *Culture bound syndromes, DSM-4 TR*, American Psychiatric Association, 2000) and the folk healers (e.g., *curanderos, yerberos, espiritistas, santeros*) to whom the families may contact for cures. Acknowledgment and acceptance of the patients' beliefs—provided that they do not negatively interfere with the course of treatment—could facilitate cooperation and acceptance of alternative treatment approaches.

As culturally competent service providers, we must begin to examine the extent to which our institutional and personal policies and practices promote and encourage equal access. Furthermore, we must examine the extent to which our practices are viewed, valued, and supported by the population we serve. Finally, we must determine the extent to which our services result in similar positive outcomes across groups.

References

American Anthropological Association (2001). *American Anthropological Association Statement on "race"* [On-line]. Available: http://www.ameranthassn.org/stmts/racepp.htm.

American Psychiatric Association (2000). *Diagnostic and statistical manual of mental dsorders* (4th edition text revision). Washington, DC: Author.

Annie E. Casey Foundation (2000). *Kids count data book*. Baltimore: Annie E. Casey Foundation.

Applewhite, S. I. (1995). Curanderismo: Demystifying the health beliefs and practices of elderly Mexican Americans. *Health and Social Work, 20*(4), 247–253.

Byrd, T. L., Mullen, P. D., Selwyn, B., et al. (1996). *Initiation of prenatal care by low-income Hispanic women in Houston.* U.S. Department of Health and Human Services: Public Health Rep 3, 536–540.

California Department of Education (2000). *Dataquest* [On-line]. Available: http://data1.cde.ca.gov/dataquest.

Cavalli-Sforza, L. L. (1995). *The great human diasporas: A history of diversity and evolution.* Reading, MA: Addison-Wesley.

Freund, W. H. (1991). *Race/ethnicity trends in degrees conferred by institutions of higher education: 1978–79 through 1988–89.* Washington, DC: National Center for Education Statistics.

García-Prieto, N. (1996). Puerto Rican families. In M. McGoldrich, J. Giordano, & J. Pearce (Eds.), *Ethnicity and family therapy.* New York: Guilford Press.

Giger, J. N., & Davidhizar, R. E. (1995). *Transcultural nursing: assessment and intervention.* St. Louis: Mosby.

Greene, V. L., & Monahan, D. J. (1984). Comparative utilization of community based long term care services by Hispanic and Anglo elderly in a case management system. *Journal of Gerontology, 39*(6), 730–735.

Gutmann, M. (1996). *The meaning of macho: Being a man in Mexico City.* Berkeley, CA: University of California Press.

Harwood, A. (1994). Acculturation in the post-modern world: Implications for mental health research. In R. G. Malgadt & O. Rodriguez (Eds.), *Theoretical and conceptual issues in Hispanic mental health* (pp. 3–17). Malabar, FL: Krieger.

Hudson, A., Hernadez Cháves, E., Bills, G. D., et al. (1995). The many faces of language maintenance: Spanish language claiming in five southwestern states. In C. Silva-Corvalán (Ed.), *Spanish in four continents* (pp. 165–183). Washington, DC: Georgetown University Press.

Iglesias, A., & Quinn, R. (1997). Culture as a context for early intervention. In S. K. Thurman, J. R. Cornwell, & S. R. Gottwald (Eds.), *Contexts of early intervention: Systems and settings.* Baltimore: Brookes.

Individuals with Disabilities Education Act 1997 Amendments. (1999). Final regulations. *Federal Register,* June 24.

Jaffe, B. F., & DeBlanc, G. B. (1972). Cleft palate, cleft lip and cleft uvula in Navajo Indians. *Cleft Palate Journal, 7,* 301–305.

Keller, C. S., & Stevens, K. R. (1997). Cultural considerations in promoting wellness. *Journal of Cardiovascular Nursing, 11,* 15–25.

Lareau, A. (2000). *Home advantage.* Ladham, MD: Rowman and Littlefield Publishing.

Maestas, A. G., & Erickson, J. G. (1992). Mexican immigrant mother's beliefs about disabilities. *American Journal of Speech-Language Pathology, 1*(4), 5–10.

Marin, G. (1989). AIDS prevention among Hispanics: needs, risk behaviors, and cultural values. *Public Health Report, 104,* 411–415.

Mathews, T. J. (1998). *Smoking during pregnancy, 1990–1996* (Vol. 47, No. 1). Hyattsville, MD: National Center for Health Statistics.

Mathews, T. J., Curtin, S. C., & MacDorman, M. F. (2000). *Infant mortality statistics from the 1998 period linked birth/infant death data set* (Vol. 48, No. 12). Hyattsville, MD: National Center for Health Statistics.

Mendoza, F. S., Ventura, S. J., Valdez, R. B., et al. (1991). Selected measures of health status for Mexican-American, mainland Puerto Ricans, and Cuban-American children. *JAMA, 265*(2), 227–232.

National Center for Education Statistics (1996a). *Dropout rates in the United States: 1994.* Washington, DC: U.S. Department of Education.

National Center for Education Statistics (1996b). *Profile of children in U.S. school districts.* Washington, DC: U.S. Department of Education.

National Center for Education Statistics (1999). *NAEP 1988 reading report card for the nation and states.* Washington, DC: U.S. Department of Education.

National Center for Health Statistics (1997). *Final nationality data.* Washington, DC: National Institutes of Health.

National Center for Health Statistics (1999). *National vital statistics.* Washington, DC: National Center for Health Statistics.

National Institutes of Health (1995). *Drug use among racial/ethnic minorities, national survey results on drug use. Monitoring the future study.* Rockville, MD: National Institutes of Health.

National Institutes of Health (1998). *Women of color health data book.* Beth- esda, MD: National Institutes of Health.

Newacheck, P. W., Hughes, D. C., & Stoddard, J. C. (1996). Children's access to primary care: Differences by race, income, and insurance status. *Pediatrics, 97,* 26–32.

Palinkas, L. A., Pierce, J., Rosbrook, B. P., et al. (1993). Cigarette smoking behavior and beliefs of Hispanics in California. *American Journal of Preventive Medicine, 9,* 331–337.

Phinney, J. S., Ong, A., & Madden, T. (2000). Cultural values and intergenerational value discrepancies in immigrant and non-immigrant families. *Child Development, 71*(2), 528–539.

Population Reference Bureau (1999). America's racial and ethnic minorities. *Population Bulletin, 54*(3), 12.

Portes, A. (1997). Immigration theory for a new century: Some problems and opportunities. *International Migration Review, 31,* 799–825.

Portes, A., & Rumbaut, R. G. (1993). *Immigrant America.* Los Angeles: University of California Press.

Powell, D. R., Zambrana, R., & Silva-Palacios, V. (1995). Including Latino fathers in parent education and support programs: Development of a program model. In R. E. Zambrana (Ed.), *Understanding Latino families*. Thousand Oaks, CA: Sage.

Salas-Provance, M. B. (1996). Orofacial, physiological, and acoustic characteristics. Implications for the speech of African American children. In A. G. Kahmi, K. E. Pollock, & J. L. Harris (Eds.), *Communication development and disorders in African American children* (pp. 155–187). Baltimore: Brookes.

Schaumann, B. F., Peagler, F. D., & Gorlin, J. (1970). Minor craniofacial anomalies among a Negro population. *Oral Surgery, Oral Medicine, and Oral Pathology, 29*, 566–575.

Scribner, R., & Dwyer, J. H. (1989). Acculturation and low birth weight among Latinos in the Hispanic HANES. *American Journal of Public Health, 79*, 1263–1276.

Sontag, J. C., & Schacht, R. (1994). An ethnic comparison of parent participation and information needs in early intervention. *Exceptional Children, 60*, 422–433.

U.S. Department of Health and Human Services. (2000). *Healthy people 2010* (2nd ed.). Washington, DC: U.S. Printing Office.

Vega, W. A. (1990). Hispanic families in the 1980s: A decade of research. *Journal of Marriage and Family, 52*, 1015–1024.

Wernette, D. R., & Nieves, L. A. (1992). Breathing polluted air: Minorities are disproportionately exposed. *Environmental Protection Agency Journal, 18*(1), 16–17.

Zayas, L. (1988). Puerto Rican familism: Consideration for family therapy. *Family Relations, 37*(4), 260–268.

Zuvekas, S. H., & Weinick, R. M. (2000). Changes in access to care, 1977–1996. The role of health insurance. *Health Services Research, 34*(1), 271–279.

Additional Resources

Delgado, M. (Ed.). (1998). *Latino elders and the twenty-first century: Issues and challenges for culturally competent research and practice*. New York: Haworth Press.

Koss-Chioino, J. (1999). *Working with Latino youth: Culture, development, and content*. San Francisco: Jossey-Bass.

Olmos, E. J. (1999). *Americanos: Latino life in the United States*. Boston: Little, Brown.

II

Communication Disorders and Development in Multicultural Populations

7

Bilingual Language Development and Language Disorders

Hortencia Ramirez Kayser

There were more than 3.4 million children with limited English proficiency in elementary and secondary schools in the United States in 1997–1998 (U.S. General Accounting Office, 2001). Schools across the United States are faced with the formidable responsibility of educating immigrant children who are speaking languages other than English. These children face the challenges of learning to speak, read, and write in English, as well as learning the content of academic subjects, while they are adjusting to the cultural and linguistic environments of American schools. When the presence of a speech or language impairment is added to the situation, the challenge becomes greater for educators and speech-language pathologists.

Many children struggle with learning English for a variety of reasons. The most common belief for children not learning English quickly and proficiently is that the child has a language disorder. When children fail in the classroom, the speech-language pathologist is frequently a member of the evaluation team to determine whether there is a language disorder or language difference. Understanding of basic principles of bilingualism and a framework in second language acquisition (SLA) will assist clinicians to make this distinction.

Bilingualism and SLA are different fields of study. Both areas have contributed principles that are of importance in the assessment and treatment of speakers of two languages who may also have a language disorder. There are several concepts related to bilingualism that must be understood before a review of SLA can be undertaken. The first concept is that bilingualism is the norm by world standards, whereas monolingualism is not the norm (Conklin & Laurie, 1983). People in many countries speak several dialects of different languages so that communication is possible with other individuals in the same region. The second concept is that persons who are bilingual are not two monolingual individuals in one (Grosjean, 1982). The bilingual is not the sum of two monolinguals; rather, the bilingual is a unique individual who cannot be easily separated into two parts. Bilingual individuals usually learn the languages in different contexts and use the languages for different purposes with different people. Expecting equal knowledge and equal abilities in two languages is not realistic (Beatens-Beardsmore, 1982). According to Haugen (1953), necessity is the mother of bilingualism, and the only common thing about bilinguals is that they are not monolingual.

There are many societal and individual variables that determine the level of bilingualism or proficiency of two languages a person may develop (Kayser, 1995). Because bilingualism is a continuum, ranging from full proficiency in two or more languages to a minimal degree of proficiency in one of the languages, it is unlikely to find two persons who are exactly alike in their use of two of the same languages (Beatens-Beardsmore, 1982; Kayser, 1995).

The purpose of this chapter is to review the literature concerning SLA as it relates to the assessment and intervention of bilingual individuals who may have speech and language disorders. The chapter begins with a conceptual framework for SLA. A discussion of the literature concerning simultaneous preschool- and school-age successive development of two languages follows. The third section concerns bilingual education. The final section reviews the literature concerning language disorders in bilingual populations.

Communicative Competence

Kessler (1984) described bilingualism in terms of the communicative competency the speaker must achieve in both languages. Children learn the grammatical, sociolinguistic, discourse, and strategic competencies necessary to successfully communicate with family and community members. *Grammatical* or *linguistic competence* refers to the mastery of phonologic, syntactic, and lexical features of a language. Sociolinguistic competency addresses the sociocultural rules for appropriate language use. This involves knowledge of the rules for who speaks, what to speak about, how to speak, and when to speak with members of the community according to their status and role. Discourse competence involves the connection of utterances to form a meaningful entity, such as in narratives and conversations. Strategic competence involves strategies that are used to compensate for breakdowns in communication when there is imperfect knowledge of the rules in the other areas of communicative competence. These strategies include paraphrasing, repetitions, circumlocutions, message modifications, hesitations, and avoidance of difficult words, phrases, or situations.

Strategic competency is an important skill in SLA, because as children develop two languages, they may not have perfect knowledge of the languages and will depend on these strategies to be effective communicators. Corder (1967) described *communicative strategies* versus *learning strategies*. Communicative strategies are used to communicate effectively, whereas learning strategies are mental processes to help construct the rules of the language. Similar to Corder's communicative and learning strategies are Wong-Fillmore's (1979) *social* and *cognitive strategies*. Social strategies include joining groups and acting as if you understand, using choice words to give the impression of expressive abilities in the language, and counting on friends for help when a topic is not understood. Cognitive strategies include the assumption that speech is related to the context, guessing, analysis of repeated phrases, and focusing on the big picture rather than the finer parts of the language. Chesterfield and Chesterfield (1985) stated that older children use several other strategies, such as imitation, deferred practice, asking informants, reading, observation, using a dictionary, silent practice, asking for repetition, and many others. This ability to develop the second language (L2) through communication strategies may be problematic to children with a language disorder. The ability must be considered in the assessment and treatment of language disorders.

Children living in environments in which two languages are used typically develop the communicative competency necessary to function in these environments. The level of language proficiency will depend on the age of acquisition, amount of exposure to the L2, the child's attitude toward or desire to learn the L2, and a number of other variables. Children have their own individual language learning differences and paths for learning the languages (Wong-Fillmore, 1979).

Second Language Acquisition

Kessler (1984), McLaughlin (1984a), and Grosjean (1982) describe three groups of children who are exposed to two languages in childhood—simultaneous bilinguals, preschool successive bilinguals, and school-age successive bilinguals. The groups are defined by the time the language is introduced to the child.

A simultaneous bilingual is a child who has learned two languages before the age of 3 years. The child may have bilingual parents or parents who speak different languages (i.e., mixed language families). A preschool successive bilingual is the child who has learned the L2 after the age of 3 years. This may be a child from a monolingual home who enters a preschool program in which the language of instruction is English. A school-age successive bilingual is a child who learns a L2 at age 5 or 6 years when entering school. The age at which children are exposed to the L2, their cognitive and linguistic development in their first language (L1), their native language skills, and any educational experiences received in the home language will impact on the development of the L2.

Simultaneous Bilinguals

The research concerning simultaneous bilinguals supports several conclusions. The first is that typically developing simultaneous bilinguals do not have any difficulty with language comprehension (Taeschner, 1983). Second, they are not different from monolinguals in reaching the milestones in language development, such as the age when first words and word combinations appear and the number of words learned. Third, linguistic context and interactions are important in the acquisition of the two languages. That is, who is using the language and how much exposure the child is receiving for each language are both important to the potential bilingualism of the child.

There is disagreement in the research related to lexical and phonologic interference and linguistic production. Lexical interference may or may not exist from the beginning of first words. Children may or may not have phonologic interference—that is, some children use the phonologic systems to distinguish the two languages and separate the languages by the sound system; others do not. Children's linguistic production also varies. Some children reared in balanced bilingual homes become bilingual; others do not.

Volterra and Taeschner (1978) observed three stages in the language development of three bilingual English-Italian–speaking children. At stage 1, the children had only one lexical system that included words from both languages. Words in English did not have equivalents in Italian and vice versa. Both languages were used indiscriminately as one would use one language. At stage 2, there was differentiation between the two lexical systems, but only one grammar. The children related the lexical items much like semantic relationships. Thus, a beginning grammar was emerging. At stage 3, there was a complete separation of the lexical and grammar systems without language mixing. Leopold (1949) and Fantini (1985) reported that complete separation of languages occurs between 3.0 and 3.5 years of age.

Leopold (1949) studied his daughter Hildegard's development of English and German. She heard English from her mother and German from her father. There was a strict separation of languages in the home. Hildegard initially mixed the languages but slowly separated the two language systems. She had an accompanying awareness of her bilingualism. She avoided the use of difficult words and constructions in her weaker language, German. She also had a complete separation of the phonologic and grammar systems but an enduring influence of the dominant language on the other in the area of vocabulary and idioms. Leopold (1949) stated that Hildegard had balanced bilingual abilities by the time she was 5 years of age. She did have a preference in languages. Children at young ages do become attached and may favor one language over the other. When Hildegard began to lose her ability to speak German, he sent the child to Germany to live with relatives for 6 months, and she quickly regained her fluency in German.

Fantini (1985) provided a sociolinguistic perspective into the simultaneous bilingualism of Mario, his son. Mario was raised in a mixed language home. Fantini, the father, spoke primarily English, whereas the mother spoke only Spanish. The language of the community was English, but Mario frequently visited Venezuela, his mother's homeland, and other Spanish-speaking countries. Although he heard both languages from birth, his first words were in Spanish at 16 months. At 20–22 months, he discriminated between the languages. Fantini described Mario as affectionate and friendly to persons who spoke in Spanish, but he was distant and would not interact with persons who spoke English. At 30 months, Mario used his first words in English. At 31–32 months, he began to mix English and Spanish. Fantini commented that the mother did not like to speak English and probably had an attitudinal influence on Mario's preference for speaking Spanish.

An interesting observation was that at 32 months Mario classified speakers by appearance. He learned that Hispanics had a certain appearance and that places such as Mexico, Venezuela, and South Texas were areas where Spanish was primarily spoken. By 36–40 months, he differentiated the language used by persons. Mario recognized that certain individuals speak English, whereas others speak Spanish. At 40 months, Mario differentiated language use by place. Spanish was used at home, but English was used on the playground. By the time he was 40 months, he marked languages with the term *Español*, and at 45 months, he used the term *English*. At 49 months, he asked for translations; when he was 50 months, he told others what languages he spoke.

Three issues are important in this age group. The first is the age at which the child is aware of the two languages; second, the typical frequency of occurrence of language mixing; and third, the typical vocabulary growth at this age.

Awareness of two languages is important so that the child can begin separating the languages and language and cognitive development (Arnberg, 1987). Quay (1995) suggests that children have the ability to differentiate between two languages before age 2 years, the presyntactic one-word stage of language acquisition. Genesee (1989) and Goodz (1994) suggest that prelinguistic infants differentiate two languages by using differences in the prosody of each language, such as intonation, stress, and rhythm as cues. According to Goodz (1994), infants hear each language as a different melody; the different languages may be as distinct as different songs to the infant.

Fantini's (1985) son showed preferences for Spanish speakers before the age of 2 years by becoming endearing to Spanish speakers and ignoring English speakers. According to Arnberg (1987), Genesee (1989), and Vihman (1985), simultaneous bilinguals become aware of the two languages by using a number of strategies. They do the following: (1) learn about the languages, (2) rely on phonetic cues to differentiate the languages, (3) relate situational variables of word use, (4) attend to adult use of language, (5) learn language use through social experiences, and (6) become increasingly sensitive to adult standards and attempt to match those standards.

Language Mixing

Language mixing, using the features of both languages, occurs up to age 3.5 years in the simultaneous bilingual. The caregiver's use of the two languages, frequency of language mixing, and type of language switching are important variables in the use of language mixing. The types of switches are intersentential switches (e.g., The baby is sick, *Tiene tos*) and intrasentential switches (e.g., The baby *tiene un* cold). Some parents of simultaneous bilingual children switch or separate the languages by speakers to assist the child in developing language awareness and, hopefully, reducing the time that the child is language mixing. Others may not regularly switch languages. Quay (1995) states that studies that interpret mixing as a lack of language differentiation do not take into account the fact that bilingual children may lack the appropriate vocabulary and may not have a choice in their language use. What this may suggest is that for some typical language-learning children, separation of the two languages and language mixing may continue for a longer period of time. The child may recognize that members of the community speak both languages, and the child may choose only one of the languages. Caregiver language models are an important variable when determining the amount of mixing that is occurring for a child.

Language mixing should decrease as the child develops language. Redlinger and Park (1980) state that language mixing may occur approximately 20–30% in Brown's stage I, 12–20% in stage II, 6–12% in stage III, and 2–6% in stages IV and V. Analysis of language samples taken over a period of time should provide evidence whether or not the child is separating the languages and that mixing the languages is decreasing.

Expressive vocabulary development is important in the understanding of bilingual language development. Researchers have attempted to determine whether the two vocabularies develop in parallel, whether specific strategies are necessary to acquire them, and whether they are quantitatively comparable to the vocabularies of monolingual children. Goodz (1994) states that early simultaneous bilingualism does not result in a delay in the appearance of first words, nor does it retard vocabulary development. There may be unequal progress in the two languages, but total vocabulary development compares favorably with the development of monolingual children in at least one language.

Volterra and Taeschner (1978) determined that their three Italian-English–speaking subjects used words belonging to both languages. When words plus the context were considered, although corresponding words were produced, the children did not consider these words as exactly corresponding to each other. Synonyms were found in their early vocabulary. Taeschner (1983) identified two stages in bilingual lexical acquisition. In the first stage, the bilingual child has no equivalents (i.e., one lexical system composed of words from both languages). In the second stage, which begins after the child has acquired approximately 50 words, the child builds a system of equivalents for those words previously mastered. The context strongly influences the child's word choice and use. Quay (1995) stated that the child begins to use equivalents immediately, in some instances using both words in one utterance. This may be a product of parent modeling. Some bilingual parents model two languages to young children. They will give both languages (e.g., doggie, *perrito*) to assure that the child is receiving both language models.

There is some evidence that although the bilingual child may have fewer words in each language than the monolingual child, when all of the words in the bilingual's two languages are counted, the child may have a slightly larger lexicon than the monolingual (Taeschner, 1983). Patterson (1998) and Pearson, Fernandez, and Oller (1993) reported that the bilingual infants' average total expressive vocabulary in Spanish and English combined was similar to the average expressive vocabulary of monolingual English-or Spanish-speaking children. Patterson (1998) stated that 100% of 26- to 27-month-old children studied used 50 words and that 90% of children who were combining words had a vocabulary of at least 50 words. These reports are only of expressive vocabulary. It is assumed that receptive vocabulary is larger than expressive language, but no reports have been available concerning bilingual children. Comprehension of both languages should be of critical importance in determining whether or not a language disorder exists.

Preschool Successive Bilinguals

Preschool successive bilinguals enter preschool at age 3–4 years speaking the home language. They usually have had at least 3 years of a monolingual native language environment. The foundations for speaking in complete sentences and asking questions have been developed. Some preschool children have older siblings who speak English and influence their development of the home language and in English. Wong-Fillmore (personal communication, 1992) has stated that children with English-speaking siblings are probably incipient bilinguals and may not be monolinguals when entering preschool programs.

The research concerning SLA in preschool children began as case studies of individual children. The descriptions were holistic and were often case studies of linguists' children who were being reared in bilingual homes. Other studies of successive bilingualism have been through cross-sectional examination of groups of children at different age levels. These studies investigated theoretical issues of SLA, such as does learning an L2 parallel that of learning the L1, how does the child separate the two languages, and when is the child aware of these two languages? More recent work is examining the development of morphologic and syntactic structures and the phases of development of these features. The results of such studies will depend on the ages of subjects, ethnic population, exposure to the languages, number of samples taken, and whether procedures are spontaneous or structure elicited. There are many other variables that will determine the external and internal validity of any such infant study of bilingualism. Table 7-1 provides a listing and the conclusive results of some studies completed with Spanish-English–speaking children.

Tabors and Snow (1994) describe a developmental sequence that preschool children follow as they develop an L2. They include (1) home language use for communication with English speakers, (2) a nonverbal stage, (3) telegraphic and formulaic phrase use in the new language, and (4) productive use of the L2.

Stage 1: Home Language Use (First Language) with English Speakers (Second Language)

Some preschool children entering English-only classrooms continue to use the home language, assuming that others will understand them or believing that others will learn their language. Some quickly recognize that continuing to use the home language does not work and that other children in the classroom do not understand them. According to

Table 7-1 Morphologic and Syntactic Structures for the Developmental Ages of Children from Bilingual English and Spanish Environments

Syntactic and Morphologic Marker	Source and Age of Development (in years.months)
Present indicative (e.g., *El muchacho hace*—The boy does)	Cohen, 4.0 Garcia, 2.0–4.5 *Gonzalez, 2.0–2.6 Maez, 1.6–2.0
First person singular (e.g., *Yo hago*—I do)	*Gonzalez, 2.6
Second person singular (e.g., *Tù haces*—You do)	*Gonzalez, 2.6
Third person singular (e.g., *Èl hizò*—He did)	*Gonzalez, 2.6
Third person plural (e.g., *Ellos hacen*—They do)	*Gonzalez, 2.6
Present progressive (e.g., *El muchacho hace*—The boy does)	Cohen, 3.0 Garcia, 2.6–4.5 *Gonzalez, 2.0–2.6
Progressive participle/gerund (e.g., *Yo estoy haciendo*—I am doing)	—
Progressive past (e.g., *Estaba haciendo*—Was doing)	*Gonzalez, 2.6–4.0
Present perfect/auxiliary present (e.g., *Ella ha hecho*—She has done)	Garcia, 4.5 *Gonzalez, 3.0–4.6
Preterit regular (e.g., *Yo hice*—I did)	Cohen, 3.0–4.0 Dale, 5.0 Garcia, 4.5 *Gonzalez, 2.0–2.6 Maez, 1.10 (third person)
Preterit irregular (e.g., *Yo supe*—I knew)	—
Imperfect indicative (e.g., *hacìa*—did)	Cohen, 4.0 Garcia, 3.0–4.5 *Gonzalez, 2.9–3.3
Future or periphrasic future (e.g., *harè/va a hacer*—I will do)	Brisk, 5.0 Cohen, 4.0 Garcia, 2.6 *Gonzalez, 2.6
Conditional (e.g., *Si el niño no lo hace, nadie lo hace*—If the boy doesn't do it, no one will)	Brisk, 5.0 Cohen, 3.5 Garcia, 3.0 (emerging) *Gonzalez, 3.0–4.0
Present subjunctive (e.g., *Quiero que Maria lo haga*—I want Maria to do it)	Cohen, 3.0–7.0 Garcia, 3.0–4.5 *Gonzalez, 2.6–4.0
Past subjunctive (e.g., *Yo haya hecho*—I would have done)	Garcia, 4.5 *Gonzalez, 3.3–4.6
Copula (e.g., *ser/estar*—is)	Garcia, 3.0 *Gonzalez, 2.0 (third person)

Table 7-1 *(continued)*

Syntactic and Morphologic Marker	Source and Age of Development (in years.months)
Imperative consisting of verb form (e.g., *haga*—do)	*Gonzalez, 2.0
	Maez, 1.6
Imperatives	
Verb + indirect object (e.g., *No lo hagas*—Do not do it)	Garcia, 4.5
Verb + indirect/direct object (e.g., *Hazlo*—do it)	Garcia, 4.5
Verb + reflexive pronoun (e.g., *Hazlo hija*—Do it daughter)	*Gonzalez, 2.6
Verb + reflexive + direct object pronoun (e.g., *Hazlo tù*—Do it yourself)	*Gonzalez, 2.9
Passives (e.g., *El vestido fue hecho por la mamà*—The dress was made by the mother)	—
Prepositions (e.g., *en, sobre, debajo, detras*—in, on, under, behind)	Garcia, 3.0
Short plurals, /s/	Dale, 5.0
Long plurals, /es/	Dale, 8.0
Possessive, constructive (e.g., *de su padre, del papà*, etc.—his father's)	*Gonzalez, 2.6–3.0
Interrogatives (e.g., *dònde, què, còmo, quièn, cuàl, por què, para que*—where, what, how, who, which, why, for what)	*Gonzalez, 2.0 (*dònde, què, por què*)
	*Gonzalez, 2.6–4.0 (*quien, cuando, còmo,* and *para què*)
Qualifying primitive adjective (e.g., *bonito*—pretty)	Garcia, 3.0–6.0
	Parra, 2.0–2.11
Possessive adjective (e.g., *En el vestido de la princesa*—On the princess's dress)	Parra, 3.0–3.11
Gender, noun adjectives, substantivization (e.g., *los caballos, las muchachas, la camisa blanca*—the horses, the girls, the white shirt)	*Gonzalez, 2.9–4.0
	Parra, 2.0–12.0
Yes and no questions in full sentence form (e.g., *No lo hizò hoy*—Used as response—He or she didn't do it today)	*Gonzalez, 2.6–4.0
Locative adverbs (e.g., *recio*—fast)	Garcia, 3.0 (emerging)
	Gonzalez, 2.9
Conjunctive (e.g., *El niño lo hizò y la muchacha no lo hizò*—The boy did it and the girl did not do it)	Garcia, 4.5
	*Gonzalez, 2.6–4.0
Negatives (*No lo haga*—Don't do it)	Garcia, 3.0
	*Gonzalez, 2.0–2.6
Pronouns (e.g., *èl, ella, ellos*—he, she, they)	Garcia, 3.0
Reflexive pronoun (e.g., *Me lo hizò*—He or she did it for me)	*Gonzalez, 2.0

*Gonzalez (1978): First age indicates age of emergence, and second age indicates established age of acquisition. All other investigators only reported established age of acquisition.
Source: Adapted from Brisk (1972, 1976); Cohen (1980); Dale (1980); Garcia (1988); Gonzalez (1978); Maez (1983); and Parra (1982).

Tabors and Snow (1994), older children (ages 4–7 years) recognize their inability to communicate with others much sooner than preschool children. Some children may choose not to learn the new language, continuing to use the home language (Hakuta, 1986; Saville-Troike, 1978).

Stage 2: Nonverbal Stage of Learning the Second Language

Krashen (1982) has described the nonverbal stage in the development of the L2 by preschool children as the *silent period*. *Nonverbal* is used here because these children do continue to communicate but not with words. The children realize that their language will not help them communicate, and, therefore, they stop talking. For some children, this nonverbal stage may last up to 8 weeks (Ervin-Tripp, 1974), whereas some may socially isolate themselves and not attempt to communicate for longer periods (Itoh & Hatch, 1978). A social consequence of their unwillingness to attempt to communicate verbally is that the English-speaking children may treat these children as infants or toddlers, or they may ignore the children (Tabor & Snow, 1994).

Stage 3: Formulaic Language

The first verbal utterances by preschool L2 learners are typically telegraphic and formulaic speech. *Telegraphic speech* is defined as content words in the utterance without function words or morphologic markers (Tabor & Snow, 1994). In the classroom, the telegraphic speech is usually about names for objects in English. The children begin to learn the English labels for concepts taught in the classroom such as numbers, the letters of the alphabet, and color names. They also learn *formulaic speech*. Formulaic speech involves the use of unanalyzed chunks or phrases such as "Hi. How are you?," "my turn," and "push me" (Wong-Fillmore, 1979). These formulaic speech patterns allow preschool children to socialize with English speakers in play situations.

Stage 4: Productive Use of the Second Language

L2 learners learn to break down the language and make comparisons of syntactic rules to become productive L2 users. They develop the finer points of the language with practice and application of the new rules they discover. Preschool children come into the L2 learning process with their own individual differences, whether social, cognitive, or communicative (Wong-Fillmore, 1979).

School-Age Successive Bilinguals

School-age successive bilinguals enter the school after age 5 years with no previous exposure to English. The advantage for a school-age successive bilingual is that he or she has a greater and more mature language and cognitive development in the L1 on which to build the L2.

Children enter the elementary and secondary school as non-English speakers at all ages. Their acquisition of English will depend on the type and amount of exposure to English, whom the child needs to communicate with, their attitudes toward the new language, their aptitude to learn an L2, and their motivation to learn the new language. The parents' attitude toward maintaining the home language may also have an influence on the development of proficiency in the L2. Two other factors that are important to consider in the acquisition of English are language loss of the home language and the educational environment or educational philosophy for English language learners.

Language Loss in Successive Bilinguals

If a child from a bilingual home is in an English-only class and the parents do not encourage the maintenance of the home language, then language loss or attrition may occur. Language loss is the weakening of an individual's L1 because of the focus on learning the L2 (Schiff-Myers, 1992). Table 7-2 summarizes the effects of language loss. Language loss can occur at any age, even in adulthood. The affect on the child's overall language development is only one aspect of language loss. The child may lose the ability to communicate with the family in the L1.

Wong-Fillmore (1991) studied language loss by children in preschool who attended English-only, home language–only, and bilingual preschool programs. Questionnaires were administered to 1,100 families who had children in English-only, bilingual, and home language–only preschool programs in 26 different states. A comparison group from 311 families who had children in the home language–only preschool programs was used. Wong-Fillmore (1991) reported negative affects on family communication patterns. She defined negative affects as the parents spoke no English and the children spoke only English. More than 64% of the parents of the children in English-only preschool programs reported the negative effect (i.e., the children spoke English only, whereas the parents continued to speak the home language only). Forty-seven percent of the parents whose children attended bilingual preschool programs reported negative effects, and 26% of the parents whose children attended home language–only programs reported similar negative effects. The comparison home language preschool programs had a reported negative effect of 10.8%. The parents reported that preschool children lost the ability to speak the home language faster than their older siblings (Wong-Fillmore, 1991). The children depended more on their peers than on the family for communication and social-emotional support systems. As the children became older, gang

Table 7-2 Language Loss Patterns

Form

Loss among forms and structures is variable

Greater number of plural over gender errors

Inconsistent use of morphologic forms and syntactic structures

Change in verb usage under influence of the L2

Change in verb usage is more likely to occur in cases in which the L1 and L2 are phonetically similar

Stylistic shrinkage: loss of one of two "same meaning" structures

Regular morphologic alternations are reduced

Reliance on less flexible word order

Preference for coordinated rather than embedded constructions

Regular morphologic alternations are reduced

Irregular patterns become regularized

Syntactic structure of the L2 is used in instances in which it would be ungrammatical in the L1

Syntax used by the individual experiencing language loss is different from developmental forms used by peers

Content

Use of L2 words for L1 words

Inconsistent use of vocabulary in the L1

Not all lexical information is equally susceptible to loss

Meaning extensions

Loan translation: an idiomatic expression from the L2 is transferred to the L1 in which it is ungrammatical

Use

Loss among individuals is variable

The individual shows signs of insecurity in language performance

The influence of the L2 is most prevalent in the causal language styles of the L1

L1 loss occurs in causal language styles before formal language styles

The amount of attention paid to speech significantly governs the outcome in L1 and L2 situations

Language loss follows the reverse developmental pattern of second language acquisition

The individual is aware of the language loss or weakness

Compensatory strategies used by children are also used by adults

Compensatory strategies used during language loss are not language bound, but they may be culturally bound

Time elapsed since emigration only becomes relevant to language loss when there is not much contact with the native language

Compensatory strategies used during the progression of language loss are also used during L2 acquisition

---

L1 = first language; L2 = second language.

Source: Reprinted with permission from Kayser, H. (Ed.) (1998). *Assessment and intervention resource for Hispanic children* (p. 60). San Diego: Singular Publishing Group.

membership became important as a social-emotional support system. If the children stop using the home language, then they may never develop full proficiency in the L2. Therefore, parents should maintain the home language so that the children will not lose their proficiency in the L1 (Hakuta, 1986).

Circumstances may be ideal and the child may still choose to speak primarily English. Such is the case with Anderson's (1999) own child. Victoria was reared in a home in which Spanish was spoken; however, she eventually lost her fluency in speaking Spanish. Victoria attended preschools in which English was the language of instruction. Victoria and her sibling used English at school and eventually used English in their play at home. The errors in language that Victoria made in Spanish over the course of the 22 months of elicitation of language samples were errors that have been reported in atypical learners of Spanish (Anderson, 1999).

Speech-language pathologists may erroneously identify children as language disordered without recognizing the possibility of language loss (Schiff-Myers, 1992). Clinicians should obtain a history of language development in the two languages, including the age at which language milestones were reached, as well as any family or sociocultural factors that may have influenced the development of the two languages. The case history should include the following: (1) the language used in the home, (2) age and conditions under which the child began to learn English, (3) ages at which the child achieved linguistic developmental milestones in the home language, (4) contacts with the homeland, and (5) motivation to become and remain proficient in each of the languages. The *Language Usage Estimate* (Skoceylas, 1971) is an instrument that has been used by researchers to estimate the amount and nature of language exposure for children in bilingual or monolingual homes. A complete language history and estimate of the home linguistic environment are important to determine whether language loss has occurred.

Bilingual Education

Bilingual education has a long history in the United States. It often occurred in private schools for languages such as Swedish, German, Finnish, Yiddish, and Spanish. For the past 30 years, the federal government has served students with limited English proficiency under Title I of the Elementary and Secondary Education Act (1965). The Bilingual Education Act of 1968 provided support to help ensure that students with limited English proficiency would master English and develop high levels of academic proficiency in academic content areas.

When the use of the native language for instruction became a federal mandate, bilingual education became a political issue that has received negative reviews by the public. There have been criticisms concerning the effectiveness of the bilingual education programs (Hakuta, 1986). The effectiveness of bilingual programs depends on several variables, including community, school, and home resources.

According to Skutnabb-Kangas (1995) school and home resources are two important factors in the success of bilingual education programs. Bilingual-trained teachers are important to the effectiveness of the instruction. Bilingual teachers must understand the pedagogy of bilingual education and use both languages to educate children. The materials the teachers use and the content of these materials must be appropriate for the children's needs. There must be relevant and cognitively demanding subject matter with opportunity to practice the L2. Therefore, there must be exposure to native speakers of the L2 in linguistically demanding formal contexts. Any non-English use in the classroom must be adapted to the students' level for comprehension. In the classroom, students should have a low level of anxiety; the teacher must be supportive, understanding, and sympathetic with reasonable objectives.

The children come into the classroom from homes that either support or do not support bilingual education. Students should come into the bilingual classroom with adequate linguistic development in their L1 and an opportunity to continue to develop the L1 outside the school in linguistically demanding formal contexts. If the parents attempt to use the L2 in the home, then the quality of interaction between parents and children will often suffer. They will spend less time interacting with the children, as well as providing an inadequate L2 model. Speech-language pathologists and teachers should encourage parents to continue to promote the development of the home language through such activities as retelling family history, stories, and using the home language (Appel & Muksken, 1987; Chamot, 1988).

There are no two bilingual programs that are exactly alike. Determining the effectiveness of bilingual education with children becomes problematic because of the many different variables to consider in the evaluation of the program (Hakuta, 1986). Unfortunately, bilingual education is the only educational philosophy or program in the public schools that is reviewed for effectiveness with all children who are learning English.

Bilingual education is an educational approach in which a student's native language is used in instruction. There are two basic approaches to bilingual education. One uses English and makes little use of the student's native language (English-based approach), whereas the other makes extensive use of the student's native language (bilingual approach). Approximately 76% of the children in bilingual education receive English-based instruction (e.g., English as a second language [ESL]); 40% receive bilingual education aimed at teaching subject matter in the child's native language; and 37% receive instruction aimed at maintaining or improving fluency in their home language (e.g., Spanish lessons for Spanish speakers.) Students in the English-based approach are expected to learn English in 2–3 years. In the bilingual approach, students are not expected to reach proficiency in 5 or more years. The time needed to attain proficiency in English can vary from child to child. It can be affected by such factors as the child's age, socioeconomic background, and the amount of formal education received in the native language. Older children who have developed language and cognitive skills in their L1 before learning English generally make faster progress in learning English than young children. For example, a study of children with limited English proficiency attending school in Fairfax, Virginia, found that students arriving in this country between ages 8 and 11 needed 5–7 years to compete with native speakers on all subject areas. However, children who arrived when they were aged 4–7 years needed 7–10 years (Collier, 1987–1988). Children from higher socioeconomic backgrounds tend to learn the L2 more easily. Other factors related to rate of learning English include the amount of exposure students have had to English, the level of parental support at home, and the classroom, school, and community environment.

The United States has several predominant curriculum designs for bilingual education. The designs include the following: (1) the maintenance model, which is designed to develop bilingualism and biliteracy; (2) the transitional model, which is designed to use the non-English language to facilitate the learning of English through curriculum content; (3) the ESL model, which is usually a component of the first two models; and (4) the high-intensity model, which is found in middle and high schools in which students are expected to learn English rapidly (Fradd, 1987).

Immersion and dual-language immersion programs are two other models of bilingual education. Immersion bilingual education programs are additive bilingual programs that have four important sociocultural factors. First, immersion programs are intended for children from the majority group language (i.e., English) who are attempting to learn a language other than English. Second, in immersion programs, teachers and administrators value and support the children's home language and culture. Third, in immersion programs, the child and parents value the home language and culture, as well as desire to learn the L2. Finally, the acquisition of the L2 by the participants and parents is regarded as a positive skill (McLaughlin, 1984b). The dual-language immersion model combines minority language speakers with English monolingual speakers in the same classroom. Dual-language immersion provides first-language instruction for children with other than English-speaking backgrounds, while simultaneously offering monolingual English-speaking children access to other languages. The purpose is to develop bilingualism in both groups (Valdes, 1997).

Transitional bilingual education is the model mandated by the reauthorized and revised Bilingual Education Act of 1974 (PL 95-561) and the *Lau v.*

Nichols (1974) decision, which held that the failure to provide English-language instruction to non-English speakers violated Title VI of the Civil Rights Act of 1964. Minority-language students are instructed in their home language until they are able to receive instruction exclusively in English (Hakuta, 1986). These children receive instruction beginning in kindergarten in the home language, and, as they progress through the grades, they are increasingly exposed to the majority language, English. When these children are determined to have adequate proficiency in English, they are transferred to English-only instruction. The home language is not maintained.

Although bilingual education is not funded to maintain the home language, there have been individual research projects that have looked at the effects of native language instruction with minority language children. The stated purpose of native language instruction has been to provide comprehensible input (Krashen, 1981) so that the child understands the nature and demands of the learning task. If the child were instructed in the unfamiliar language, then the child's level of learning of the curriculum would be expected to be compromised by the child's lack of comprehension. Research studies suggest that bilingual children who develop their proficiency in both languages experience intellectual and academic advantages over monolingual children. In other words, instruction by means of a minority language in early grades is not just promoting proficiency in the surface manifestations of that language, but it is also promoting the deeper cognitive and academic skills that underlie the development of literacy in both the bilingual's languages. Additionally, children between 9 and 12 years also make more rapid progress in academic aspects of their L2 than do children between 5 and 8 years (Appel & Muksken, 1987). The Office of Civil Rights reviewed the length of time children with limited English proficiency needed to become proficient in English. Among the findings was that no clear consensus exists on the length of time that children with limited English proficiency need to become proficient in English. The factors related to the time needed to reach English proficiency through bilingual education are numerous. Proficiency is reached in 2–3 years of bilingual education using English-based approaches and is much longer for approaches based on extensive use of the child's home language. Children may reach proficiency in basic interpersonal communication skills and conversational skills within 2 years; however, they may not achieve the language skills necessary to perform on par with native English speakers in cognitive academic language proficiency necessary for academic subjects from 5–7 years of instruction in English (U.S. General Accounting Office, 2001; Cummins, 1992). Basic interpersonal communication skills involve face-to-face communication in which the conversational participants can actively negotiate meaning and have a shared reality. They are the language skills used in everyday conversation. Supported by a wide range of meaningful, situational, and paralinguistic gestures, cognitive academic language proficiencies involve understanding and using the fundamentals of written language and literacy necessary for the academic tasks of writing essays on abstract topics, analyzing literature, and making arguments. A child may have conversational language skills but not be able to perform the language tasks necessary to be on par with his age peers (Cummins, 1992).

Language Disorders in Bilingual Children

One of the more difficult tasks for a speech-language pathologist in providing clinical services to children and adults learning English as an L2 is to determine whether the child has a communication disorder or whether the behavior observed is the result of the impact of development of the L2 on the L1. Factors in SLA such as language loss and mixing and code switching make this an especially challenging process. These services can best be provided by a speech-language pathologist who is competent to provide services in the native language of the client. According to the American Speech-Language-Hearing Association (1989),

> Speech-language pathologists who present themselves as bilingual for the purposes of providing clinical services must be able to speak their primary language and to speak (or sign) at least one other language with native or near-native proficiency in lexicon (vocabulary), semantics (meaning), phonology (pronunciation), morphology/syntax (grammar) and pragmatics (uses) during clinical management. To provide bilingual assessment and remediation services in the client's language, the bilingual speech-language pathologist or audiologist should possess: (1) the ability to describe the process of normal speech and language acquisition for bilingual and monolingual individuals and how those processes are manifested in oral (or manually coded) and written language; (2) the ability to administer and interpret formal and informal assessment procedures to distinguish between communication differences and communication disorders in oral (or manually coded) and written language; (3) the ability to apply intervention strategies for treatment of communication disorders in the client's language; and (4) the ability to recognize cultural factors that affect the delivery of speech-language pathology and audiology services to the client's language community. (p. 93)

Information on the assessment of speech and language in children learning English as an L2 is discussed in Chapter 13. In providing services to individuals who are developing English proficiency, speech-language pathologists should follow the guidelines, competencies, and definitions outlined in the *Position paper: Social dialects and implications of the position on social dialects* (ASHA, 1983) and the *Clinical management of communicatively handicapped minority language populations* (ASHA, 1985).

Assessment

Determining whether a language disorder exists in a child learning an L2 would not be difficult if the child were monolingual in either language. The confounding variables of native language loss and normal language development while developing a L2 make determining the presence of a speech or language disorder difficult. Assessment of competence in the linguistic characteristics of a language cannot be determined unless the speech-language pathologist is knowledgeable of the linguistic features of the language and the normal development of these features in the language. Voice quality, loudness, pitch, and the production of clicks or glottal stops make it difficult to rule out vocal pathology when the speech-language pathologist is not familiar with the vocal characteristics of the language. Hesitations, false starts, and filled and silent pauses may be used, whether due to lack of familiarity with the language or characteristics of dysfluency.

There are three principles concerning the speech and language evaluation of bilingual children. First, both languages should always be evaluated, even when the child only understands the home language. Second, if one of the languages is within low normal limits, then a language disorder probably does not exist. Third, a concomitant disorder may exist, such as oral motor disorder, developmental apraxia of speech, phonologic impairment, or developmental delay. There may be significant factors in the case history, such as a significant birth history (e.g., congenital infection, birth weight less than 1,500 g, head trauma, and so forth) or hearing impairment. Table 7-3 summarizes the characteristics that have been reported for bilingual children who were identified as language disordered. Most of these data were developed without the case history or recognition of language loss as a factor, and, therefore, caution is recommended to its application to children learning two languages.

Intervention

Once a child has been identified as language disordered, the issue is whether the child should receive services in one or both lan-

Table 7-3   Reported Language Difficulties in Bilingual Children with Language Impairments

Form
Inability to discriminate tones, phonemes, and morphemes
Inability to produce phonemes /s/, /L/, /r/, and /rr/
Substitutes, omits, or distorts sounds
Reverses the order of sounds in words
Uses incorrect word order
Substitutes schwa for articles, pronouns, and other grammatical structures
Content
Comprehension of who, what, when, and why questions
Word retrieval difficulties
Inability to associate sounds with objects or experiences
Inappropriate verbal labels for common objects, actions, and persons
Poor vocabulary
Use
Poor conversational skills
Poor topic maintenance
Poor turn-taking
Perseverates on a topic
Comments inappropriately
Difficulty with retelling stories
Difficulty with narrating personal experiences
Difficulty with classifying events with verbal labels
Friendships may be limited to low achievers
Limited group interactions with classmates
Uses gestures
Behaviors
Short attention span
Distractibility
Daydreams
Demands immediate gratification
Disorganized
Unable to stay on task
Appears confused

Source: Adapted from Ambert (1986a, 1986b); Damico, Oller, and Story (1983); Kayser (1990); Langdon (1983); Linares-Orama and Sanders (1977); Maldonado (1984); Merino (1983); Ortiz and Maldonado-Colon (1986); Roseberry-McKibbin, (1995); and Taylor (1986).

guages. Despite such legal mandates as the Individuals with Disabilities Education Act, misconceptions remain about the ability of children with language impairments to learn more than one language and about the use of the L1 in helping minority-language children acquire English as an L2. Many speech-language pathologists and educational professionals believe that minority-language children who are experiencing difficulty in mastering language skills should receive intervention only in English. The argument has been that these children need to learn English to be able to communicate in the predominant language used in the school and the community. Ortiz (1984) and Gutierrez-Clellen (1999) stated that there is a belief that children are confused when English and the home language are used for instruction. There is an assumption that bilingualism is difficult and not attainable for the individual with a language disorder. Therefore, these children are thought better served in English-only education and language intervention.

Research suggests that this assumption is flawed. Bruck (1982) reported that a group of native English-speaking children with language impairments who attended 2 years of French immersion programs achieved cognitive, first-language, and academic test scores comparable to a control group of English-speaking children with language impairments who received English-only language instruction. Thus, these children had no deleterious effects from 2 years of instruction in an L2. The children in this study were from middle-class homes in which the home language and culture were valued by all parties and the home language was maintained in the home.

Research in speech-language pathology supports the hypothesis that the native language is instrumental in helping minority-language children with language impairments develop skills in the native and the majority language (Kiernan & Swisher, 1990; Perrozzi, 1985; Perozzi & Chavez-Sanchez, 1992). Experimental single-subject designs by Kiernan and Swisher (1990) and Perozzi (1985) support the use of the L1 before instructing in the L2 and suggest that a bilingual curriculum is better than teaching only in English.

Role of the Speech-Language Pathologist in Providing Services to Bilingual or Limited English-Proficient Individuals

There are bilingual individuals who are proficient in English or have native or near-native proficiency in English. For these individuals, it is not necessary for clinical services to be provided in the native or L1 of the client. Some bilingual English-proficient individuals may seek the services of a speech-language pathologist to improve pronunciation of English. Speech-language pathologists should follow the guidelines established by the *Position paper: Social dialects and implications of the position on social dialects* (ASHA, 1983).

In 1998, the American Speech-Language-Hearing Association adopted the following position statement on the role of the speech-language pathologist in providing services to persons learning ESL (ASHA, 1998).

> It is the position of the American Speech-Language-Hearing Association that speech-language pathologists who possess the required knowledge and skills to provide English as a second language (ESL) instruction in school settings may provide direct ESL instruction. ESL instruction may require specialized academic preparation and competences in areas such as SLA, comparative linguistics, and ESL methodologies, assessment and practicum. Speech-Language pathologists who do not possess the requisite skills should not provide direct instruction in ESL but should collaborate with ESL instructors in providing pre-assessment, assessment and/or intervention with English as a Second Language speakers in school settings (ASHA, 1998).

Speech-language pathologists play an important role in identifying whether children with limited proficiency in English have an underlying communication disorder. The child's proficiency in English must be distinguished from language development in the L1s and L2s and a true disorder. When the child is determined not to have a speech-language disorder, instruction in developing English as an L2 should be provided by a professional with competence in methodology of ESL. The speech-language pathologist may consult with the ESL instructor at the preassessment, assessment, and intervention stages of ESL services. According to the position paper, in the preassessment stage, the speech-language pathologist may: (1) collaborate with the ESL instructor on issues such as language development and code switching in children who are developing English proficiency, and (2) provide information to and gather data from the ESL instructor on the child's socialization patterns of L1 and L2 development and language use in the classroom and at home.

In the assessment stage, the speech-language pathologist may (1) consult with the provider of ESL instruction on the child's performance on testing completed by the speech-language pathologist and the ESL instructor, and (2) collaborate with the ESL instructor in developing an intervention plan that includes adapting the curricula to meet the child's needs.

During intervention with children and youth with communication disorders, the speech-language pathologist should continue to consult with and collaborate with the ESL instructor. Collaboration between both professionals is an essential aspect of the educational and rehabilitation process and allows both professionals to share in planning, implementation, and evaluation.

Conclusion

Children are capable of learning two languages. Each child brings to the language-learning experience his or her own social, cognitive, and linguistic aptitudes and abilities. No two children are alike because of the multitude of variables that make each child an individual in two language worlds. The age of L2 learning, the environment of language learning, and the educational system that supports or does not support the use of two languages are all part of the language experiences for the bilingual child.

The critical recommendation that the speech-language pathologist can provide to the bilingual family is to maintain the home language through oral language and literacy. The child will learn English in the community and school. The parent is the model for the home language. The foundation that the parent provides in the home language will be the foundation for language learning and literacy in English.

References

Ambert, A. N. (1986a). Identifying language disorders in Spanish-speakers. *Journal in Reading, Writing and Learning Disabilities International,* 2(1), 32–41.

Ambert, A. N. (1986b). Identifying language disorders in Spanish-speakers. In A. C. Willig & H. F. Greenberg (Eds.), *Bilingualism and learning disabilities* (pp. 15–36). New York: American Library Publishing Co., Inc.

American Speech-Language-Hearing Association (1983). Position paper: Social dialects and implications of the position on social dialects, *ASHA, 25*(9), 23–27.

American Speech-Language-Hearing Association (1985). Clinical management of communicatively handicapped minority language populations. *ASHA, 27*(6), 29–32.

American Speech-Language-Hearing Association (1989). Bilingual speech-language pathologists and audiologists. *ASHA, 31,* 93.

American Speech-Language-Hearing Association (1998). Provision of English-as-a-second-language instruction by speech-language pathologists in school settings: position paper and technical report. *ASHA, 40*(Suppl. 18).

Anderson, R. (1999). Impact of first language loss on grammar in a bilingual child. *Communication Disorders Quarterly, 21,* 1, 4–16.

Appel, K., & Muksken, P. (1987). *Language contact and bilingualism.* London: Edward.

Arnberg, L. (1987). Learning two languages: Simultaneous and successive bilingualism. In L. Arnberg (Ed.), *Raising children bilingually: The pre-school years* (pp. 66–73). Philadelphia: Multilingual Matters, LTD.

Beatens-Beardsmore, H. (1982). *Bilingualism: Basic principles.* Boston: College-Hill Press.

Brisk, M. E. (1972). *The Spanish syntax of the preschool Spanish-American: The case of New Mexican five-year-old children.* Unpublished doctoral dissertation, University of New Mexico, Albuquerque, NM.

Brisk, M. E. (1976). The acquisition of Spanish gender by first-grade Spanish-speaking children. In G. D. Keller, R. V. Teschner, & S. Viera (Eds.). *Bilingualism in the bicentennial and beyond* (pp. 143–160). Jamaica, NY: Bilingual Review Press.

Bruck, M. (1982). Language impaired children's performance in an additive bilingual education program. *Applied Psycholinguistics, 3,* 45–60.

Chamot, A. (1988). Bilingualism in education and bilingual education: The state of the art in the United States. *Journal of Multilingual and Multicultural Development, 9*(1), 11–35.

Chesterfield, R., & Chesterfield, K. B. (1985). Natural order in children's use of second language learning strategies. *Applied Linguistics, 6,* 45–59.

Cohen, S. W. (1980). *The sequential order of acquisition of Spanish verb tenses among Spanish-speaking children aged 3–7.* Unpublished doctoral dissertation, University of San Francisco.

Collier, V. (Winter 1987–88). The effect of age on acquisition of a second language for school. *New Focus.*

Conklin, N. F., & Laurie, M. A. (1983). *A host of tongues: Language communities in the United States.* New York: The Free Press.

Corder, S. P. (1967). The significance of learners' errors. *IRAL, 5,* 161–170.

Cummins, J. (1992). The role of primary language development in promoting educational success for language minority students. In C. Leyba (Ed.), *Schooling and language minority students: A theoretical framework.* Los Angeles: California State University.

Dale, P. (1980). *Acquisition of English and Spanish morphological rules by bilinguals.* Unpublished doctoral dissertation, University of Florida, Gainesville.

Damico, J. S., Oller, J. V., Jr., & Storey, M. E. (1983). The diagnosis of language disorders in bilingual children: Surface oriented and pragmatic criteria. *Journal of Speech and Hearing Disorders 48,* 385–394.

Elementary and Secondary Education Act of 1968. *Title VII (also known as the Bilingual Education Act),* Sections 701 et seq., 20 U.S.C.A., Sections 880b et seq. P.L. 90-247, 81 Stat. 783 (Jan. 2, 1968).

Elementary and Secondary Education Act of 1965. Sections 20 U.S.C. 2701 et seq.

Ervin-Tripp S. M. (1974). Is second language learning like learning the first? *TESOL Quarterly, 8*, 111–127.

Fantini, A. E. (1985). *Language acquisition of a bilingual child: A sociolinguistic perspective.* Clevedon, England: Multilingual Matters.

Fradd, S. H. (1987). The changing focus of bilingual education. In S. H. Fradd, & W. J. Tikunoff (Eds.), *Bilingual education and bilingual special education: A guide for administrators* (pp. 1–44). Boston: College-Hill Press.

Garcia, E. (1988). Effective schooling for language minority students. *Focus, 1*, 1–10.

Genesee, F. (1989). Early bilingual development: One language or two? *Child Language, 16*, 161–179.

Goodz, N. S. (1994). Interactions between parents and children in bilingual families. In F. Genesee (Ed.), *Educating second language children: The whole child, the whole curriculum, the whole community* (pp. 61–81). New York: Cambridge University Press.

Gonzalez, G. (1978). *The acquisition of Spanish grammar by native Spanish-speaking children.* Rosslyn, VA: National Clearing House for Bilingual Education.

Grosjean, F. (1982). *Life with two languages: An introduction to bilingualism.* Cambridge, MA: Harvard University Press.

Gutierrez-Clellen, V. F. (1999). Language choice in intervention with bilingual children. *American Journal of Speech-Language Pathology 8*(4), 291–302.

Hakuta, K. (1986). *Mirror of language: The debate on bilingualism.* New York: Basic Books, Inc.

Haugen, E. (1953). *The Norwegian language in America: A study in bilingual behavior* (2 vols.). Philadelphia: University of Pennsylvania Press.

Individuals with Disabilities Education Act (PL 101-476) (1990). 20 U.S.C. 1400.

Itoh, H., & Hutch, E. (1978). Second language acquisition: A case study. In E. Hatch (Ed.), *Second language acquisition: A book of readings* (pp. 76–90). Rowley, MA: Newberry House Publishers.

Kayser, H. (1990). Social communicative behaviors of language disorders Mexican-American students. *Child Language Teaching Therapy, 6*(3), 255–269.

Kayser, H. (1995). *Bilingual speech-language pathology: An Hispanic focus.* San Diego: Singular.

Kessler, C. (1984). Language acquisition in bilingual children. In N. Miller (Ed.), *Bilingualism and language disability* (pp. 26–54). San Diego: College-Hill Press.

Kiernan, B., & Swisher, L. (1990). The initial learning of novel English words: Two single-subject experiments with minority-language children. *Journal of Speech and Hearing Research, 33*, 707–716.

Krashen, S. (1981). *Principles and practice in second language acquisition.* Elmsford, NY: Pergamon Press.

Krashen, S. (1982). *Second language acquisition and second language learning.* New York: Pergamon Press.

Langdon, H. W. (1983). Assessment and intervention strategies for the bilingual language disordered student. *Exceptional Children, 50*(1), 37–46.

Lau v. Nichols, 414 U.S. 563, 39 L. Ed. 2n 1, 94 S. Ct. 786 (1974).

Leopold, W. F. (1949). *Speech development of a bilingual child: A linguist's record* (4 vols.). Evanston, IL: Northwestern University Press.

Linares-Orama, N., & Sanders, L. J. (1977). Evaluation of syntax in three-year-old Spanish-speaking Puerto Rican children. *Journal of Speech and Hearing Research, 20*(2), 350–357.

Maez, L. F. (1983). The acquisition of noun and verb morphology in 18–24 months old Spanish-speaking children. *NABE Journal, 7*, 53–68.

Maldonado, E. (1984). *Profiles of Hispanic students placed in speech, hearing, and language programs in a selected school district in Texas.* Unpublished doctoral dissertation, University of Texas at Austin, Austin.

McLaughlin, B. (1984a). *Second-language acquisition in childhood: Vol. 1 Preschool children* (2nd ed.). Hillsdale, NJ: Lawrence Erlbaum.

McLaughlin, B. (1984b). *Second-language acquisition in childhood: Vol. 2 School-age children* (2nd ed.). Hillsdale, NJ: Lawrence Erlbaum.

Merino, B. (1983). Language development in normal and language handicapped Spanish speaking children. *Hispanic Journal of Behavioral Sciences, 5*(4), 379–400.

Ortiz, A. A. (1984, Spring). Choosing the language of instruction for exceptional bilingual children. *Teaching Exceptional Children,* 208–212.

Ortiz, A., & Maldonado-Colon, E. (1986). Reducing inappropriate referrals of language minority students in special education. In A. C. Willig & H. F. Greenberg (Eds.), *Bilingualism and learning disabilities* (pp. 37–52). New York: American Library.

Parra, R. (1982). *The sequential order of acquisition of categories of Spanish adjectives by Spanish-speaking children of age 2 to 12 years.* Unpublished doctoral dissertation, University of San Francisco.

Patterson, J. L. (1998). Expressive vocabulary development and word combinations of Spanish-English bilingual toddlers. *American Journal of Speech-Language Pathology, 7*, 46–56.

Pearson, B. Z., Fernandez, S. C., & Oller, D. K. (1993). Lexical development in bilingual infants and toddlers: Comparison to monolingual norms. *Language Learning, 43*, 93–100.

Perozzi, J. A. (1985). A pilot study of language facilitation for bilingual, language handicapped children: Theoretical and intervention implications. *Journal of Speech and Hearing Disorders, 50*, 403–406.

Perozzi, J. A., & Chavez-Sanchez, M. L. (1992). The effect of instruction in L1 on receptive acquisition of L2 for bilingual children with language delay. *Language, Speech, and Hearing Services in Schools, 23*, 348–352.

Quay, S. (1995). The bilingual lexicon: Implications for studies of language choice. *Journal of Child Language, 22*, 369–387.

Redlinger, W. E., & Park, T. Z. (1980). Language mixing in young bilinguals. *Journal of Child Language, 7*, 337–352.

Roseberry-McKibbin, C. (1995). Distinguishing language difference from language disorder in linguistically and culturally diverse students. *Multicultural Education, 4*, 12–16.

Saville-Troike (1978). *Guide to culture in the classroom.* Roslyn, VA: National Clearinghouse for Bilingual Education.

Schiff-Myers, N. B. (1992). Considering arrested language development and language loss in assessment of second language learners. *Language, Speech, and Hearing Services in the Schools, 23*, 28–33.

Skoceylas, R. B. (1971). *Language usage estimate.* Albuquerque, NM: University of New Mexico.

Skutnabb-Kangas, T. (1995). Multibilingualism and the education for minority children. In O. Garcia & C. Baker (Eds.). *Policy and practice in bilingual education: Extending the foundations* (pp. 40–62). Clevedon, UK: Multilingual Matters Ltd.

Tabors, P. O., & Snow, C. E. (1994). English as a second language in preschool programs. In F. Genesee (Ed.), *Educating second language children: The whole child, the whole curriculum, the whole community* (pp. 103–125). New York: Cambridge University Press.

Taeschner, T. (1983). *The sun is feminine: A study on language acquisition in bilingual children.* New York: Springer-Verlag.

Taylor, O. (1986). Historical perspectives and conceptual framework. In O. Taylor (Ed.), *Nature of communication disorders in culturally and linguistically diverse populations* (pp. 1–18). San Diego: College-Hill Press.

U.S. General Accounting Office. (2001). *Meeting the needs of students with limited bilingual proficiency.* Washington, DC: United States General Accounting Office.

Valdes, G. (1997). Dual-language immersion programs: A cautionary note concerning the education of language-minority students. *Harvard Educational Review 67*(3), 391–429.

Vihman, M. M. (1985). Language differentiation by the bilingual infant. *Journal of Child Language, 12,* 297–324.

Volterra, V., & Taeschner, T. (1978). The acquisition and development of language by bilingual children. *Journal of Child Language, 5,* 311–326.

Wong-Fillmore, L. (1979). Individual differences in second language acquisition. In C. Fillmore, D. Kempler, & W. S. Wang (Eds.), *Individual differences in language ability and language behavior* (pp. 203–228). New York: Academic Press, Inc.

Wong-Fillmore, L. (1991, September). The no cost study on LEP families with children who have been in preschool programs. *Early Childhood Research Quarterly.*

8

Multicultural Issues in the Management of Neurogenic Communication and Swallowing Disorders

John D. Tonkovich

In this century, speech-language pathologists in the United States will face many new opportunities as a result of the changing composition of the American population. We are gradually becoming a country inhabited by persons with a great deal of diversity relative to traits such as ethnicity, race, and religion. Not everyone speaks English, nor is everyone monolingual. Further, those who have studied diversity issues in our country generally agree that there is heterogeneity within each so-called multicultural group. For instance, Spanish speakers and those of Spanish-speaking descent are often categorized as *Hispanic*. Some of these individuals are Mexican, Caribbean, Puerto Rican, Spainish, and from a variety of other countries and national origins who may concomitantly possess different combinations of African, Indian, and European influences (Kayser, 1998). That individuals or their relatives, or both, speak Spanish does not make them a homogeneous group. Clearly there is diversity among each subcategory of Hispanic individuals as well. Baker (2000) also reminds us that culture does not necessarily correspond with racial or ethnic background, and within each broad cultural group are variations resulting from factors such as age, gender, socioeconomic status, educational level, and individual differences that cut across cultural backgrounds.

The American Speech-Language-Hearing Association (2001) noted that 7.5% of its member speech-language pathologists represented membership in a racial or ethnic minority group, compared with 17.7% in the population of the United States. It is also interesting to note that the speech-language pathologists in this country are overwhelmingly women. Projections from the U.S. Bureau of the Census (2001) for the first decade of this century suggest that there will be increases in the proportion of non-Hispanic black and Asian and Pacific Islander Americans, Hispanic Americans, and foreign-born individuals living in the United States. During this time frame, the proportion of non-Hispanic American Indian residents is expected to remain relatively constant, whereas the proportion of non-Hispanic white Americans will decline.

Interestingly, during the next several decades, there will be a dramatic increase in the proportion of individuals in the United States who are elderly. Consequently, it is anticipated that the demand for speech-language pathology services for adults with neurogenic communication and swallowing disorders will increase dramatically as well.

Attention to diversity issues is now routinely considered a part of the standards adopted by professional organizations and other accrediting bodies. The American Speech-Language-Hearing Association has standards for clinical certification in speech-language pathology and for accreditation of graduate programs in speech-language pathology that require practicum and courses dealing with multicultural issues across the life span. The Association's position paper on social dialects (ASHA, 1983) clarified that dialectal variations of the English language are not communication disorders. In 1985, the Association identified competencies that were necessary for the delivery of speech-language pathology services to those from culturally and linguistically diverse populations (ASHA, 1985). There are also medical rehabilitation accreditation standards that require health care organizations to demonstrate sensitivity to the cultural and religious practices of the persons they serve (Commission on Accreditation of Rehabilitation Facilities, 2001). The profession is challenged, therefore, to prepare culturally competent professionals to meet the communication and swallowing needs of a growing number of individuals from a variety of backgrounds, religions, and beliefs.

It is highly likely that speech-language pathologists will see an increase in the number of elderly clients with neurogenic communication and swallowing disorders and who may require special accommodations for their cultural and linguistic diversity. Therefore, it is imperative that clinicians have a mechanism for taking into account the variety of influences that might affect service delivery. One of the challenges in particular for speech-language pathologists is to determine the extent to which their clients from multicultural backgrounds differ or deviate from their multicultural peer group. This may be particularly important when assessing individuals who have suffered communication and swallowing losses as a result of cerebrovascular accidents or other neurologic disorders. Speech-language pathologists need to determine not only the best approaches for assessment but also suitable treatment approaches considering each client's unique ethnic, cultural, and religious background.

Some have advocated for the use of interpreters and translators in the provision of speech-language pathology services to those from culturally and linguistically diverse groups (Kayser, 2001; Wallace, 1997). Interpreters are those who interpret one language or dialect into a second one orally, whereas translators are those who interpret one language or dialect into a second in writing. There may be benefits and hindrances to the use of interpreters. These individuals can be assets to the speech-language pathologist, not only in assisting with removing language barriers, but they may also serve as resources for cultural issues. On the other hand, sometimes interpreters fail to convey accurate information because something is lost in the interpretation, or they may convey too much information to the client in the ways they communicate, cues, hints, or even answers. Sometimes interpreters are paid paraprofessionals who might engage in activities such as screening of speech, language, or hearing, treatment activities that don't require clinical decision making, chart recording, clinical record maintenance, preparation of clinical materials (Kayser, 2001), and feeding of dysphagic patients. Although the use of paid paraprofessionals and interpreters may be advantageous and sometimes occurs in school settings, it is rare to see such individuals employed in the health care settings in which services are delivered to those with adult clients with neurogenic communication and swallowing disorders. Most health care institutions in recent years have experienced dramatic reductions in reimbursement for rehabilitation services, and it would be rare that interpreter fees would be budgeted. It is incumbent on speech-language pathologists in health care settings to rely on other resources to meet the demands of their clients from multicultural groups.

A number of recent works have addressed specifically the potential influences on neurogenic communication and swallowing service delivery to African Americans (Wallace & Tonkovich, 1997), Asian Americans (Cheng, Breakey, & Wallace, 1997), Pacific Islander Americans (Mashima, Goo-Yoshino, & Wallace, 1997), Native Americans (Wallace, Inglebret, & Friedlander, 1997), and Hispanic Americans (Reyes & Peterson, 1997), among other groups. Authors of these works have attempted to identify prominent cultural mores, communication patterns, spiritual orientation, and food preferences for specific cultural groups. In general, they have advocated for a model that takes into account the ways in which a particular client from a culturally or linguistically diverse group differs from what might be expected in someone from the so-called majority population. As mentioned previously, it is clear that even within a particular racial or ethnic group, there is no homogeneity. For example, many African American individuals identify themselves as members of Protestant religions (Wallace & Tonkovich, 1997), but some are Catholic, Jewish, Muslim, and some practice other religions. These affiliations might affect dietary customs, views of life, illness, death, and the will of a higher power. It is interesting to know what some members of multicultural groups feel and think and do. Although it is important to consider these factors when diagnosing and treating communication disorders, it would be impossible and beyond the scope of this chapter to identify every possible combination of ethnic, racial, cultural, socioeconomic, and religious identity and attempt to speculate about how individuals with those attributes should be treated. It is difficult, if not unreasonable, to implement a treatment model that focuses solely on the ways in which clients who identify with a particular multicultural group *differ* from the majority population, when these clients likely differ also from members of their own groups.

In addition to focusing treatment for communicatively disordered clients from culturally and linguistically diverse backgrounds with sensitivities to their differences, it would appear to be of benefit to consider how these clients are *similar* to communicatively disordered individuals from the majority population and other groups. That is to say, individuals who suffer a cerebrovascular accident involving the left hemisphere will often have similar aphasic attributes, regardless of their multicultural identity (or lack thereof). There may be some speech-language pathology interventions and procedures that transcend ethnic, racial, and religious parameters. Some may be better suited for individuals from *all* backgrounds by virtue of their effect on communication or swallowing outcomes.

This chapter, therefore, offers a framework for the delivery of speech-language pathology services to individuals from a variety of ethnic, racial, cultural, and religious backgrounds. Central to this framework are the notions that individuals from multicultural groups may present with symptoms that are different *and* similar to others from other groups. Discussion in this chapter takes into consideration the fact that a number of diagnostic and treatment practices currently used by speech-language pathologists might be culturally biased and might be viewed as alienating individuals from some multicultural groups. However, there are some innovative and contemporary diagnostic and treatment methodologies that might actually transcend membership in a particular multicultural group, and these methodologies are identified and discussed.

Multicultural Considerations

When managing clients from culturally or linguistically diverse groups, speech-language pathologists must ascertain which of several differences might be relevant to service delivery. These might include cultural, linguistic, religious, nonverbal communication, and, for dysphagic clients, food preference issues. Sensitivity to relevant issues such as these will maximize the effectiveness of the speech-language pathology interventions and will improve the functional outcomes of these interventions. The extent to which particular issues are relevant might be ascertained best by clinicians through an extensive and detailed case history. Case history information should include, but is not limited to (1) languages or dialects used; (2) relative preference for one language or dialect over the other; (3) communication contexts, topics, and partners; (4) the client's role in the family and in the community; (5) the client's educational level, socioeconomic status, vocational, and avocational interests; and, for dysphagic clients, (6) food preferences.

The discussion now focuses on identifying *some* of these issues that may be relevant for adults from multicultural groups with neurogenic communication and swallowing disorders. It is not intended to be a detailed listing of *all* of the issues that could potentially affect service delivery but should serve as a guide to clinicians about factors to consider in planning assessment and treatment activities for adults with neurogenic communication and swallowing difficulties.

Cultural Issues

Speech-language pathologists should be particularly attentive to possible influences of cultural factors that might influence how they deliver services to those adults with neurogenic communication and swallowing difficulties. One of the first things clinicians should attempt to determine is the extent to which their clients were acculturated to the mainstream American society. Many Americans who were born in other countries readily adapt to and take on American cultural characteristics, whereas many others do not. Many African Americans assimilate into the mainstream American culture, whereas many others do not. When clinicians overlook important cultural factors, clients may appear to be more impaired than they actually are.

For instance, speech-language pathologists working with those from culturally and linguistically diverse groups should be particularly sensitive to materials and tasks that introduce cultural biases into clinical management activities. On the *Boston Naming Test* (Kaplan, Goodglass, & Weintraub, 2001), for example, one of the pictured items that must be identified is "asparagus." The cue that is provided for this item when it is missed is "something to eat." Abdelal (1997) stated that asparagus is not known as an edible plant in Arabic culture. In fact, a type of plant that looks like asparagus sometimes grows as a parasite and is managed as a weed by Arabic farmers. Bilingual aphasics from Arabic countries would never consider that asparagus would be "something to eat." This example underscores a need for speech-language pathologists to have some *a priori* knowledge about the cultural backgrounds of their clients.

Many Native Americans (i.e., American Indians and indigenous Alaskans) live on federal Indian reservations or indigenous Alaskan villages. Many of those living on these set-aside lands have limited access to adult rehabilitation services, and many live in poverty (Wallace, Inglebret, & Friedlander, 1997). A proportion of reservation Indians live in dwellings without running water, indoor toilet facilities, or electricity, and most do not have cellular telephones or telephones in their homes. Also, for many tribal and native groups, silence is an integral part of the culture and the communication process and may be evidenced by longer latencies when answering questions. These latencies may reflect the individual's demonstration of respect for the communication partner, organization of one's thoughts, or maintenance of privacy, among other reasons (Wallace, Inglebret, & Friedlander, 1997). Many standardized assessment tools for aphasia and for cognitive-communication dysfunction require responses that may lie outside the realm of experience for many American Indian and indigenous Alaskan clients. Clinicians unfamiliar with the culture of these clients might mistake longer response latencies for impaired performance and penalize clients accordingly as they score these assessment instruments.

Kayser (2001) suggested some ways in which test instruments and procedures might be modified to more accurately reflect communication performance of those from multicultural groups and to minimize cultural biases. One way involves administering a test using standardized procedures, then re-administering it by altering procedures to accommodate the needs of the client (e.g., longer response latencies allowed, rewording and rephrasing instructions). Another suggestion was to adapt the test instrument so that it becomes culturally appropriate for a particular target population. For instance, instead of requesting that aphasic clients with Arabic backgrounds name the item "asparagus" on visual confrontation, the item "date" (the fruit) might be substituted.

Other issues may relate to the way in which elders are treated within particular multicultural groups. Many African Americans, Asian Americans, and Hispanic Americans place a high value on obedience and revere parents and elders for their wisdom and hindsight. For this reason, speech-language pathologists should refrain from using the first names of elderly clients unless asked to do so and should refer to older clients using formal titles such as "Mr.," "Mrs.," and "Reverend" (Cheng, Breakey, & Wallace, 1997; Pena, 1998; Reyes & Peterson, 1997; Wallace & Tonkovich, 1997). Speech-language pathologists refrain from confusing the titles "Miss" and "Mrs." so as not to insult some older Hispanic women (Pena, 1998). Clinicians talking to older Native Americans may wish to show respect by listening intently with the head down and without direct eye contact or risk being interpreted as being disrespectful (Wallace, Inglebret, & Friedlander, 1997). Strong ties to family characterize many cultural groups. Consequently, speech-language pathologists may wish to engage family members actively in the treatment process to capitalize on those relationships and to facilitate generalization of newly acquired communication or swallowing behaviors, or both.

Cheng, Breakey, and Wallace (1997) remind clinicians that well-educated Asian American clients might be offended by materials and procedures that are viewed as childlike or childish. This admonition is applicable for members across cultural groups. When possible, clinicians might wish to incorporate materials that have particular relevance for the individuals they treat.

It is often customary in many Asian American and other homes for people to remove their shoes before entering the home. Speech-language pathologists providing home-based speech-language pathology services, to meet health department requirements and to be respectful of clients, might wish to bring a pair of slippers or disposable shoe coverings to prevent offending clients and their families.

In summary, clinicians should be cognizant of cultural factors that might affect their service delivery to those from multicultural groups. Lack of attention to these factors might lead to mistaken diagnoses or to the risk of offending clients and their families. Clients and their families will appreciate adaptations to testing and treatment procedures to accommodate relevant cultural issues of clients.

Linguistic Issues

A number of linguistic issues that are unrelated to a neurogenic communication disorder may affect speech-language pathology service delivery. For bilingual clients with communication disorders, clinicians should attempt to discern the extent to which each language was spoken. For example, Ortiz (1993) estimated that approximately 65% of Hispanic Americans are bilingual. Of these individuals, it is estimated that 19.0% use Spanish exclusively, 56.0% use both languages but prefer Spanish, 12.5% use both languages but prefer English, and 12.5% use English only. Code switching, the alternating use of two languages, is a phenomenon commonly observed in many bilingual Hispanic American communities. It occurs in other cultural groups as well, including code switching between Standard English and African American Vernacular for some African American clients. Code switching should be assessed and managed in those with neurogenic communication disorders (Reyes & Peterson, 1997). Code switching is influenced by a variety of situational variables, including the conversational participants, setting, and topic. Code-switching goals may be appropriately included in the treatment plans of aphasic clients who code switched before the onset of aphasia but have difficulty post-onset.

Many Asian languages and Chinese languages in particular, as well as some Native American languages, are tonal. That is, there may be several words with the same segmental composition but that differ in suprasegmental aspects (Ryalls & Behrens, 2000). A word may be misspoken because of an incorrect tonal pattern and not because of the segmental production. This is often particularly challenging for speech-language pathologists who are not fluent in tonal languages to assess, even when an interpreter is used (Cheng, 1997).

Tonal influences might be particularly noticeable when speakers of the tonal language are dysarthric, as suprasegmental aspects of speech production might be altered. In these situations, speech-language pathologists must rely on the assistance of interpreters or family members. When clients mispronounce a word (because of impaired tonal patterning), speech-language pathologists may need to compare the mispronunciation with the interpreter's or family member's correct production of the targeted word and then compare the auditory perceptual contrasts between the two. This procedure might enable the clinician to intervene in a way that facilitates correct production of these tonal differences.

Linguistic prosody may be relevant for other clients as well. Many African American clients use African American Vernacular, an English dialect that has distinctive phonologic, semantic, syntactic, and pragmatic features and one that is rich in prosodic variety. In contrast, the prosodic patterns of West Indian American clients may reflect pronunciations and speech rhythm patterns that are unlike those in African American Vernacular. African natives who speak English and some African language(s) may have yet another characteristic set of prosodic patterns. Clinicians should attempt to incorporate relevant linguistic prosody variables into treatment plans as appropriate.

Not all African American clients use African American Vernacular, and some may only use some features of the dialect in specific contexts. Speech-language pathologists should not make the assumption that all clients speak the vernacular. Some persons, particularly those with acquired Broca's aphasia, may delete grammatical morphemes that they used before the onset of aphasia.

For bilingual speakers, clinicians should also take into account linguistic features of the native language that may have some influence on production in English. Arabic speakers, for example, customarily place adjectives and possessive pronouns after the nouns they modify. Prepositional use may differ from that in English, and there is no indefinite article (Abdelal, 1997). Clinicians should not mistake syntactic differences in aphasic clients as syntactic errors, and should consider the linguistic rules of the native language before diagnosing syntactic aphasic disturbances.

Bilingual clients and those who speak more than one English dialect require additional consideration by speech-language pathologists. During assessments, clinicians must determine the extent to which English (or standard English dialect) was used or preferred, the degree to which the client was able to code switch, and linguistic rules and patterns that may have influenced pronunciation and usage before the onset of the neurogenic communication disorder to accurately determine the client's communicative proficiency post-onset.

Religious Issues

Speech-language pathologists need to be particularly sensitive to religious influences on service delivery. For clients with dysphagia, for example, religious influences might affect when services can be delivered, as well as the foods that can be used during trial feedings.

Some Catholic clients may be restricted from eating meat on Ash Wednesday and on Fridays during the Lenten season before Easter. Many Jewish clients, particularly those who observe Orthodox Judaism, are bound by dietary laws and observances that prohibit certain foods, including pork and shellfish products. In addition, Jewish clients who keep kosher may not be able to eat foods that have not been certified as being kosher for Passover during the Passover season each spring. Some Jewish clients may not wish to participate in treatment sessions that fall on their Sabbath—from sundown on Friday to sundown on Saturday—and some Christian clients may not wish to receive treatment on Sundays.

Several factors may need to be considered in the delivery of speech-language pathology services to Muslim clients who have communication or swallowing deficits, or both. Many Muslims or followers of Islam may prefer to be treated by clinicians of the same gender (Wallace & Tonkovich, 1997). This may pose a unique challenge for male clients, given that most speech-language pathologists are women. Some Islamic clients observe daily prayer times or participate in *jum'a*—a special noontime prayer on Friday, their holy day (Campbell, 2001)—and speech-language pathology treatments should not be scheduled during this time. Islamic clients celebrate *E'id*, or Ramadan, a month-long period of fasting during daylight hours. It is the ninth month of the Muslim calendar, and, during this time, Muslims cannot eat or drink anything (including water) and may not even chew gum. Speech-language pathologists treating Muslim clients with dysphagia may need to conduct sessions after sundown during Ramadan, when intake of food and liquids is permissible.

The celebration of Ramadan is based on the lunar calendar, and it falls 10 days earlier each year. In addition to fasting, Muslims must take time out to pray five required prayers each day. Provisions for prayer time should be made in the schedules of Muslim clients with neurogenic communication and swallowing difficulties, particularly those who are hospitalized on inpatient rehabilitation units. To qualify for inpatient medical rehabilitation, clients are typically expected to receive at least 3 hours of therapy (i.e., physical therapy, occupational therapy, speech-language therapy) per day. Modifications in scheduling may accommodate those who must pray. It may also be important for Muslim aphasic clients to have a nonaphasic family member or friend join them in prayer. Muslim clients may also prefer not to have home-based speech-language pathology services, because the home is regarded as a private place (Campbell, 2001).

A number of assessment instruments and commercially available workbook activities include some items that relate to holidays that are customarily celebrated in the United States. Members of the Jehovah's Witnesses religion do not celebrate holidays or birthdays and may lack sufficient experience to respond to these items appropriately. Some Native American tribes view the owls and witches at Halloween as omens and may not wish to respond to them (Campbell, 2001).

Some Christian African American clients may view illnesses such as Parkinson's disease and cerebrovascular accidents as arising from divine punishment, as God's reaction to a sinful act (Wallace & Tonkovich, 1997). This notion may pose unique challenges to speech-language pathologists wishing to intervene with these individuals. These persons and their family members may not seek rehabilitation for what has been perceived as "God's will." It is sometimes useful, with permission of the client and family, to speak to the client's clergy to assist in counseling.

Speech-language pathologists should not underestimate the importance of religious influences on service delivery to those with neurogenic communication and swallowing disorders. These factors may affect not only how and when treatment sessions will be conducted but may also have ramifications about the extent to which clients and their families believe that the speech-language pathology treatments will help them.

Nonverbal Communication Issues

Speech-language pathologists need to be aware of nonverbal aspects of communication that might typify some members of culturally diverse groups. An awareness of these nonverbal behaviors will aid speech-language pathologists in interacting with clients and their families, and clinicians will be less likely to misinterpret these nonverbal signals.

Pena (1998) noted that some Hispanic bilingual male patients may characteristically glance at women during treatment rather than make continuous eye contact. In traditional Asian cultures, direct eye contact is not typical (Cheng, Breakey, & Wallace, 1997). The Qur'an commands Muslim men not to look intently at women, and vice versa, so that both genders can avoid arousal and temptation (Ali, 1993). Speech-language pathologists need to be careful not to mistake this lack of eye contact for inattention, particularly in clients who have suffered right hemisphere damage or traumatic brain injuries.

Many Asian Americans bow, smile, and nod reassuringly out of respect for the opinions and statements of the clinician, even when they don't understand or agree with what was said (Cheng, Breakey, & Wallace, 1997). These behaviors not only show respect but also serve as an attempt not to offend or cause conflict. Out of politeness, Arab clients may show agreement with the clinician even though they disagree and then not follow through with the intervention (Shariefzadeh, 1992). Clinicians should make certain that clients and their families understand and agree with what has been said.

In Arab cultures, touching during conversation is acceptable only between members of the same gender. Clinicians might implement treatment approaches that involve touching or hand holding such as melodic intonation therapy (Sparks, 2001) and unknowingly risk offending or alienating clients. Similarly, the clinician should not hold his or her hand out to shake hands with a member of Arabic culture unless that member initiates the handshaking (Abdelal, 1997).

Wallace, Inglebret, and Friedlander (1997) suggested that Native Americans may be offended at having to perform tasks that have no apparent meaning for them (e.g., sticking out the tongue, repeating syllables for diadochokinetic testing). This is particularly true when the clinician is younger than the patient.

A number of nonverbal aspects of communication may be different for some members of various multicultural groups. Speech-language pathologists should familiarize themselves with these issues to ensure that they do not misdiagnose reduced eye contact during conversations and that they do not offend clients and their families, among other things.

Food Preference Issues

Dysphagic clients from multicultural groups may pose unique challenges to speech-language pathologists, particularly when pureed foods are indicated. Some Japanese clients prefer noodles and fish at breakfast, and Caribbean clients may prefer fish at breakfast as well (Campbell, 2001). These may be difficult to prepare in a pureed consistency. Some clients from Hispanic cultures may prefer pureeing home-prepared foods instead of using commercially pureed baby foods (Palacio, 2000). Clinicians may need to be creative in recommending foods that would be pleasing to clients, as most pureed foods lack aesthetic appeal as it is.

Many African Americans have preferences for foods that are high in fat and salt content, and this is viewed as one factor contributing to the higher incidence of cerebrovascular accidents observed among them. Even though the diet of these individuals might include vitamin-rich cooked greens, they are often seasoned with pork fat or bacon (Wallace & Tonkovich, 1997). These factors might play a role in the selection of foods for persons with dysphagia and for any stroke prevention education activities.

In Native American communities, food is commonly shared with others. Consequently, some individuals might not understand receiving food to be consumed individually during dysphagia treatment sessions. Speech-language pathologists providing home-based dysphagia treatments for Native Americans may be obligated to accept food and drink when it is offered (Higheagle, 1995). Doing so will serve to establish rapport between the speech-language pathologist and clients and their families.

To summarize, in assessing clients from multicultural groups, speech-language pathologists should make certain that they have attended to relevant cultural, linguistic, religious, nonverbal communication, and food preference issues. Attention to these issues will result in more accurate assessment of the extent of impairment and will likely help to establish a bond between the clinician and clients and their families.

A Framework for Clinical Management

Once speech-language pathologists have ascertained the extent to which their clients from multicultural groups differ from those of the mainstream American society and have conducted evaluations, it is necessary to develop clinical interventions that address the neurogenic communication or swallowing disorders, or both. Some interventions might be more appropriately used with clients from multicultural groups and may be more effective and efficient.

Speech-language pathology interventions have a number of philosophic bases that guide them, and speech-language pathologists generally focus interventions relative to those philosophic bases. These philosophies include the degree to which a person's level of functioning can be restored to premorbid levels, the degree of external assistance or supervision needed, and the presumed impact on the person's quality of life, among other factors. Unfortunately, many neurogenic communication and swallowing disorders are not completely reversible, so individuals that have them must deal with chronic, residual effects. They may be dependent on others in the environment to assist them to maintain a reasonable quality of life.

The Joint Commission on Accreditation of Healthcare Organizations (1999) attempted to identify some of these philosophic bases and specified a definition of rehabilitation outcomes. Rehabilitation outcomes were defined as restoration, improvement, or maintenance of the patient's optimal level of functioning, self-care, self-responsibility, independence, and quality of life. Speech-language pathology interventions for those with neurogenic communication and swallowing disorders, regardless of cultural identity, have focused disproportionately on attempts to *restore* individuals to prior levels of functioning, instead of focusing on attempts to *improve* the level of functioning in spite of the chronic residual effects. By their very nature, restorative interventions have focused heavily on didactic and repetitive task interventions. There is reason to believe that these interventions may not be appropriate for those from some multicultural groups.

In recent years, a new model that is applicable also to specifying the philosophic bases of neurogenic communication and swallowing disorder interventions has increased in popularity. This model specifies distinctions among *impairments, activities,* and *participation* (World Health Organization, 1997). In the context of health conditions, *impairments* refer to loss or abnormalities of body structures or physiologic or psychological functions. *Activities* relate to the nature and degree of functioning at the level of the person and may be limited in nature, duration, and quality. *Participation* refers to the nature and extent of a person's involvement in life situations relative to impairments, activities, health conditions, and contextual factors. Most speech-language pathology interventions for those with neurogenic etiologies have focused on impairments and activities, and there have been obscure generalization processes to reduce participation restrictions (Worrall, 2000). Such interventions rely on formal tests and treatment probes to determine the level of deficit and degree of change after therapy (Simmons-Mackie, 2001). Holland (1994), advocating for a model that reduced participation restrictions for aphasic individuals, suggested methods that worked directly within the social context of communication, in spite of impairments and activity limitations.

Process Orientation to Treatment

It is necessary to identify those treatment approaches that lead to a reduction of participation restrictions. Myers (1999) contrasted two speech-language pathology treatment approaches, a task-oriented one and a process-oriented one. Task-oriented treatments focus on improving a specific activity and are designed to focus on the symptoms of a communication or swallowing disorder as opposed to the cause. These approaches are often highly individualized to the client and often are of immediate functional use. The speech-language pathologist typically delivers task-oriented treatment directly, in an individual session that is devoid of context or other communication partners. For persons with anomic aphasia, for example, it might be determined that the person has difficulty saying words associated with making food choices. Task-oriented treatment for this aphasic person might focus on visual confrontation naming of photographs of various food choices. When the person is able to retrieve the words associated with the pictured items with reasonable consistency, task-oriented treatment might focus on the visual confrontation naming of photographs from some other semantic category. That the aphasic person is able to say the names of pictured food items does not necessarily imply that the person will be able to say the names of other food items not trained or request those foods when ordering in a restaurant. The underlying assumption in task-oriented treatment is that discrete trials in performing the treatment task will somehow generalize to some sort of functional use of the task behavior. The use and practicality of task-oriented treatment may not be apparent to and particularly alienating for those from multicultural groups and for those non-English speakers. Clinicians providing task-oriented treatments also face a greater likelihood of introducing culturally biased vocabulary or other assumptions into the treatment regimen.

Process-oriented treatment approaches address the mechanisms that are underlying disabilities and, as such, focus primarily on the cause rather than the symptoms. As such, they are likely to have direct impact on the reduction of participation restrictions. Process-oriented treatments address several functions indirectly and simultaneously and have greater potential for generalization. Often, process-oriented treatments provide some sort of contextual framework or other conversational partners, or both. Persons with anomic aphasia receiving process-oriented treatments, for instance, might be provided with a number of word retrieval strategies that facilitated access to the mental lexicon. Significant others in the lives of these aphasic persons also might be instructed about these strategies, so that they may assist when the aphasic persons have word retrieval difficulties. Once aphasic persons and significant other communicative partners know how to use the strategies, presumably the strategies will work for all word classes. Inclusion of others from the client's social and familial milieus facilitates generalization and helps minimize the effects of cultural bias in the treatment.

Process-oriented treatment approaches are appropriately used with clients from multicultural groups who have neurogenic communication or swallowing disorders. They have greater potential for generalization and work to reduce participation restrictions. In the following discussion, we will identify some process-oriented treatment approaches for those with aphasia, cognitive-communication disorders, dementia, dysarthria, and dysphagia. These approaches take into account similarities about the disorders that transcend membership in a culturally or ethnically diverse group.

Aphasia Treatment Methodologies

Traditional treatment models for aphasia have been derived from a medical model, because clinicians plan and control treatment because of their expertise, with little participation from clients who are passive and dependent (Pyypponen, 1993; Simmons-Mackie, 2001). When treatment efforts that have focused on *restoring* communication functioning to premorbid levels have been exhausted and individuals have not made complete recoveries, speech-language therapy is discontinued, and these individuals are left to cope with the residual effects (Hersh, 1998). Several aphasia treatment methodologies would appear to be advantageous in engaging the client and significant others actively and preparing them to cope with residual effects.

Simmons-Mackie (2000, 2001) advocated for a social model of aphasia management that is designed to reduce the social consequences of aphasia, promote the individual's participation in a social world, and reduce participation restrictions. She stated that although aphasia therapy efficacy research often pointed to improved modification of behavior in task-oriented approaches, the importance of these findings was irrelevant if the changes failed to make a difference in the lives of the persons being treated.

Pressures from third-party payers and increasingly decreased funding for speech-language therapy for aphasic individuals have provided some of the impetus for a social approach to aphasia therapy (Gonzales-Rothi, 1996). More significant influences have come from interviews with aphasic persons and their families. Individuals with aphasia have reported discrimination against them because of impaired communication, social isolation, loss of access to work, education and leisure pursuits, and a reduction of community supports (Parr, 1996; Simmons-Mackie, 2000).

Table 8-1   Principles of a Social Model of Aphasia Management

Communication is designed to meet the dual goals of social interaction and transaction of messages.
Communication is a flexible, dynamic, multidimensional activity.
Aphasia management should emphasize authentic, relevant, and natural contexts.
Conversation should be considered as a primary site of human communication.
Communication is a collaborative achievement.
Aphasia management activities should focus on the social and personal consequences of aphasia.
Aphasia management activities should focus on adaptations rather than impairments.
Aphasia management activities should emphasize the perspectives of the person with aphasia.
Clinicians should embrace qualitative as well as quantitative outcome measures.

Source: Adapted from Simmons-Mackie, N. N. (2000). Social approaches to the management of aphasia. In L. E. Worrall & C. M. Frattali (Eds.), *Neurogenic communication disorders: A functional approach* (pp. 162–188). New York: Thieme.

Simmons-Mackie (2000, 2001) outlined the principles underlying the social approach to aphasia management, and these are provided in Table 8-1. Communication serves dual goals, one involving the exchange of information or transaction and the other involving the fulfillment of social needs or interaction. For aphasia management to be successful, it must focus on both of these goals. That communication is flexible and dynamic takes into account the fact that nonaphasic individuals often have communicative exchanges in which the phonologic, semantic, syntactic, or pragmatic aspects, or all, of messages deviate from an idealized norm. It is assumed that aphasia treatment with a social focus would take this into account and evaluate performance not in terms of how accurate an utterance is, but the extent to which it achieves social or communicative goals, or both.

Instead of evaluating the performance of individuals with aphasia relative to an unnatural "therapy" context, the social model promotes judging success made in authentic, natural contexts that are relevant to the aphasic person. Social approaches emphasize natural conversation between the aphasic person and others so that it is a collaborative achievement.

A social approach to aphasia management also takes into account the social consequences of aphasia. Simmons (1993) reported that aphasic clients failed to use learned compensatory strategies when the behaviors would be "stigmatizing" within their social communities. Sometimes social and personal consequences for persons with aphasia outweigh their ability to use communication strategies successfully. Social approaches to aphasia management also focus on adaptive behaviors. Some bilingual speakers, for instance, might experience a word retrieval difficulty in one language and produce the proffered word in the other language, using this to alert the conversational partner that a word search is in progress.

The social approach to aphasia management is respectful of the perspective of the person with aphasia. The author recently treated an elderly African American man with severe global aphasia. He was able to communicate his needs adequately via drawing, yet he and his wife perceived this as a social stigma. He preferred to remain silent rather than face embarrassment as a non-oral communicator. The social approach to intervention, instead of abandoning the idea of having the man use drawing as a communication modality, might focus on identifying the social barriers that inhibit the use of drawing outside of therapy and then address those barriers (Simmons-Mackie, 2000).

In a social model of aphasia intervention, there is a focus on qualitative as well as quantitative measures. Instead of having the clinician identify how the aphasic person is doing objectively, the client subjectively evaluates his or her own progress.

Social approaches to aphasia intervention focus on conversation and not on production of discrete responses to specific stimuli. It may be necessary for clients to learn compensatory strategies to manage their aphasic deficits. Tonkovich (1998) identified some strategies for managing word retrieval difficulties, and these are identified in Table 8-2. These strategies enable the aphasic client to compensate for difficulties with word retrieval and to keep conversations moving. For strategies that may be unlike those used by their nonaphasic conversational partners, it may be necessary to engage the nonaphasic partners in using interactive drawing (Lyon, 1995) or pantomime (Demchuk, 1996).

Simmons-Mackie and Damico (1997) suggested that, in selecting compensatory strategies, clinicians consider factors such as the amount of communicative burden placed on the nonaphasic partner (e.g., guessing what a gesture is); stigma associated with the strategy (e.g., amount of attention called to it); naturalness; time constraints; effect on the flow of the interaction; and appropriateness in a specific context (e.g., cultural norms). It becomes crucial therefore for clinicians to include training for communicative partners of aphasic clients.

Partners learn concrete strategies to use when aphasia interferes, helps the aphasic client use augmentative communication tools, and encourages communicative interactions with aphasic speakers. One approach that has been used in this manner is supported conversation training for aphasia (Kagan, 1998; Kagan & Gailey, 1993; Kagan et al., 2001). This approach relies on the use of community volunteers who are specifically interested in talking to people with aphasia and helping them with their communication. Volun-

Table 8-2   Word Retrieval Strategies for Aphasia

Try to use another word that means the same thing. For example, say "sofa" if you can't think of "couch."

Try to describe the word. For example, say "a black and white smelly animal" if you can't think of the word "skunk."

Try to think of the first letter of the word.

Try to think of the first sound of the word.

Try to write the word.

Try to gesture or pantomime the word. For example, show with your hand how you would play a ukulele, even if you can't think of the word "ukulele."

Try to draw a picture of the word you are trying to say.

Try to say what the word is not. For example, "It's not a tiger, it's not a leopard, it's not a lion. . . . "

Use the first word that comes to mind, even if it's the wrong word. Sometimes the word you think of will be similar to the one you are trying to say, like "caramel" for "carousel."

Try to find the item, and show it to someone.

Wait and stop thinking about the word. Sometimes it will come to you on its own.

Source: Reprinted with permission from Tonkovich, J. D. (1998). Management of communicative and swallowing disorders in non-acute settings. In A. F. Johnson & B. F. Jacobson (Eds.), *Medical speech-language pathology: A practitioner's guide.* New York: Thieme.

teers are trained in using resources, question forms, gesture and pantomime, interactive drawing, responding to receptive problems, alerting to topic initiation and change, giving adequate processing time, use of simultaneous multimodal input, and reflection of messages (Kagan & Gailey, 1993; Kagan et al., 2001). One additional advantage of using this approach is that it also facilitates communication with people who speak another language.

The training of conversational partners is crucial to process-oriented interventions for aphasic clients. Speech-language pathologists might recruit and train partners from the client's community, thereby decreasing the social participation restrictions of the aphasic clients. Partners can learn strategies for facilitating expression by learning to encourage the use of pantomime, drawing, or writing. Some strategies partners might learn to facilitate comprehension are listed in Table 8-3. When partners use these strategies effectively they are of immediate functional gain to the aphasic client.

Aphasia interventions that focus on processes necessary for successful communicative interactions help keep the aphasic client communicating. They also help family members and friends learn how to communicate with the aphasic client. These interventions transcend membership in a particular multicultural group and serve to minimize the participation restrictions associated with aphasia.

Table 8-3   Auditory Comprehension Strategies for Conversational Partners of Aphasic Patients

Keep your sentences short and simple.

Repeat what you say two or three times.

Use gestures and pointing to supplement what you are saying.

Write down the key words about the topic you are talking about. For example, if you want to let your partner know that you have to go to the store to get some milk, you might write the words "store" and "milk" when you say them. Point to the printed words and say them again to help your partner understand what you're saying.

When you ask a yes or no question, try asking it a different way and see if your partner responds the same way. For instance, if you ask "Do you want the channel changer?" and he/she says "no," then ask, "Do you want to turn the TV off?" and see if he/she still says "no." Often people who have difficulty understanding following a stroke say "yes" more often than "no," even when they mean "no." Sometimes they say "no" when they mean "yes." Asking questions several different ways will help you figure out what your partner really wants.

Make sure you have his/her attention before speaking to him/her. You might try letting him/her know you have something to say to him/her by calling his/her name or prefacing your remarks with an alerting sentence like "Here's something for you."

Source: Reprinted with permission from Tonkovich, J. D. (1998). Management of communicative and swallowing disorders in non-acute settings. In A. F. Johnson, & B. F. Jacobson (Eds.), *Medical speech-language pathology: A practitioner's guide.* New York: Thieme.

Methodologies for Cognitive-Communication Disorders

Process-oriented treatment approaches for individuals with cognitive-communication disorders stemming from right hemisphere cerebrovascular accidents or traumatic brain injuries also focus on providing clients and their communicative partners with strategies to maximize the likelihood of successful interactions. Cherney and Halper (2000) identified the *cognitive* impairments in cognitive-communication disorders as including the processes of attention, perception, memory, organization, reasoning and problem solving, and the chief *communication* impairment in pragmatic aspects of communication. Traumatically brain-injured clients often have concomitant word retrieval difficulties.

Larkins, Worrall, and Hickson (2000) advocated integrating treatment activities for those with cognitive-communication disorders into real-life experiences such as shopping and social interaction. Such interventions might focus on compensatory strategy training, functional skills training, and environmental adaptation.

Compensatory strategy training consists of teaching clients ways to compensate for the impairment caused by the brain damage. Clients might be trained in the use of external memory aids (e.g., memory notebook, alarm watches) or internal aids (e.g., self-cueing, use of mental associations to facilitate comprehension or retrieval). The family members and others relevant in the lives of these clients might also be trained about how the strategies are applied so that they can provide external verbal guidance to the client when necessary. Functional skills training is based on the assumption that functional skills can be improved through repeated practice in the environments in which they naturally occur (Hartley, 1995). For example, Cherney and Halper (2000) suggested that, for clients with visual scanning deficits, paper and pencil scanning tasks might be less relevant than allowing the client to scan and select items in a vending machine in a hospital cafeteria. Compensatory strategy training might be paired with the functional skills of training, so that the client might be aided by self-cued verbal strategies (e.g., "I need to look all the way to the left," "I need to take my time").

Environmental adaptations focus on changing the environment so that the individual can perform adequately in spite of his or her impairments. For instance, Hartley (1995) suggested establishing a quiet study area so that the person with attention deficits is not distracted or posting a morning checklist so that clients have a detailed listing of all of the morning grooming activities that need to be accomplished (e.g., showering, shaving).

To manage the pragmatic aspects of communication that may be impaired after right-hemisphere cerebrovascular accidents or traumatic brain injuries, speech-language pathologists might engage communicative partners into the interventions. Clients need to learn self-initiated strategies for conversational skills such as topic maintenance, social appropriateness, and appropriate use of presupposition. Conversational partners can learn to support the use of these strategies and provide external verbal guidance when necessary.

Process-oriented interventions for clients with cognitive-communication disorders serve to reduce participation restrictions. This is accomplished by training clients to use external and internal compensatory strategies, practice performing functional skills in the context in which they occur, and modifying the environment to maximize cognitive-communication successes. By engaging family members and relevant others into treatment sessions, speech-language pathologists will help the client succeed in executing the pragmatic aspects of communication that are typically impaired in this clinical population.

Interventions for Dysarthria

Process-oriented interventions for dysarthria vary as a function of the severity of the dysarthria. Speech-language pathologists should use treatment approaches that focus on speech intelligibility for those with mildly to moderately dysarthric speech, speech intelligibility and speech augmentation for those with moderately to severe dysarthric speech, and alternate communication systems for those with severely to profoundly dysarthric speech.

Speech intelligibility interventions for those with mildly dysarthric speech require clinicians to teach the client appropriate strategies for maximizing articulatory precision. Strategies for accomplishing this goal might include decreasing the speech rate by any of several techniques (e.g., vowel prolongation, one word at a time, longer pauses between words); increasing vocal intensity, particularly for those with flaccid, unilateral upper motor neuron, and hypokinetic dysarthrias; or exaggerating articulatory movements, or all (Tonkovich, Boettcher, & Rambow, 2001). Clinicians should teach clients the strategies, get them to verbalize the strategies, and practice using the strategies in conversation. Garcia, Cannito, and Dagenais (2000) suggest that beat gestures might be an effective accompaniment to training, teaching the client to tap out the beat of each syllable or word with a finger.

A number of speech-language pathologists seem to engage in the practice of offering clients task-oriented treatments for dysarthria that include the use of repetitive oral-motor exercises. Presumably, such activities are designed to "strengthen" muscle movements, despite the fact that there are no empirical data to support how these exercises strengthen the oral musculature (Tonkovich, Boettcher, & Rambow, 2001), as well as empirical evidence to suggest that intelligible speech is possible with little residual strength of the oral musculature (Barlow & Abbs, 1983). Dysarthric clients from multicultural groups and their families might not understand how these repetitive oral movements relate to speech production and may not wish to engage in them. Clinicians should refrain from using them.

As mentioned previously in this chapter, speakers of tonal languages who are dysarthric may require some additional interventions that relate to modifying not only segmental but also suprasegmental aspects of speech production. Family members and others relevant in the lives of these clients may be able to assist the clinician is determining what exactly those modifications might be.

Yorkston et al. (1999) suggested a number of strategies for improving speech intelligibility in dysarthric speakers for speakers and for their communicative partners, and these are presented in Table 8-4. What is interesting about this approach and what makes it a good example of process-oriented treatment is that it assumes that improved communication is enhanced not only by modifying the behaviors of the speaker but also requires modification of listener behavior. One strategy for caregivers that is particularly interesting to note is the one that relates to the hearing sensitivity of care-

Table 8-4   Dysarthric Speaker Strategies and Strategies for Conversational Partners

---

Dysarthric speaker strategies
    Provide your communication partner context for what you are saying
    Don't shift topics abruptly
    Use turn-taking signals
    Get your listener's attention
    Use complete sentences
    Use predictable types of sentences
    Use predictable wording
    Watch the tone of your voice
    Rephrase your message
    Accompany speech with simple gestures when appropriate
    Take advantage of situational cues
    Make the environment as "friendly" as possible
    Avoid communication over long distances
    Use alphabet board supplementation
    Communicate emotional messages
    Have a handy backup system
Dysarthric partner strategies
    Make sure you know the general topic of the conversation
    Watch for turn-taking signals
    Give your undivided attention
    Choose the time and place for communication
    Watch the speaker
    Piece together the cues
    Make the environment work for you
    Avoid communication over long distances
    Make sure your hearing is as good as possible
    Decide on and incorporate strategies for resolving communication breakdowns
        Signal as soon as you don't understand
        Let the speaker know the parts you did understand
        Let the speaker repeat misunderstood words one at a time

---

Source: Reprinted with permission from Yorkston, K. M., Beukelman, D. R., Strand, E. A., & Bell, K. R. (1999). *Management of motor speech disorders in children and adults* (2nd ed.). Austin, TX: PRO-ED.

givers. A number of elderly clients who are dysarthric actually modify their speech adequately, but they are not understood by their communicative partners who are hearing impaired. This may provide an opportunity for the speech-language pathologist to provide guidance about hearing losses and referral to audiologists for the communicative partners.

Moderately to severely dysarthric speech interventions might focus on some of the techniques for improving articulatory precision discussed previously but might also focus on ways that the dysarthric client can augment speech production. One approach that augments speech production is an alphabet strategy described by Yorkston et al. (1999). This strategy involves the dysarthric speaker saying a word and, if it is not understood, saying the word again while pointing to the first letter of the word on an alphabet board. Hustad (1999) and Hustad and Beukelman (2001) presented data to suggest that moderately to severely dysarthric speakers could maximize their speech intelligibility by using an augmentative alphabet board in conjunction with a topic supplementation board. Topic supplementation provides the dysarthric speaker's listener with the broad general topic of the conversation (e.g., family, meal, recreational activity), and the speaker uses speech production as well as alphabet board supplementation. Another way to augment speech production for this group of dysarthric speakers might be to teach them iconic gestures to use as speech is produced (Garcia, Cannito, & Dagenais, 2000). Whenever augmentative methodologies are chosen, clinicians should be careful to make sure that the client and relevant others in that person's life understand the rationale for the use of the augmentative methods and that he or she feels comfortable using them.

Severely to profoundly impaired dysarthric speakers might best be served by providing them with training in the use of an alternate communication system. This might take a simple form, such as using an alphabet board or a homemade picture or word board that the client can use to convey basic needs to more sophisticated electronic communication systems or gestural systems. One advantage to using alternative systems with persons from multicultural groups is that they can be customized to reflect the dysarthric speaker's native language or preferred dialect pattern.

Soto (2000) suggested that communicatively impaired individuals and their families from traditionally underserved American minorities often do not have access to information on augmentative and alternative communication (AAC) devices and services. Soto (2000) advocated frank and respectful discussions with clients and their families about AAC devices and sensitivity and respect for the perspective of these individuals. Bridges (2000) described a bilingual/bidialectal system developed for a Lumbee Indian client and advocated selecting devices with digitized speech output capabilities so that dialectal patterns of speech could be recorded and used with the device. Others have described AAC interventions for those from low-income Latino families (McCord & Soto, 2000) and from African American communities (Harris, 2000). There is general agreement that families should be actively engaged in the intervention process and that clinicians be sensitive and respectful of their cultural beliefs and perspectives.

In summary, it is clear that process-oriented methodologies serve to reduce the participation restrictions of dysarthric speakers from multicultural groups. Whether the focus of the intervention is on speech intelligibility, speech augmentation, or alternate communication, family members and relevant others should be incorporated into the treatment activities. The more that these individuals can be accepting of the communication modifications necessary for their dysarthric loved one, the more that barriers to communication can be reduced.

Interventions for Dementia

The use of process-oriented treatments for persons with dementia is obvious. For clients with dementia to continue communicating at their maximal level, it is necessary to use strategies that they and those who interact with them will use successfully. Lubinski and Orange (2000) stated that it is the speech-language pathologist's job to identify what strategies caregivers and dementia patients can use to facilitate communication. They advocated caregiver education; environment design or redesign (e.g., adequate lighting and noise reduction); and modeling of strategies that promote interaction. Interestingly, these authors offered the suggestion of using intergenerational communication opportunities (that would complement the respect for elders valued by many multicultural groups) and encouragement of dementia patients to observe or participate in social and cultural events that are appropriate to factors such as their racial, ethnic, and religious interests.

A unique training program for caregivers of patients with dementia is the FOCUSED program (Ripich, 1996). The key components of this training program are presented in Table 8-5. In this program, caregivers are trained to perform modifications in their communication interactions to maximize the likelihood of communicative successes with their loved one. Ripich stated that family members often want to ask "test questions" of the client with dementia (e.g., "What day is it today?," "Where are we going later?"). A good rule of thumb for caregivers is that if they already know the answer to the question, then it is probably of little value to ask it of the client with dementia. Hopper and Bayles (2001) described the use of recruiting volunteers to work with dementia patients. This approach might be particularly useful for recruiting volunteers from a client's cultural or ethnic community, enhancing the communication opportunities for the person with dementia and reducing barriers to participation.

The family members and relevant others in the lives of clients with dementia from multicultural groups will likely need education about

Table 8-5 FOCUSED Strategies for Communicating with Persons with Dementia

---

F = FACE THE PERSON, call his/her name, touch him/her; establish and maintain eye contact if appropriate.

O = ORIENT THE PERSON TO THE TOPIC, repeat key words several times, repeat and rephrase instructions, use nouns and specific names rather than pronouns.

C = CONTINUE THE CONVERSATIONAL TOPIC, restate the topic throughout the conversation, tell the person with dementia when you are going to change topics.

U = "UNSTICK" INCORRECT WORD USAGE BY PROVIDING THE CORRECT WORD, repeat the sentence that the person with dementia said and use the correct word, ask person with dementia "Did you mean . . . ?"

S = STRUCTURE QUESTIONS, provide two-alternative forced-choice questions (e.g., Do you want to get dressed before breakfast or after breakfast?), use yes or no questions (e.g., Are you hungry?).

E = EXCHANGE IDEAS IN CONVERSATIONS, keep conversations going by smiling, nodding, and making comments such as "that's nice" and "I know what you mean," avoid asking test questions (e.g., Where is it that you're sitting right now?), give clues and hints to help the person answer your questions.

D = DIRECT, SHORT SIMPLE SENTENCES ARE BEST, put the subject at the beginning of the sentence, use and repeat nouns, avoid the use of pronouns, use gestures, pictures, printed words, and facial expressions to supplement your speech.

Source: Adapted from Ripich, D. (1996). *Communicating with persons with Alzheimer's disease: The FOCUSED program for caregivers.* Austin, TX: The Psychological Corporation.

dementia and the concomitant communication and memory losses. It is also important for clinicians working with these individuals to be sensitive to the beliefs and attitudes of these individuals and to attempt to come to agreement about *why* particular communication strategies for dementia are useful and facilitating.

Interventions for Dysphagia

Many individuals with neurogenic dysphagia are restricted from eating and drinking and are fed via percutaneous endoscopic gastrostomy tubes. Others may be permitted to have peroral nourishment but may be restricted to pureed foods and thickened liquids. It is incumbent on speech-language pathologists who work with dysphagic clients from multicultural groups to make certain that clients and their families understand the consequences of violating swallowing safety precautions.

Process-oriented treatment approaches for dysphagia include client and family instruction about the nature of the dysphagia. If the client is permitted to have peroral nourishment, treatment should also address the foods and food consistencies required, as well as any swallowing safety precautions that must be followed. The speech-language pathologist should instruct family members and any other caregivers about how to provide external verbal guidance to those clients who need it.

Client and family instruction about dysphagia might include a review of the clients' videofluoroscopic swallowing study, pictures and diagrams about how food or liquids might enter the lungs instead of the stomach, and, if available, written instructions in the native language. Clinicians may find it useful for clients and family members to restate what they understand about dysphagia so that the clinician can help clarify any points that have been missed.

If clients require thickened liquids, then clinicians should assess how well clients and family members can use thickening agents to prepare liquids to the required consistency. The author recently provided a home-based speech-language pathology visit to a bilingual Mexican American client with dysphagia who needed liquids thickened to honey consistency. The clinician asked the client's daughter to prepare some honey-thick liquid so that he could observe how the client managed it. The daughter got a glass of water and added a large spoonful of honey to it. Although it was clear that the daughter had been instructed about the need for honey-thick liquids in the acute care setting, it was apparent that nobody had ascertained if she knew what that meant.

Clients who need to use swallowing safety precautions that minimize aspiration risks need to be trained to use them. Techniques such as chin tuck, double swallow, head turn, and post-swallow cough often reduce the risk of aspiration, and the efficacy of these techniques has often been confirmed objectively by previous videofluoroscopic study.

Clients who are unable to take peroral nourishment due to confirmed aspiration or silent aspiration pose unique challenges to speech-language pathologists. McCullough et al. (1999) identified that speech-language pathologists reported widespread use of oral and pharyngeal exercises in treating oral-pharyngeal dysphagia, yet there is little, if any, empirical evidence to support their use. Hallowell and Chapey (2001) reported that many managed care organizations emphasize "evidence-based medical necessity" clauses that require practitioners to present a solid body of well-controlled research to support the efficacy of such interventions. If unable to provide support of this type, practitioners may not be reimbursed for the services delivered. Speech-language pathologists should avoid providing dysphagia treatment procedures that lack scientific evidence, as these methods may give false hope to clients about their potential recovery and may have no rehabilitative value.

Recently, it has been determined that clients at risk for aspiration of thin liquids might be able to drink water without significant increased risk of aspiration pneumonia (Garon, Engle, & Ormiston, 1997; Panther, 1998).

Speech-language pathologists, after consultation with the client's physician, may determine that a water protocol might be introduced safely for the client. In addition to providing dysphagic clients with a more "normalized" fluid intake, the water protocol may, in fact, reduce the dehydration complications associated with thickened liquids.

Food plays a major role in the lives of many individuals from multicultural groups. When clients from these groups are prohibited from eating and drinking, there may be increased participation restrictions, particularly related to family celebrations. Commenting on functional swallowing measures that have been developed to date, Sonies (2000) stated that limitations in roles of family, work, or recreation have not been addressed. Dysphagia interventions should teach clients and their families strategies that are required for the safe oral intake of nutrition and hydration. When oral intake is not indicated, clinicians should provide instruction about the dangers of aspiration. They should also provide empathy about the social and emotional ramifications of the dysphagia that the client is experiencing.

Summary

In this chapter, an attempt has been made to offer speech-language pathologists some guidance in planning interventions for neurogenic communication and swallowing disorders in individuals from multicultural groups. As our American society becomes more multicultural and older in the near future, clinicians need to be sensitive to the many possible cultural, linguistic, religious, nonverbal communication, and food preference issues that may be relevant to the delivery of speech-language pathology interventions. Clinicians should be careful not to assume that there is homogeneity in broad categories of cultural, ethnic, racial, or religious groups. And, although it is important to take the differences into consideration, clinicians should not lose sight of the fact that individuals with particular communication or swallowing disorders have similarities that transcend membership in a multicultural category.

Process-oriented treatment approaches that teach strategies not only to the client but also to the family members and relevant others are preferred over traditional task-oriented treatments. Process-oriented treatments have a greater potential for generalization and have a greater impact on reducing the participation restrictions of the clients in their communities of choice. In working with family members, clinicians need to be respectful of differing opinions that may (or may not) have cultural, ethnic, religious, or socioeconomic underpinnings. They need to collaborate with families to develop interventions that effect a positive change in clients so that they can function in society at their maximum, most independent level. To do anything less would be a disservice to the clients we serve.

Acknowledgments

The author wishes to acknowledge Ahmed Mohamed Abdelal, Sadi Alzahrani, and Jennifer D. Williams for their assistance in the preparation of this chapter.

References

Abdelal, A. M. (1997). *Examining for bias in assessment instruments used by speech-language pathologists to evaluate individuals from Arabic and Spanish cultures.* Unpublished Master's thesis, Worcester State College, Worcester, MA.

Ali, A. Y. (1993). *The meaning of the holy Qur'an* (5th ed.). Brentwood, MD: Amana Corporation.

American Speech-Language-Hearing Association (1983). Position paper: Speech-language on social dialects. *ASHA, 27,* 23–25.

American Speech-Language-Hearing Association (1985). Clinical management of communicatively handicapped minority language populations. *ASHA, 31,* 93.

American Speech-Language Hearing Association (2001). *Omnibus survey.* Rockville, MD: American Speech-Language-Hearing Association.

Baker, R. (2000). The assessment of functional communication in culturally and linguistically diverse populations. In L. E. Worrall & C. M. Frattali (Eds.), *Neurogenic communication disorders: A functional approach* (pp. 81–100). New York: Thieme.

Barlow, S., & Abbs, J. (1983). Force transducers for the evaluation of labial, lingual, and mandibular motor impairments. *Journal of Speech and Hearing Disorders, 48,* 616–621.

Bridges, S. (2000). Delivery of AAC Services to a rural American Indian community. *Augmentative and Alternative Communication, 9*(2), 6–9.

Campbell, D. (2001). Multicultural competency. *ADVANCE for Speech-Language Pathologists and Audiologists, 11,* 9, 7–8.

Cheng, L. L. (1997). Asian American cultures. In D. Battle (Ed.), *Communication disorders in multicultural populations* (pp. 38–77). Boston: Andover.

Cheng, L. L., Breakey, L. K., & Wallace, G. L. (1997). Asian Americans: Culture, communication and clinical management. In G. L. Wallace (Ed.),

Multicultural neurogenics: A resource for speech-language pathologists providing services to neurologically impaired adults from culturally and linguistically diverse backgrounds (pp. 227–242). San Antonio: Communication Skill Builders.

Cherney, L. R., & Halper, A. S. (2000). Assessment and treatment of functional communication following right hemisphere damage. In L. E. Worrall & C. M. Frattali (Eds.), *Neurogenic communication disorders: A functional approach* (pp. 276–292). New York: Thieme.

Commission on Accreditation of Rehabilitation Facilities (2001). *2001 Medical rehabilitation standards manual.* Tucson, AZ: Commission on Accreditation of Rehabilitation Facilities.

Demchuk, M. (November 1996). Creative communication in aphasia. Paper presented at the annual meeting of American Speech-Language-Hearing Association, Seattle.

Garcia, J. M., Cannito, M. P., & Dagenais, P. A. (2000). Hand gestures: Perspectives and preliminary implications for adults with acquired dysarthria. *American Journal of Speech-Language Pathology, 9,* 107–115.

Garon, B. R., Engle, M., & Ormiston, C. (1997). A randomized control study to determine the effects of unlimited oral intake of water in patients with identified aspiration. *Journal of Neurological Rehabilitation, 11,* 139–148.

Gonzales-Rothi (1996). The compromise of aphasia treatment: Functional and practical but realistic. *Aphasiology, 10,* 483–485.

Hallowell, B., & Chapey, R. (2001). Delivering language intervention services to adults with neurogenic communication disorders. In R. Chapey (Ed.), *Language intervention strategies in aphasia and related neurogenic communication disorders* (4th ed.) (pp. 173–193). Philadelphia: Lippincott Williams & Wilkins.

Hartley, L. (1995). *Cognitive-communication abilities following brain injury: A functional approach.* San Diego: Singular.

Harris, O. (2000). An AAC training program at an historically black university. *Augmentative and Alternative Communication, 9,* 2, 12–13.

Hersh, D. (1998). Beyond the "plateau": Discharge dilemmas in chronic aphasia. *Aphasiology, 12,* 207–218.

Higheagle, B. M. (1995). *Guidelines for obtaining and disseminating information in Native American communities: A survey of speech-language pathologists and audiologists.* Unpublished Master's thesis, Washington State University, Pullman, WA.

Holland, A. L. (1994, September). A look into the cloudy crystal ball for specialists in neurogenic language disorders. *American Journal of Speech-Language Pathology,* 34–36.

Hopper, T., & Bayles, K. A. (2001). Management of neurogenic communication disorders associated with dementia. In R. Chapey (Ed.), *Language inter-*

vention strategies in aphasia and related neurogenic communication disorders (4th ed.) (pp. 829–846). Philadelphia: Lippincott Williams & Wilkins.

Hustad, K. C. (1999). Effects of context on intelligibility and comprehensibility of severely dysarthric speech. Unpublished doctoral dissertation, University of Nebraska, Lincoln, NE.

Hustad, K. C., & Beukelman, D. R. (2001). Effects of linguistic cues and stimulus cohesion on intelligibility of severely dysarthric speech. *Journal of Speech Language Hearing Research, 44*(3), 497–510.

Joint Commission on the Accreditation of Healthcare Organizations (1999, May/June). Ensuring consistency in rehabilitation standards. *Joint Commission Perspectives, 14.*

Kagan, A. (1998). Supported conversation for adults with aphasia. Clinical Forum. *Aphasiology, 12,* 816–830.

Kagan, A., Black, S. E., Duchan, J. F., et al. (2001). Training volunteers as conversation partners using "Supported Conversation for Adults with Aphasia" (SCA): A controlled trial. *Journal of Speech Language Hearing Research, 44*(3), 624–628.

Kagan, A., & Gailey, G. (1993). Functional is not enough: Training conversational partners for aphasic adults. In A. Holland & M. Forbes (Eds.), *Aphasia treatment: World perspectives* (pp. 199–226). San Diego: Singular.

Kaplan, E., Goodglass, H., & Weintraub, S. (2001) *Boston Naming Test* (2nd ed.). Philadelphia: Lippincott Williams & Wilkins.

Kayser, H. (1998). Hispanic cultures and language. In D. Battle (Ed.), *Communication disorders in multicultural populations* (2nd ed.) (pp. 157–196). Boston: Butterworth–Heinemann.

Kayser, H. (2001). Service delivery issues for culturally and linguistically diverse populations. In R. Lubinski & C. Frattali (Eds.), *Professional issues in speech-language pathology and audiology* (2nd ed.) (pp. 389–400). San Diego: Singular.

Larkins, B. M., Worrall, L. E., & Hickson, L. M. (2000). Functional communication in cognitive communication disorders following traumatic brain injury. In L. E. Worrall & C. M. Frattali (Eds.), *Neurogenic communication disorders: A functional approach* (pp. 206–219). New York: Thieme.

Lubinski, R., & Orange, J. B. (2000). A framework for the assessment and treatment of functional communication in dementia. In L. E. Worrall & C. M. Frattali (Eds.), *Neurogenic communication disorders: A functional approach* (pp. 220–246). New York: Thieme.

Lyon, J. (1995). Drawing: Its value as a communication aid for adults with aphasia. *Aphasiology, 9,* 33–94.

Mashima, P., Goo-Yoshino, S., & Wallace, G. (1997). Pacific Islander Americans: Culture, communication and clinical management. In G. L. Wallace (Ed.), *Multicultural neurogenics: A resource for speech-language pathologists providing services to neurologically impaired adults from culturally and linguistically diverse backgrounds* (pp. 243–260). San Antonio: Communication Skill Builders.

McCord, S., & Soto, G. (2000). Working with low-income Latino families: Issues and strategies. *Augmentative and Alternative Communication, 9*(2), 10–12.

McCullough, G. H., Wertz, R. T., Rosenbek, J. C., & Dineen, C. (1999). Clinicians' preferences and practices in conducting clinical/bedside and videofluoroscopic swallowing examinations in an adult neurogenic population. *American Journal of Speech-Language Pathology, 8*, 149–163.

Myers, P. S. (1999). *Right hemisphere damage: Disorders of communication and cognition.* San Diego: Singular.

Ortiz, M. (1993). *The Hispanic challenge: Opportunities confronting the church.* Downers Grove, IL: InterVarsity Press.

Palacio, M. (2000). Home care advantage. *ADVANCE for Speech-Language Pathologists and Audiologists, 10, 51, 21.*

Panther, K. (1998). Should patients who aspirate thin liquids be given water? *ASHA, 40*(3), 12–13.

Parr, S. (1996). Everyday literacy and aphasia: radical approaches to functional assessment and therapy. Clinical Forum. *Aphasiology, 10*, 469–503.

Pena, B. (1998). Tips for working with Hispanic bilingual patients. *Communication Disorders and Sciences in Culturally and Linguistically Diverse Populations, 7*(3).

Pyypponen, V. (1993). The point of view of the clinician. *Aphasiology, 7*, 579–581.

Reyes, B., & Peterson, C. S. (1997). Hispanic Americans: Culture, communication and clinical management. In G. L. Wallace (Ed.), *Multicultural neurogenics: A resource for speech-language pathologists providing services to neurologically impaired adults from culturally and linguistically diverse backgrounds* (pp.165–192). San Antonio: Communication Skill Builders.

Ripich, D. (1996). *Communicating with persons with Alzheimer's disease: The FOCUSED program for caregivers.* Austin, TX: The Psychological Corporation.

Ryalls, J., & Behrens, S. J. (2000). *Introduction to speech science: From basic theories to clinical applications.* Needham Heights, MA: Allyn & Bacon.

Shariefzadeh, V. S. (1992). Families with Middle Eastern roots. In E. W. Lynch & M. J. Hanson (Eds.), *Developing cross-cultural competence: A guide for working with young children and their families* (pp. 319–351). Baltimore: Brookes.

Simmons, N. (1993). *An ethnographic investigation of compensatory strategies in aphasia.* Ann Arbor, MI: University Microfilms International.

Simmons-Mackie, N. N. (2000). Social approaches to the management of aphasia. In L. E. Worrall & C. M. Frattali (Eds.), *Neurogenic communication disorders: A functional approach* (pp. 162–188). New York: Thieme.

Simmons-Mackie, N. (2001). Social approaches to aphasia intervention. In R. Chapey (Ed.), *Language intervention strategies in aphasia and related neurogenic communication disorders* (4th ed.) (pp. 246–268). Philadelphia: Lippincott Williams & Wilkins.

Simmons-Mackie, N., & Damico, J. (1997). Reformulating the definition of compensatory strategies in aphasia. *Aphasiology, 8,* 761–781.

Sonies, B. C. (2000). Assessment and treatment of functional swallowing in dysphagia. In L. E. Worrall & C. M. Frattali (Eds.), *Neurogenic communication disorders: A functional approach* (pp. 262–275). New York: Thieme.

Soto, G. (2000). "We have come a long way. . . . " AAC and multiculturalism: From cultural awareness to cultural responsibility. *Augmentative and Alternative Communication, 9(2),* 1–3.

Sparks, R. (2001). Melodic intonation therapy. In R. Chapey (Ed.), *Language intervention strategies in aphasia and related neurogenic communication disorders* (4th ed.) (pp. 703–717). Philadelphia: Lippincott Williams & Wilkins.

Tonkovich, J. D. (1998). Management of communicative and swallowing disorders in non-acute settings. In A. F. Johnson & B. F. Jacobson (Eds.), *Medical speech-language pathology: A practitioner's guide.* New York: Thieme.

Tonkovich, J. D., Boettcher, T. L., & Rambow, M. W. (2001). *Dysarthria rehabilitation* (2nd ed.). Austin, TX: PRO-ED.

U.S. Bureau of the Census (2001). *Projections of the resident population by race, Hispanic origin, and nativity: Middle series, 1999 to 2100.* Washington, DC: U.S. Bureau of the Census.

Wallace, G. L. (1997). Working with interpreters and translators. In G. L. Wallace (Ed.), *Multicultural neurogenics: A resource for speech-language pathologists providing services to neurologically impaired adults from culturally and linguistically diverse backgrounds* (pp. 39–56). San Antonio: Communication Skill Builders.

Wallace, G. L., Inglebret, E., & Friedlander, R. (1997). American Indians: Culture, communication and clinical management. In G. L. Wallace (Ed.),

Multicultural neurogenics: A resource for speech-language pathologists providing services to neurologically impaired adults from culturally and linguistically diverse backgrounds (pp. 193–226). San Antonio: Communication Skill Builders.

Wallace, G. L., & Tonkovich, J. D. (1997). African Americans: Culture, communication and clinical management. In G. L. Wallace (Ed.), *Multicult ural neurogenics: A resource for speech-language pathologists providing services to neurologically impaired adults from culturally and linguistically diverse backgrounds* (pp. 133–164). San Antonio: Communication Skill Builders.

World Health Organization (1997). *ICIDH-2 International classification of impairments, activities, and participation.* Geneva: World Health Organization.

Worrall, L. E. (2000). A conceptual framework for a functional approach to acquired neurogenic disorders of communication and swallowing. In L. E. Worrall & C. M. Frattali (Eds.), *Neurogenic communication disorders: A functional approach* (pp. 3–18). New York: Thieme.

Yorkston, K. M., Beukelman, D. R., Strand, E. A., & Bell, K. R. (1999). *Management of motor speech disorders in children and adults* (2nd ed.). Austin, TX: PRO-ED.

Additional Resources

http://aphasia.on.ca

This is the website for the Aphasia Institute (incorporating the Pat Arato Aphasia Centre). It contains information about aphasia, resources, and training in supported conversation techniques for aphasia.

9

Fluency Disorders

Tommie L. Robinson, Jr., and Thomas A. Crowe

Disorders of fluency are probably the most recognized communication disorder. For years, researchers and scholars have struggled to understand the nature of fluency disorders and their characteristic and have tried to come to some consensus on terminology and definitions. A review of the literature indicates the use of terms such as *fluency, dysfluency, stuttering, cluttering,* and *stammering.* Cooper and Cooper (1998) refer to *fluency disorders* as an umbrella term under which the preceding terms fall. The term *stuttering* is probably the most frequently used term. Nevertheless, its definition is not inclusive of the other terms. Stuttering is a multidimensional disorder of speech characterized by dysfluencies, secondary behaviors, and attitudinal or cognitive issues. For the purpose of this chapter, the term *stuttering* will be used, because it represents most of the clinical cases presented.

Universality of Stuttering

Like most disorders that affect the human condition, stuttering is not restrained by geographic demarcations. Stuttering appears on every continent, in every country, in every corner of the globe. The evidence for the universality of stuttering is summarized effectively by Van Riper (1982) and by Bloodstein (1995).

The universality of stuttering pertains to cultures as well as continents and countries. There is strong evidence that stuttering appears in all cultures, or, to put it more conservatively, there is no compelling evidence for any culture that indicates stuttering does not exist within it. Cultural groups that have been studied include the following:

Native Americans: Clifford, Twitchell, & Hull, 1965; Johnson, 1944a,
     1944b; Lemert, 1953; Snidecor, 1947; Stewart, 1960; Zimmerman,
     Liljeblad, Frank, & Cleeland, 1983
African Americans: Anderson, 1981; Brutten & Miller, 1988; Conrad,
     1985, 1987; Ford, 1986; Goldman, 1967; Leith & Mims, 1975;
     Nathanson, 1969; Robinson, 1992; Robinson & Crowe, 1987, 1998;
     Robinson, Davis, & Crowe, 2000
Asians: Lemert, 1962; Toyoda, 1959; Wakaba, 1983
Hispanics: Bernstein-Ratner & Benitez, 1985; Dale, 1977; Jayaram,
     1983; Nwokah, 1988; Travis, Johnson, & Shover, 1981
West Indians: Ralston, 1981
Africans: Aron, 1962; Goodhall & Brobby, 1982; Kirk, 1977; Morgen-
     stern, 1953, 1956; Nwokah, 1988

Results of these studies generally suggest that cultural differences
influence speech fluency and that there are differences in perceptions,
beliefs, values, and norms about speech fluency and stuttering among various cultural groups. One possible significance of these suggestions is that
cultural factors might appreciably affect the outcomes of clinical intervention with stuttering.

There has been controversy about the universality of stuttering. The
argument that stuttering is not universal was based on sparse, largely anecdotal data that for the most part was later refuted. The best-known case of
this was the assertion by Johnson (1944a, 1944b) and two of his students,
Snidecor (1947) and Stewart (1960), that stuttering did not exist in the Utes,
Bannock, and Shoshone American Indian tribes. This idea was based on the
researchers' findings that no stuttering was reported in interviews with
members of the tribes, that social pressures on communication appeared to
be minimal within the tribes, and that no word in the tribal languages
could be found for stuttering. Evidence was later presented (Zimmerman et
al., 1983) that stuttering does exist in these American Indian tribes and
that there were many descriptions of stuttering. The earlier researcher
failed to establish trust with the American Indian tribes; therefore, their
qualitative research was flawed. Johnson, Snidecor, and Stewart did not
realize that the subjects were not being truthful from fear of being blamed
for the cause of stuttering.

Prevalence of Stuttering among Cultures

The idea that stuttering may not exist in some cultures is
given little credence today. The thought that social demand on communi-

cation and stuttering might be positively correlated is one possible explanation for varying prevalence of stuttering across cultural groups. Cooper and Cooper (1998) stated, ". . . universally accepted definitions do not exist regarding what constitutes the fluency disorders that the English terms *stuttering* and *stammering* and their equivalents in other languages have come to encompass and symbolize." They also indicate a great deal of variability in the data collection process across cultures. In a review of the literature, Van Riper (1982) and Bloodstein (1995) indicated that the prevalence of stuttering in the general population is approximately 0.8%, whereas the incidence of stuttering is between 5% and 10% based on a series of studies done by various researchers over the past years. See Tables 9-1 through 9-5 depicting prevalence research in various cultural groups.

Cultural Factors in Assessment and Treatment

The relevance of cultural factors in the assessment and treatment of communication disorders has been discussed in the literature (Battle, 1997; Taylor, 1986; Terrell & Hale, 1992; Van Kleeck, 1994). For assessment to be accurate and meaningful and for treatment to be maximally effective, both should be conducted with regard to the client's cultural identity, cultural assimilation, cultural environment, and cultural system (Crowe, Di Lollo, & Crowe 2000; Robinson & Crowe, 1998). Clinicians and researchers have attempted to address culturally appropriate clinical services by providing models for service delivery in various clinical settings and with various cultures (Seymour, 1986; Seymour & Seymour, 1977; Taylor, 1986, 1987; Taylor & Payne, 1983; Taylor &

Table 9-1 Stuttering Prevalence in African American Populations

Author(s)	n	Findings
Waddle (1934)	1,582	1.7:1.0 ratio in children
Carson & Kanter (1945)	NA	60% higher than white children
Neely (1960)	NA	No differences
Prichett (1966)	NA	1.3:1.0 ratio African American to white children
Goldman (1967)	694	2.4:1.0 ratio African American male to female children
Gillespie & Cooper (1973)	5,054	2.8%
Conrad (1980)	1,271	2.7% African American adults 2:1 ratio male to female

NA = not available.

Table 9-2   Stuttering Prevalence in African Populations

Author(s)	n	Findings
Morgenstern (1953, 1956)	5,618	2.67% of Ibo school children
Aron (1962)	6,581	1.26% of Bantu school children
Kirk (1977)	NA	High incidence of dysfluent speech (non-pathologic) among children from Ghana
Goodall & Brobby (1982)	NA	5.5% prevalence in Dakar school children 3.5% prevalence in Accra district
Nwokah (1988)	NA	Incidence in Nigerians and West Africans may be the highest in the world

NA = not available.

Samara, 1985; Vaughn-Cooke, 1983, 1986). These models, for the most part, have been discussed relative to nonbiased assessment and treatment of speech articulation and language disorders with little reference to the treatment process.

Recently, attention has been given to the influence of cultural factors on the evaluation and treatment of stuttering (Cooper & Cooper, 1998; Crowe, Di Lollo, & Crowe, 2000; Robinson & Crowe, 2000; Watson & Kayser, 1994). Consideration of cultural variables in the treatment of stuttering should begin when clients or their families make the first clinical contact to schedule an evaluation or to obtain information. Clinical intervention for treatment of stuttering should be structured within the context of each client's *cultural system* and *cultural environment*, after determining the client's *cultural identity* and *degree of assimilation* into the culture, for therapy to be maximally effective and also for therapy to be efficient in regard to time spent setting and achieving goals. The clinician's attention to the cultural dimensions of the clinical relationship will increase the probability that

Table 9-3   Stuttering Prevalence in Caribbean Populations

Author(s)	n	Findings
McCartney (1971)*	NA	1.07–4.46% prevalence in Bahamians
Ralston (1981)	1,999	4.7% prevalence in Caribbean children
Leith & Gibson (1991)	1,217	3.6% prevalence in children in Nassau

NA = not available.
*Cited in Leith & Gibson (1991).

Table 9-4   Stuttering Prevalence in Hispanic Populations

Author(s)	n	Findings
Leavitt (1974)	10,455	0.84% prevalence in New York City Puerto Ricans
Leavitt (1974)	10,499	1.50% prevalence in Puerto Ricans in San Juan
Ardila, Bateman, & Nino (1994)	1,879	2% prevalence among Spanish-speaking university students from Bogotá, Colombia

counseling for the treatment and prevention of stuttering will be effective (Crowe, 1995).

Cultural systems pertain to all that comprises the belief systems of clients. Cultural systems include values, attitudes, perceptions, and myths, as well as other cultural variables. This is often referred to as the *phenomenal field*. Phenomenal field refers to the comprehensive experiences and belief systems of individuals. To a large extent, culture-based factors determine the perceived reality in which clients operate. The client's perceptions of reality may or may not match the clinician's. If perceptions of the client do not match those of the clinician, then there is a strong likelihood that therapy, and especially counseling, will not be maximally effective. Cultural variables account for only one of the many reasons that the client and clinician's phenomenal fields may not match, but having different cultural systems is a frequent reason why they do not match.

The client's cultural environment is also important to consider when structuring a plan for counseling in fluency intervention. This includes all aspects of the client's environment, including the client's phenomenal field, access to experience, semantic environment, relationships with significant others, and language environment. In the case of child clients, it is important for clinicians to remember that parents and primary caregivers are the chief

Table 9-5   Stuttering Prevalence in Asian Populations

Author(s)	n	Findings
Toyoda (1959)	140,000	0.82% prevalence in Japanese school children
Ozawa (1960)	7,600	0.90% prevalence in Japanese school children
Lemert (1962)	NA	More stuttering among Japanese than among Polynesians

NA = not available.

architects of their child's environment. Parents and primary caregivers should be counseled to be active in designing an environmental gestalt for the child that is conducive to speech fluency and normal personality development (Crowe, 1994). The environment of the child with dysfluencies should be conducive to him or her developing the coping use of ego functions that might, in turn, help prevent the development of defensive reactions to speech dysfluency and therapy. In the case of adult clients, it is important for clinicians to remember that the family and spouse are participants in the client's environment. However, the participation of the family and spouse in assessment, intervention, and counseling may be governed by cultural values or perception of role and family social structures.

A general model for inclusion of these cultural factors in assessment and therapy planning for individuals who stutter is discussed later in this chapter. Also discussed later are techniques for identifying aspects of the client's cultural identity, cultural assimilation, cultural environment, and cultural system, as well as the influence of culture on beliefs and behavior related to stuttering.

Factors That Influence Stuttering in Cultural Groups

Researchers have reported a number of factors that may influence all aspects of speech and language. A number of these factors have been discussed earlier in this text and have been highlighted over the years by researchers and scholars as having great impact on the service delivery to clients and patients and their families. Specific to the area of stuttering, such influences have been linked to attitudes, myths, beliefs, religion, nonverbal behaviors, and events in the life cycle.

Attitudes

An attitude is a state of mind, feeling, orientation, or disposition (*American Heritage Dictionary of the English Language*, 1996). For years, researchers and clinicians have examined the relationship between stuttering and attitude. It has been determined that attitude plays a major role in the diagnostic and treatment processes. The beliefs that accompany stuttering are a major component of the stuttering syndrome. Starkweather (1980) indicated that treating one aspect of stuttering and ignoring the others doom any therapeutic approach to failure.

From a cultural perspective, attitudes toward communication disorders and, specifically, stuttering are different for various cultural groups. Harris

(1986) indicated that attitudes evolve from individuals' value systems and culture. She further states,

> These value systems are often so ingrained in a person's mind that his or her values become truth, usually not only for that particular person but for all humans. Practitioners must acknowledge the potential for differences in perception of the causes and meaning of disabilities, the elements necessary for differences in the value of rehabilitation, and the differences between their own belief systems and those of their clients. (p. 229)

Myths and Beliefs

It is important for clinicians to be familiar with the myths and beliefs of the culture group relative to etiologic factors and approaches to intervention for stuttering. It is also important to note that some myths and beliefs are evidenced in the fact that, in some cultures, families do not see the value of speech-language services. Clinicians must take these myths very seriously, because they represent the parents' honest understanding of stuttering. For example, families may be reluctant to seek the advice of the speech-language pathologist if they believe that they can cure stuttering by hitting the child or adult in the mouth with a dishtowel.

Religion

Some cultural groups have very strong religious beliefs and practices. Clinicians should be mindful that sometimes religious practices might greatly influence the family's acceptance of the stuttering intervention process. In some cultures, for instance, clinicians may find that some families may view stuttering as a curse from God. In other cultures, seeking clinical service in general may be against religious practices. For example, those who practice voodoo may seek the help of the voodooist rather than the speech-language pathologist.

Nonverbal Behaviors in Stuttering

Clinicians, during their interactions with children and adults, should be mindful of nonverbal behaviors such as silence, eye contact, and physical activity levels (e.g., excessive gross motor behavior, constant body movements, out-of-seat behavior, extraneous hand movements, and so forth). These behaviors are often misconstrued as secondary mannerisms or avoidance behaviors when they are, in fact, cultural nonverbal behaviors. For example, in some cultures, it is inappropriate to use eye contact during conversation with a person of more status. Or clinicians may find that the eye contact of some African American clients may be less than that of the mainstream population, depending on the age, race, gender, and communication style of the listener. In these cases, it would be inappropriate for clinicians to establish eye contact as a treatment goal.

Cycle of Life

Stuttering has been linked to a number of holidays, family activities, and events in the lives of patients and clients, in that it has been reported that stuttering severity increases during these events. It is important for clinicians to obtain as much information in this while taking the case history. However, implications are made here, especially for the treatment process. Clinicians find themselves developing clinical strategies to address the stressors that may develop from these events. Furthermore, clinicians also see correlation with the degree of stuttering in regard to these events. It is important to know, depending on the cultural background of an individual, the events that might be important from group to group. For example, a Jewish person who stutters might find it stressful to read from the Torah during synagogue service, whereas, with a Central American family, a young lady who stutters might have exceptional difficulty with her speech at the time of her *quincianera* (celebration on the fifteenth birthday symbolizing womanhood). These examples represent a correlation between cultural events and the communication demands placed on individuals during these events.

A Decision Model for Inclusion of Multicultural Variables in Stuttering Intervention Programming

Robinson and Crowe (1998) presented a decision model for inclusion of multicultural variables in stuttering intervention. In this model, depicted in Figure 9-1, six levels are presented: pre-intervention, intake, evaluation, parent and client counseling, treatment, and carryover and generalization. In this model, decisions are made at each intervention level as to the relevance of cultural variables in the intervention process. In the schematic, the solid arrows represent the possible directions through the intervention

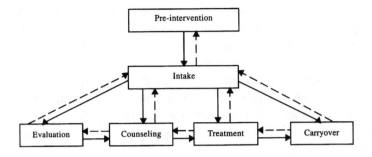

Figure 9-1   A decision model for inclusion of multicultural variables in stuttering intervention.

Decision Level I: Pre-Intervention
• Cultural identification
• Age and gender
• Communication norms

Decision Level II: Intake
• General disorder typing
• Specific cultural variables relative to stuttering
• Myths
• Attitudes
• Terminology
• Beliefs

Decision Level III: Evaluation
• Cultural adjustment/modification
  1. Nonverbal behaviors
  2. Verbal language/Interaction
  3. Visual stimuli
• Cognitive learning styles
• Parental-child interaction styles
• Client clinical interaction styles

Decision Level IV: Parent/Client Counseling
• Rules for interaction
• The family unit
  1. Relative to cultural identity
  2. Relative to residential history
  3. Relative to generational factors
• Importance of language spoken in the home

Decision Level V: Treatment
• Build culture-based factors into therapy goals/techniques

Decision Level VI: Carryover/ Generalization
• Utilize the home unit
• Utilize peers
• Utilize the client

process. The broken arrows indicate that a client's progress through the levels is not necessarily linear, in that previous levels may often need to be revisited to address additional cultural factors. At each level, decisions are made regarding which cultural factors should be addressed at that level.

Culture-Related Issues in Assessment and Treatment

Cultural Identity and Cultural Assimilation

Making assumptions about a client's cultural identity is risky. Clinicians must be mindful that cultural identity goes beyond the race of individuals, and just because a culture has been assigned to the client, it does not mean that the client identifies with that particular culture. Second, after the cultural identity of the client has been determined, age and gender must also be considered before evaluation, because in some cultures, these variables influence the communication norms that are expected by clients or parents of clients. At this point, clinicians will have enough information to make generalizations regarding the culture-based beliefs and values about communication that the clients and their significant others bring to the clinical setting (Watson & Kayser, 1994).

A factor that should be considered when gathering cultural background information about a client is his or her degree of cultural assimilation. Although clients may identify with a given culture, they may not be fully assimilated into the culture. The degree of assimilation in a particular culture may vary from client to client.

Assessment

Most standardized assessment programs often do not consider cultural information, so clinicians should add this information to the clinical protocol. First of all, clinicians should consider areas such as the cultural identity, cultural assimilation, cultural environment, and cultural system (i.e., attitudes and beliefs). Crowe, Di Lollo, and Crowe (2000) provide a format that can be used to guide clinicians' discovery in these areas (see Appendix 9-1).

Next, clinicians may find it necessary to modify test items or testing procedures to make them more culturally appropriate. Clinicians should also note that, when working with children who stutter, parent-child interaction is an important part of the data-gathering process. Clinicians should consider differences based on cultural backgrounds. Particular attention should be given to issues such as directive behaviors, child-rearing practices, and verbal expectations, which often influence parent-child interaction (Conrad, 1985, 1987). With adults, clinicians must note culturally specific pragmatic and social interaction styles, such as who is allowed to speak and when, what the rules are for interruptions, how are topics introduced, and so forth. Finally, commercial programs are often used during the evaluation process. They are often standardized, based on normative data or items that were developed with the mainstream population in mind. Clinicians should feel comfort in knowing that modifications to these testing instruments can and should be made with the client's cultural background in mind.

Culture-Specific Test Items

During the evaluation process, clinicians should consider the cultural experiences of the parents and clients. When using commercial programs as a means for evaluating speech fluency, it is important to take this notion under consideration. For example, a clinician may want to review the suggested "topics to elicit conversation" when using the *Stuttering Prediction Instrument for Young Children* (Riley, 1981) with an urban Hispanic child. In the review, the clinician needs to determine the experiences that the child has had. If a child has never had a traditional American birthday party or planted a garden, as suggested, then it may be difficult to expect a response in this regard. The "story plates" used in this instrument depict middle-class white America at a birthday party, planting a garden, and so forth. Clinicians should substitute these story plates for ones that reflect the child's culture and experiences.

Similar test modification can be easily made for adults. Conversational samples should reflect their experiences and culture rather than the experience and expectations of the clinician. Speech samples and conversational topics should be of interest to the client to obtain a representative sample of the client's speech fluency behavior. Although these procedures may be implemented to address the specific needs of the individuals, clinicians are responsible for assuring that the integrity of the assessment instrument is not at risk; that is, the instrument still needs to measure what it purports.

Parent-Child Interaction

An important aspect of conducting a speech fluency evaluation on preschool and early school-age children is observation of parent-child interaction. It is crucial that clinicians are aware of the interaction styles that are specific to different cultures. There is nothing more demeaning to parents than being told their child-rearing practices and interaction skills are causing their child to stutter. This can be spearheaded if the clinician has selectively sought to understand the cultural dynamics of the family. During the evaluation process, clinicians should take caution in conveying this information to the parent and should also seek to research and understand the culture's interaction style. Rules that govern when children are allowed to talk, how conversations are initiated with children, who initiates the conversation, emotionality, nonverbal cues, and so forth within the culture should be examined.

Pragmatic and Social Interaction Style

Social language behavior also plays a major role in speech fluency behavior, especially with adults who stutter. Often times during the evaluation process, clinicians observe and evaluate the client's level of interaction as it pertains to verbal behaviors (interruptions, initiating conversation, turn-taking, vying for the floor, and so forth) and nonverbal behaviors (hand, facial, head, and whole body movements, eye contact, and so forth). In cases in which there is no understanding of the culture, clinicians can easily diagnose behaviors as abnormal in these areas. In reality, these observations should be evaluated as differences rather than disorders.

Intervention

Clinical intervention for stuttering and other fluency disorders should be based on factors previously discussed such as values, beliefs, attitudes, religion, interaction styles, and so forth. Strategies should be developed and incorporated to minimize cultural bias and to assure clients and families of the value in their beliefs. Here again, clinicians should make an effort to modify stimuli so that they represent the client's cultural background. In addition, clinicians should focus on ways to enhance the clinician-child interaction; clinician-family interaction, where necessary; cognitive learning styles with children (Robinson & Crowe, 1998); and the social interaction styles of the adults. Some suggestions for each area are below.

Clinician-Child Interaction

1. Use culturally relevant and culturally appropriate topics during discussion. This will aid the clinician in not only getting to understand the client, but also making culture an ongoing focus in the treatment process. Selecting the right topic for discussion makes the client believe that the focus of therapy has his or her interest at heart. This also helps with motivation factors with adolescents and adults.

2. Incorporate the physical activity levels of the individuals. This technique is important in working with children whose physical activity levels are high and whose cognitive learning style is different. Teaching children to maintain speech fluency control during high-energy movements is more feasible than trying to change physical behaviors. That is, taking a client's natural state (i.e., energy level and cognitive style) and teaching new communication skills are easier and more meaningful than trying to change the client's energy level, cognitive style, and communication skills. In this way, the likelihood of carryover is greater.

3. Monitor the client's secondary mannerisms to distinguish them from "normal" behaviors. During the therapy process, it is important for clinicians to devote time to ongoing assessment of secondary mannerisms. In some cultures, expressive verbal communication may be accompanied by nonverbal movements that may be reflected in facial contortions, extraneous body movements, hand gestures, eye contact, and so forth. Clinicians should provide ongoing study of these behaviors to rule out cultural influence. This can be done through observing others in the culture (i.e., parents, significant others, and community), interviewing individuals from the culture, reading information that has been printed on the specific culture, and so forth. Clinicians should attempt to change or modify only those behaviors that are not culturally related.

4. Expand the treatment program by using peers and the family unit as a part of remediation. If culturally appropriate, clinicians may find peers and family members to be very useful during the therapy process. To have friends and family members as a part of the treatment process will provide the patient or client with a support system to aid in building self-esteem and to encourage carryover. Culturally, some groups are more comfortable with the extended family units, and clinicians will find that the family works better in this regard.

Clinician-Family Interaction

1. Understand myths and offer alternatives when appropriate. It is important for clinicians to be familiar with the myths of the culture group, relative to etiologic factors and approaches to therapy for stuttering. Clinicians must take these myths very seriously, because they represent the client and family's honest understanding of stuttering. Clinicians should be able to offer alternative approaches to the myths relative to treatment or aid the family in understanding the origin of the myths, or both. A word of caution is offered here as well. For this to work effectively, the clinicians must establish a strong relationship and trust with the family. Then, and only then, will it be appropriate to approach this issue.

2. Incorporate parents, spouse, caregivers, and significant others in the intervention process when culturally appropriate. Depending on the cultural group, some parents feel more a part of the treatment process if they are "hands-on" participants. Nevertheless, with another group, more expectations are placed on the clinician as the change-agent. Clinicians should also take into consideration such characteristics as literacy skills, educational level, employment, and other variables when giving assignments and modeling techniques for parents.

Cognitive Learning Style

1. Develop functional and hands-on activities. Clinicians should be mindful of the need to make treatment activities as engaging and exciting as possible. With individuals from diverse backgrounds, clinicians must determine whether their learning style is relational or analytic and develop activities accordingly. Hilliard (1976) and Hale-Benson (1987) described relational learning styles in opposition to the analytic learning styles. They indicated that analytical cognitive style might include characteristics such as stimulus-centered concentration; parts-specific style; long attention span; Standard English language styles; formal and stable rules for language organization; and long concentration span. Aspects of relational cognitive style may include self-centeredness; global understanding; fine descriptive characteristics; fluent spoken language; short attention span; short concentration span; gestalt learning; and language dependent on unique context, interactional characteristics of the communicant's time and place, inflection, muscular movements, and other nonverbal cues. African American children tend to use relational learning styles. Although this is one example, our clinical encounters lead us to a variety of cultures; for each, these characteristics should be considered.

Stuttering therapy activities should be based on real life events. In other words, treatment strategies should be incorporated into events and activities necessary for the clients to assume a culturally competent verbal interaction, while maintaining speech fluency.

Understanding the learning style of the individual will also help determine the frequency of variability activities. From a cultural standpoint, if the individual is a relational style learner, then she or he will need engaging speech fluency activities that will take under consideration the individual's attention span and concentration span.

2. Make treatment programs reflective of the cultural experiences of the clients. This concept has been emphasized throughout this chapter. It is a factor that should be given to each clinical encounter, so that individuals from diverse cultures are not penalized for experiences that have not been a part of their lives. It is important for clinicians to conduct extensive interviews, interactions, and observations, as well as keep an open line of communication with all individuals involved in the patient's or client's environment. When developing speech fluency goals and activities, the clinician should include experiences that the patient or client has had as a part of the activities.

When using a commercial fluency treatment program that involves specific activities and materials, clinicians may have difficulty developing strategies to enhance the cultural sensitivity of the program. However, the concepts of the program may be preserved and used with other activities for cultural enrichment. For example, a component of *The Fluency Development System for Young Children* (Meyers & Woodford, 1992) can be adjusted to substitute characters familiar to the client rather than the "Tortoise and Hare" fable as a basis for establishing the cognitive linguistic components of the therapy program. A culturally relevant story or fable can be substituted for the story in the commercial program. For programs that do not require adherence to specific activities and materials, modification for inclusion of culturally sensitive materials can be made easily. For example, when using the *Fluency Rules Therapy Program for Young Children* (Runyan & Runyan, 1986) or the *Stuttering Therapy for Children* (Gregory & Hill, 1980) with an African American school-age child, clinicians can use sports activities to adjust for physical activity level and can easily incorporate narrative discourse activities.

Social Interaction Style

1. Learn how the individual communicates in his or her culture. Clinicians should be mindful of attributes such as silence, interruptions, topic maintenance, verbal expectations, and so forth. These are important to consider in dealing with children and adults who stutter. Often, clients and their families are penalized for interaction styles that clinicians judge to be inappropriate. What the client evidences may in fact be a culturally specific interaction style that may have no deleterious effect on speech. For example, silence may be interpreted as a stuttering behavior when it may actually be a nonverbal communication style in the client's culture. Another example would be for the American Indian and Hispanic cultures in which there may be long periods of silence before responding to a question or a comment.

2. Create mock social interactions. Clinicians may find use in creating social settings that can be used to prepare the client for actual events. Creating scenarios such as ordering in a restaurant, talking on the telephone, asking someone out on a date, making a class presentation, and so forth are pragmatic in a functional communication process. These also prove to be invaluable to meeting the social needs of patients and clients. Using this approach also allows for individuality of goals and objectives and allows the clinician the opportunity to work with the unique cultural nature of the client. For example, as with a case mentioned earlier, a goal in therapy was to aid a young man preparing for his bar mitzvah by helping him to read the Torah fluently. Another example involves helping a young Roman Catholic child who stutters to recite the rosary or prayers before confirmation.

3. Use verbal conflict as a therapy tool. For cultural groups that place high regard on being verbal, it is important that clinicians incorporate much verbal activity in the therapy session. An effective way to accomplish this is by keeping the client in verbal conflict. This is done by taking an opposing viewpoint

on an issue of discussion between the client and the clinician. Using this strategy helps the client prepare to engage in conversation and verbal exchange with peers and family members. However, there are some cultures in which this activity would be inappropriate. For example, in some Asian cultures, it is inappropriate to be in conflict with the person in authority.

The Arc of Counseling

Although counseling is an ongoing process, it should definitely begin at the speech fluency evaluation. This is an especially important level in clinical intervention with multicultural clients, because it is here that "the stage" is set for therapy, ideally with the complete comprehension and support of clients and their support of others. Clinicians should be mindful of the three aspects of counseling. The first aspect is that counseling should begin, when possible, before stuttering develops for prevention purposes and definitely before stuttering becomes severe. This becomes a challenge to clinicians, especially because there are cultural myths and beliefs about the necessity of the intervention process.

The second aspect of counseling concerns the interpretation of test results to clients, definition of the disorders and treatment, and explanation of prognosis. Clinicians should remember to observe rules for cultural interaction. Rules, such as for verbal, nonverbal, and social interaction, should be observed. This will remove potential sources of miscommunication between clients and clinicians. For example, a miscommunication can occur if the clinician addressed the client inappropriately or violated the personal space of the client.

The third aspect of counseling addresses personal adjustments of the clients and significant others as an ongoing part of the treatment process. Here it is important that the clinician explore the possible significance of cultural identity, residential history, and generational factors (i.e., age and maturity).

It is also important that clinicians understand rules or interacting with individuals from diverse backgrounds. Important attributes such as touching, establishing eye contact, and observing levels of emotion are crucial to the counseling session. Clinicians must be able to adjust to cultural differences to win the trust of clients and parents so that counseling with them will be maximally effective.

Need for Research

There still remains a dearth of information relative to examining speech fluency and stuttering in populations other than in the mainstream population groups. A review of the literature indicated limited research pertaining to cultural groups, and clinical experience indicates that there is a need for future study. Specifically, there is a need for study of cultural influences in the following areas:

Stuttering development. There still exists the need to study the development of stuttering in various cultures. Limited information is known about the course that stuttering takes in multicultural groups. Perhaps there are developmental differences that might warrant a course of intervention in some cultures that is quite different from our current offerings. Such studies might examine the development of stuttering in various populations, as well as parent-child interaction, family-child interaction, and general characteristics.

Manifestation. There is also the need to explore those attributes that mark speech stuttering in various cultures and linguistic groups. It has been suggested that there are differences in interaction styles, attitudes, secondary mannerisms, dysfluency types, beliefs, and other variables. There is now a need to provide empirical data that support these hypotheses and suggestions.

Intervention. The intervention process continues to be the most challenging area for clinicians in the treatment of stuttering. Given the diversity of the individuals who seek clinical services and those who do not, applying the cookie-cutter approach to intervention is not sufficient. There is a need to further explore the evaluation and therapy processes to maximize service delivery options for persons in various cultural and linguistic groups.

Finally, as discussed in Chapter 15, a word of caution is in order. It is important that contemporary research moves away from comparing cultural groups in research protocols and begins to examine and explore persons within groups for their own uniqueness, as well as explore carefully defined groups for their own characteristics. There is no clinical value in comparing individuals from different cultural groups to the mainstream population. There is value in recognizing the heterogeneity within cultural groups, as well as the homogeneity of individuals within any group.

References

American heritage dictionary of the English language (3rd ed.) (1996). Boston: Houghton Mifflin.

Anderson, B. (1981). *An analysis of the relationship of age and sex to type and frequency of disfluencies in lower socioeconomic preschool Black chil-*

dren. Unpublished doctoral dissertation, Northwestern University, Evanston, IL.

Ardila, A., Bateman, J. R., & Nino, C. R. (1994). An epidemiologic study of stuttering. *Journal of Communication Disorders, 27,* 37–48.

Aron, M. (1962). The nature and incidence of stuttering among a Bantu group of school going children. *Journal of Speech and Hearing Disorders, 27,* 116–128.

Battle, D. (1997). Multicultural considerations in counseling communicatively disordered persons and their families. In T. A. Crowe (Ed.), *Applications of counseling in speech-language pathology and audiology* (pp. 118–141). Baltimore: Williams and Wilkins.

Bernstein-Ratner, N., & Benitez, M. (1985). Linguistic analysis of the bilingual stutterer. *Journal of Fluency Disorders, 10,* 211–219.

Bloodstein, O. (1995). A handbook on stuttering (5th ed.). San Diego: Singular Publishing.

Brutten, G., & Miller, R. (1988). The disfluencies of normally fluent Black first graders. *Journal of Fluency Disorders, 13,* 291–299.

Carson, C., & Kantner, C. E. (1945). Incidence of stuttering among white and colored children. *Southern Speech Journal, 10,* 57–59.

Clifford, S., Twitchell, M., & Hull, R. (1965). Stuttering in South Dakota Indians. *Central States Speech Journal, 16,* 59–60.

Conrad, C. (1980). *An incidence study of stuttering among black adults.* Unpublished research project, Northwestern University, Evanston, IL.

Conrad, C. (1985). *A conversational act analysis of Black mother-child dyads including stuttering and nonstuttering children.* Unpublished doctoral dissertation, Northwestern University, Evanston, IL.

Conrad, C. (1987). Fluency in multicultural populations. In L. Cole & V. Deal (Eds.), *Communication disorders in multicultural populations.* Unpublished manuscript. Rockville, MD: American Speech-Language-Hearing Association.

Cooper, E. B., & Cooper, C. S. (1998). Fluency disorders. In D. Battle (Ed.), *Communication disorders in multicultural populations* (pp. 189–211). Boston: Andover Medical Publishers.

Crowe, T. (1994). Preventative counseling with parents at risk. In C. W. Starkweather & H. F. M. Peters (Eds.), *Proceedings of the first World Congress on fluency disorders* (pp. 232–235). Nijmegen, The Netherlands: University Press.

Crowe, T. A. (1995, December). *Counseling for fluency disorders: Rationale, strategy and technique.* Paper presented as part of a short course (with W. Manning and G. W. Blood) at the American Speech-Language-Hearing Association Convention, Orlando.

Crowe, T. A., Di Lollo, A., & Crowe, B. (2000). *Crowe's protocols: A comprehensive guide to stuttering assessment.* San Antonio: The Psychological Corporation.

Dale, P. (1977). Factors related to dysfluent speech in bilingual Cuban-American adolescents. *Journal of Fluency Disorders, 2,* 311–314.

Ford, S. (1986). *Pragmatic abilities in Black disfluent preschoolers.* Unpublished master's thesis, Howard University, Washington, DC.

Gillespie, S. K., & Cooper, E. B. (1973). Prevalence of speech problems in junior and senior high schools. *Journal of Speech and Hearing Research, 16*(4), 739–743.

Goldman, R. (1967). Cultural influences on the sex ratio in the incidence of stuttering. *American Anthropology, 69,* 78–81.

Goodall, H. B., & Brobby, G. W. (1982). Stuttering, sickling, and cerebral malaria: A possible organic basis for stuttering. *Lancet, 8284,* 1279–1281.

Gregory, H., & Hill, D. (1980). Stuttering therapy for children. *Seminars in Speech, Language and Hearing, 1*(4), 351–363.

Hale-Benson, J. E. (1987). *Black children: Their roots, culture, and learning styles.* Baltimore: The Johns Hopkins University Press.

Harris, L. (1986). Barriers to the delivery of speech, language, and hearing services in Native Americans. In O. L. Taylor (Ed.), *Nature of communication disorders in culturally and linguistically diverse populations* (pp. 219–236). San Diego: College-Hill Press.

Hilliard, A. (1976). *Alternative to IQ testing: An approach to the identification of gifted minority children (Final report).* Sacramento, CA: California State Department of Education.

Jayaram, M. (1983). Phonetic influences on stuttering in monolingual and bilingual stutterers. *Journal of Communication Disorders, 16,* 287–297.

Johnson, W. (1944a). The Indians have no word for it: I. Stuttering in children. *Quarterly Journal of Speech, 30,* 330–337.

Johnson, W. (1944b). The Indians have no word for it: II. Stuttering in adults. *Quarterly Journal of Speech, 30,* 456–465.

Kirk, L. (1977). Stuttering and quasi-stuttering. *Georgia Journal of Communication Disorders, 10,* 109–126.

Leavitt, R. R. (1974). *The Puerto Ricans: Cultural change and language deviance.* Tucson, AZ: University of Arizona Press.

Leith, W. R., & Gibson, A. (1991). *The prevalence of stuttering among school children in Nassau, the Bahamas.* Unpublished manuscript, Wayne State University, Detroit.

Leith, W. R., & Mims, H. A. (1975). Cultural influences in the development and treatment of stuttering: A preliminary report on the Black stutterer. *Journal of Speech and Hearing Disorders, 40,* 459–466.

Lemert, E. M. (1953). Some Indians who stutter. *Journal of Speech and Hearing Disorders, 18,* 168–174.

Lemert, E. M. (1962). Stuttering and social structure in two Pacific societies. *Journal of Speech and Hearing Disorders, 27,* 3–10.

McCartney, T. O. (1971). *Neurosis in the sun.* Nassau, Bahamas: Executive Ideas of the Bahamas.

Meyers, S. C., & Woodford, L. L. (1992). *The fluency development system for young children.* Buffalo, NY: United Educational Services.

Morgenstern, J. J. (1953). *Psychological and social factors in children's stammering.* Doctoral dissertation, University of Edinburgh, Edinburgh, Scotland.

Morgenstern, J. J. (1956). Socioeconomic factors in stuttering. *Journal of Speech and Hearing Disorders, 21,* 25–53.

Nathanson, S. (1969). *A study of the influence of race, socioeconomic status and sex on the speech fluency of 200 nonstuttering fifth graders.* Unpublished doctoral dissertation, Northwestern University, Evanston, IL.

Neely, M. M. (1960). *An investigation of the incidence of stuttering among elementary school children in the parochial schools of Orleans Parish.* Master's thesis, Tulane University, New Orleans.

Nwokah, E. (1988). The imbalance of stuttering behavior in bilingual speakers. *Journal of Fluency Disorders, 13,* 357–373.

Ozawa, Y. (1960). Studies of misarticulation in Wakayama district. *Journal of Medicine, University of Osaka, 5,* 319.

Prichett, M. (1966, November). *The role of the East St. Louis schools: A study of the effectiveness of multi-approach in stuttering therapy.* Proceedings of the Annual Meeting of the Illinois Speech Association, Chicago.

Ralston, L (1981). Stammering: A stress index in Caribbean classrooms. *Journal of Fluency Disorders, 6,* 119–133.

Riley, G. D. (1981). *Stuttering prediction instrument.* Austin, TX: PRO-ED.

Robinson, T. L., Jr. (1992). *An investigation of speech fluency skills in African American preschool children during narrative discourse.* Unpublished dissertation, Howard University, Washington, DC.

Robinson, Jr., T. L., & Crowe, T. A. (1987). A comparative study of speech disfluencies in nonstuttering black and white college athletes. *Journal of Fluency Disorders, 12,* 147–156.

Robinson, Jr., T. L., & Crowe, T. A. (1998). Culture-based considerations in programming or stuttering intervention with African American clients and their families. *Language Speech and Hearing Services in the Schools, 29,* 172–179.

Robinson, Jr., T. L., & Crowe, T. A. (2000). Multicultural issues in speech fluency. In T. Coleman (Ed.), *Clinical management of communication disorders in culturally diverse children* (pp. 251–269). Boston: Allyn & Bacon.

Robinson, Jr., T. L., Davis, J. G., & Crowe, T. A. (2000). Disfluency in non-stuttering African-American preschoolers during conversation and narrative discourse. *Contemporary Issues in Communication Science and Disorders, 27*, 64–171.

Runyan, C. M., & Runyan, S. E. (1986). A fluency rules therapy program for young children in the public schools. *Language, Speech and Hearing Services in Schools, 17*, 276–284.

Seymour, H. N. (1986). Clinical principles for language intervention. In O. L. Taylor (Ed.), *Nature of communication disorders in culturally and linguistically diverse populations* (pp. 115–133). Austin, TX: PRO-ED.

Seymour, H. N., & Seymour, C. M. (1977). A therapeutic model for communication disorders among children who speak Black English vernacular. *Journal of Speech and Hearing Disorders, 42*, 247–256.

Snidecor, J. C. (1947). Why the Indian does not stutter. *Quarterly Journal of Speech, 33*, 493–495.

Starkweather, C. W. (1980). A multiprocess behavioral approach to stuttering therapy. *Seminars in Speech, Language and Hearing, 1*, 327–337.

Stewart, J. L. (1960). The problem of stuttering in certain North American Indian societies. *Journal of Speech and Hearing Disorders* (Monograph Supplement 6), 87.

Taylor, O. L. (1986). Historical perspectives and conceptual framework. In O. L. Taylor (Ed.), *Nature of communication disorders in culturally and linguistically diverse populations* (pp. 1–17). Austin, TX: PRO-ED.

Taylor, O. L. (1987). Clinical practice and a social occasion. In L. Cole & V. R. Deal (Eds.), *Communication disorders in multicultural populations*. Unpublished manuscript. Rockville, MD: American Speech-Language-Hearing Association.

Taylor, O. L., & Payne, K. T. (1983). Culturally valid testing: A proactive approach. *Topics in Language Disorders, 3*, 8–20.

Taylor, O. L., & Samara, R. (1985). *Communication disorders in underserved populations: Developing nations.* Paper presented at the National Colloquium on Underserved Populations, American Speech-Language-Hearing Association, Washington, DC.

Terrell, B. Y., & Hale, J. E. (1992). Serving a multicultural population: Different learning styles. *American Journal of Speech-Language Pathology: A Journal of Clinical Practice, 1*, 5–8.

Toyoda, B. (1959). A statistical report. *Clinical Paediatrica, 12*, 788.

Travis, L. E., Johnson, W., & Shover, J. (1981). The relationship of bilingualism to stuttering. *Journal of Speech Disorders, 2*, 185–189.

Van Kleeck, A. (1994). Potential cultural bias in training parents as conversational partners with their children who have delays in language development. *American Journal of Speech-Language Pathology: A Journal of Clinical Practice, 3*(1), 67–78.

Van Riper, C. (1982). *The nature of stuttering* (2nd ed.). Englewood Cliffs, NJ: Prentice-Hall.

Vaughn-Cooke, F. B. (1983). Improving language assessment in minority children. *Asha, 25,* 29–34.

Vaughn-Cooke, F. B. (1986). The challenge of assessing the language of non-mainstream speakers. In O. L. Taylor (Ed.), *Treatment of communication disorders in culturally and linguistically diverse populations* (pp. 23–48). Austin, TX: PRO-ED.

Waddle, Y. (1934). A comparison of speech defectives among colored and white children. Master's thesis, University of Iowa, Iowa City, IA.

Wakaba, Y. (1983). Group therapy for Japanese children who stutter. *Journal of Fluency Disorders, 8,* 93–118.

Watson, J. B., & Kayser, H. (1994). Assessment of bilingual/bicultural children and adults who stutter. *Seminars in Speech and Language, 15,* 149–164.

Zimmerman, G., Liljeblad, S., Frank, A., & Cleeland, C. (1983). The Indians have many terms for it: Stuttering among the Bannock-Shoshone. *Journal of Speech and Hearing Research, 26,* 315–318.

Additional Resources

American Speech-Language-Hearing Association. (1996). *Issues in assessing and treating speech fluency behaviors.* Rockville, MD: American Speech-Language-Hearing Association.

Bullen, A. K. (1945). A cross-cultural approach to the problem of stuttering. *Child Development, 16,* 1–88.

Cooper, E. B., & Cooper, C. S. (1985). *Cooper personalized fluency control therapy-revised.* Allen, TX: DLM.

Robinson, Jr., T. L., & Crowe, T. A. (1994, November). *A model for inclusion of multicultural variables in fluency intervention programming.* Paper presented at the American Speech-Language-Hearing Association Annual Convention, New Orleans.

Stuttering Foundation of America, Memphis, TN. http://www.stuttering-homepage.com.

□ □ □
□ □ □
□ □ □

Appendix

Sample Assessment Forms

Appendix 9-1

Sample assessment form to aid in determining the cultural factors relevant to the treatment of a child client.

Date of assessment _____

Client's name _____

Name of person completing form _____

Relationship to the child _____

|CULTURAL FACTORS

Instructions: Answer each question by writing your response in the space provided or by circling the most accurate response on the scale provided for some of the questions.

Cultural Identity

1. With what culture does the child primarily identify?_____

    _____

2. Please list all other cultures with which the child might identify. _____

    _____

Cultural Assimilation

1. To what extent is the child in touch with the customs, traditions, beliefs, food, music, and art of the culture?

0	1	2	3	4	5	6
Not at All	Slightly	Less Than Half	About Half	More Than Half	Nearly Completely	Completely

2. To what extent is the child in touch with his/her secondary culture(s)?

0	1	2	3	4	5	6
Not at All	Slightly	Less Than Half	About Half	More Than Half	Nearly Completely	Completely

3. Does the child have the opportunity to participate in social activities other than those that represent his/her primary culture?

0	1	2	3	4	5	6
Never	Occasionally	Less Than Half the Time	About Half of the Time	More Than Half of the Time	Often	Always

4. How often does the child participate in social activities other than those that represent his/her primary culture?

0	1	2	3	4	5	6
Never	Occasionally	Less Than Half the Time	About Half of the Time	More Than Half of the Time	Often	Always

Cultural Environment

1. What is the primary language spoken in the child's home? _____

    _____

    _____

continued

2. Name all other languages spoken in the child's home on a daily basis._____

_____

_____

3. What language(s) does the child use most on a daily basis? _____

_____

4. How many generations of family live in the child's household? _____

_____

5. Do all the people living in the child's household share the same culture? _____ Yes _____ No
   If no, name the cultures represented in the household as well as the relationship to the child
   of each person who represents a culture other than the child's primary culture.

_____

_____

6. What is the child's native country?_____

   What is the native country of each person living in the child's home, if different from the child's?

_____

_____

7. How many of the child's friends share the same primary culture as the child? _____

_____

8. To what extent do you feel the child's primary culture is a distinguishing or determining
   characteristic of his/her

   a. neighborhood

0	1	2	3	4	5	6
Not at All	A Little	Somewhat	Moderately	A Lot	Nearly Completely	Completely

   b. school

0	1	2	3	4	5	6
Not at All	A Little	Somewhat	Moderately	A Lot	Nearly Completely	Completely

   c. education

0	1	2	3	4	5	6
Not at All	A Little	Somewhat	Moderately	A Lot	Nearly Completely	Completely

   d. social life

0	1	2	3	4	5	6
Not at All	A Little	Somewhat	Moderately	A Lot	Nearly Completely	Completely

   e. religious life

0	1	2	3	4	5	6
Not at All	A Little	Somewhat	Moderately	A Lot	Nearly Completely	Completely

continued

Cultural System

▌ATTITUDES

1. How are people who stutter regarded within the child's primary culture?

_____

_____

_____

_____

2. How much does the child's primary culture influence family attitudes about stuttering?

0	1	2	3	4	5	6
Not at All	A Little	Somewhat	Moderately	A Lot	Nearly Completely	Completely

Please explain your response.

_____

_____

_____

3. Are the child's attitudes toward stuttering different from those of other people who live in his/her home?

____ Yes ____ No   If yes, please explain. _____

_____

_____

▌BELIEFS

1. Is there a belief in the child's primary culture about the cause of stuttering?

____ Yes ____ No   If yes, please explain. _____

_____

_____

_____

2. Is there a belief in the child's primary culture about the cure or control of stuttering?

____ Yes ____ No   If yes, please explain. _____

_____

_____

_____

3. Is there ever conflict in the child's home among the different generations or people living there about cultural beliefs?

____ Yes ____ No   If yes, please explain. _____

_____

_____

_____

continued

4. If you answered yes, are these conflicts ever about stuttering or speaking abilities and behaviors?

    ____ Yes   ____ No   If yes, please explain. _____

    _____

    _____

    _____

    _____

5. How much does the family's primary culture influence their beliefs about stuttering?

0	1	2	3	4	5	6
Not at All	A Little	Somewhat	Moderately	Very Much	Nearly Completely	Completely

Appendix 9-2

Sample assessment form to aid in determining the cultural factors relevant to the treatment of an adult client.

Date of assessment _____

Client's name _____

Name of person completing this form _____

Relationship to the client _____

|CULTURAL FACTORS

Instructions: Answer each question by writing your response in the space provided or by circling the most accurate response on the scale provided for some of the questions.

Cultural Identity

1. With what culture do you primarily identify?

   _____
   _____
   _____
   _____

2. Name all other cultures with which you identify.

   _____
   _____
   _____
   _____

Cultural Assimilation

1. To what extent do you feel in touch with your primary culture (customs, traditions, food, music, art, beliefs)?

0	1	2	3	4	5	6
Not at All	Slightly	Less Than Half	About Half	More Than Half	Nearly Completely	Completely

2. To what extent do you feel in touch with your secondary culture(s)?

0	1	2	3	4	5	6
Not at All	Slightly	Less Than Half	About Half	More Than Half	Nearly Completely	Completely

3. Do you have the opportunity to participate in social activities other than those that represent your primary culture?

0	1	2	3	4	5	6
Never	Occasionally	Less Than Half the Time	About Half of the Time	More Than Half of the Time	Often	Always

4. How often do you actually participate in social activities other than those that represent your primary culture?

0	1	2	3	4	5	6
Never	Occasionally	Less Than Half the Time	About Half of the Time	More Than Half of the Time	Often	Always

continued

Cultural Environment

1. What is the primary language spoken in your home?

   _____

   _____

2. Name all other languages spoken in your home or by you on a daily basis.

   _____

   _____

   _____

3. What languages do you use most on a daily basis?

   _____

   _____

   _____

4. How many generations live in your household? _____

5. Do all the persons living in your household share the same culture? _____ Yes _____ No
   If no, name cultures represented in your household and the relationship to you of each person
   who represents a culture other than your own primary culture.

   _____

   _____

   _____

   _____

6. What is your native country? _____
   What is (are) the native country(ies) of all persons living in your home, if different than your own?

   _____

   _____

   _____

   _____

7. How many of your friends and social acquaintances are of the same primary culture as you?

0	1	2	3	4	5	6
None	A Few	Less Than Half	About Half	More Than Half	Almost all	All

8. How many of your professional colleagues or friends are of the same primary culture as you?

0	1	2	3	4	5	6
None	A Few	Less Than Half	About Half	More Than Half	Almost all	All

9. To what extent do you feel your primary culture is a distinguishing or determining characteristic
   of your

   a. Neighborhood

0	1	2	3	4	5	6
Not at All	A Little	Somewhat	Moderately	A Lot	Nearly Completely	Completely

continued

b. Job/Career

0	1	2	3	4	5	6
Not at All	A Little	Somewhat	Moderately	A Lot	Nearly Completely	Completely

c. Education

0	1	2	3	4	5	6
Not at All	A Little	Somewhat	Moderately	A Lot	Nearly Completely	Completely

d. Social Life

0	1	2	3	4	5	6
Not at All	A Little	Somewhat	Moderately	A Lot	Nearly Completely	Completely

e. Religious Life

0	1	2	3	4	5	6
Not at All	A Little	Somewhat	Moderately	A Lot	Nearly Completely	Completely

Cultural System

1. Attitudes

   a. How are persons who stutter regarded within your culture?

   _____

   _____

   _____

   _____

   _____

   b. How much does your culture influence your attitudes about stuttering?

0	1	2	3	4	5	6
Not at All	A Little	Somewhat	Moderately	A Lot	Nearly Completely	Completely

   Please explain your response. _____

   _____

   _____

   _____

   _____

   _____

   c. Are your attitudes toward stuttering different than those of other persons who live in your home?

   _____ Yes _____ No   If yes, please explain._____

   _____

   _____

   _____

   _____

   _____

   _____

continued

2. Beliefs

   a. What do you believe to be the cause of stuttering?

   _____

   _____

   _____

   _____

   _____

   Is this a general belief within your culture? _____ Yes _____ No

   b. Do you believe that stuttering can be cured or controlled? _____ Yes _____ No

   If yes, please explain how you think stuttering can be cured or controlled.

   _____

   _____

   _____

   _____

   _____

   If you answered no, please explain why you think stuttering cannot be cured or controlled.

   _____

   _____

   _____

   _____

   _____

   c. Are your answers to question b general beliefs within your culture about the cure or control

   of stuttering? _____ Yes _____ No

   d. Is there ever conflict in your home among the different generations or persons living there

   about cultural beliefs? _____ Yes _____ No

   If you answered yes, do these conflicts ever concern stuttering or speaking abilities and behaviors?

   _____ Yes _____ No If you answered yes, please explain. _____

   _____

   _____

   _____

   _____

   _____

   e. How much does your culture influence your beliefs about stuttering?

0	1	2	3	4	5	6
Not at All	A Little	Somewhat	Moderately	A Lot	Nearly Completely	Completely

10

Voice and Voice Disorders

R. Wayne Holland and Glenda DeJarnette

Voice reflects the health status of the body through its connection with neurologic and endocrinologic systems. Moreover, the health status of subglottal and supraglottal systems is often reflected in the voice. To the trained and untrained ear, the voice suggests a person's age, gender, and emotional state. Speech-language pathologists are trained to consider these traditional aspects of the voice in clients. As of this writing, clinical protocols do not presuppose that racial, ethnic, or cultural factors contribute to the quality of voice. In fact, few acoustic and physiologic data exist that compare laryngeal structure and function across racial, ethnic, and cultural groups. A few perceptual studies exist that allude to the fact that culturally determined linguistic patterns color the tone of voice of speakers and influence the listener's perception of voice tone.

The perception of the voice is not restricted to the phonatory apparatus and its functioning. Indeed, the perceived aerodynamic and torque interactions of the phonatory system with respiratory and resonatory systems provide the greatest appreciation of voice. Thus, a full examination of multicultural issues affecting normal and abnormal voice function ultimately must consider the variables that affect these combined systems to generate the vocal product. Throughout this chapter, information is shared that pertains to the respiratory system, laryngeal system, and supralaryngeal resonatory systems, because it is believed that quality assessment of voice disorders and intervention must consider the interactions of these systems.

There is a paucity of information on the impact of multicultural variables on the production of normal and abnormal voice. This chapter presents the information that is available regarding voice in culturally diverse groups. Specifically, the chapter examines (1) incidence of voice-related pathologies in minority groups in the United States; (2) health issues related to voice dysfunction; (3) racial and ethnographic factors related to voice; and (4) the role of the speech-language pathologist in prevention, assessment, and intervention. The reader is cautioned that the categorization of minority groups is an artificial contrivance in that several groups (e.g., Asian and Hispanic groups) have racially, ethnically, or culturally distinct subgroups.

Incidence of Voice-Related Pathologies in Minority Groups in the United States

A review of the literature concerning the epidemiology of voice-related pathologies in minority groups yields insufficient data on the national distribution of all disorders. In some instances, the incidence reports extend beyond the United States to suggest racial distributions. Subsequently, studies of the incidence of the various voice-related pathologies among minority groups in the United States await epidemiologic investigation on a national scale. The available literature scans a few of the pathologies related to the vocal cords and the nasal and oropharyngeal ports. This literature is reviewed in Incidence of Oral and Nasopharyngeal Pathologies and is followed by an examination of health information that reiterates the need for increased research of voice-related pathologies in culturally diverse populations in the United States.

Incidence of Vocal Cord Pathologies

Incidence of all vocal cord disorders among minority groups in the United States is difficult to ascertain, because no studies currently exist that are cross-sectional for race or ethnicity. This section discusses a recent report of the incidence of laryngeal cancer in the United States, with a focus on African American and white adults. A second report is presented that examines the incidence of laryngeal pathologies in Asian, African American, and white children.

Yang, Thomas, and Davis (1989) reported the incidence of laryngeal cancer by subsite for adult blacks and whites across gender, with ages ranging from younger than 29 years to 79 years. Blacks constituted 10% of the subject pool. Medical records for 1973–1982 were used to report the data. Subjects were identified through the National Cancer Institute's Surveillance, Epidemiology, and End Results (SEER) program. Comparative ratios for incidence of squamous cell carcinoma revealed that black and white men exhibited a higher incidence than women for all subsites. The rate ratios were largest between the genders for the glottis subsite, as compared with the supraglottis and subglottis. The investigators indicated that anatomic and physiologic differences between the genders might have accounted for the disparity in the incidence rates. Although Yang and colleagues (1989) did not comment on the differences in incidence between the races, the data reflect that, compared with white men, black men had a higher incidence of all subsite laryngeal cancers, most notably cancer of the glottis. Likewise, compared with white women, black women had a higher incidence of all subsite laryngeal cancers, except for the glottis. Recent national statistics also show that African American and Native American women are at greater risk for laryngeal cancer and have a lower 5-year survival rate than white women (American Cancer Society, 1998; Landis, Murray, Bolden, & Wingo, 1998).

The incidence of laryngeal pathologies in children was investigated by Dobres and colleagues (1990), who used medical chart inspection as the method of data collection. A portion of the medical charts was marked for race. Asian children constituted 0.02% of the subjects, black children constituted 5%, and white children constituted 79%. Thirty laryngeal pathologies were noted in the data. Overall, the incidence of laryngeal pathologies was greater among men than women, and subglottic stenosis showed the highest incidence. The investigators suggested that the distribution of laryngeal pathologies across the races mirrored the overall finding for the total sample. Asians had the greatest male-to-female incidence ratio (4.3 to 1.0), whites had the second greatest (1.8 to 1.0), and blacks had the lowest (1.4 to 1.0). It is unclear whether the results for age-related incidence in the total sample is the same across the races, because the age breakdown for race was not shared. Moreover, visual inspection of the data suggests that there might be proportional differences in the distribution of the pathologies, as well as some gender-related differences across race groups. For all groups, the occurrence of subglottic stenosis was the highest. Subsequent pathologies, however, showed patterns for minority groups that differed from that of the white children. Although vocal nodules were clearly more prevalent in white men as compared with white women, vocal nodules were only slightly more prevalent in Asian men compared with Asian women. Among the black children, the women showed a higher incidence of vocal nodules as compared with men.

In the case of laryngomalacia, a pattern difference occurred as well in that neither the Asian nor the black children followed the gender ratio distribution that was observed in the white children (Dobres et al., 1990). The incidence of laryngomalacia was higher among white men than among white women; however, the pattern among blacks was the reverse. The incidence was higher among black women. Laryngomalacia was equally dispersed among Asian men and women. Only 5 of the 30 pathologies [i.e., subglottic stenosis, vocal nodules, laryngomalacia, dysphonia (normal larynx), and vocal fold paralysis] were clearly evidenced across all groups. Of course, as Dobres and colleagues (1990) suggested, the minority sample sizes were small, making definitive comparisons difficult.

Incidence of Oral and Nasopharyngeal Pathologies

Other than cleft palate, the incidence of oral and nasopharyngeal pathologies in minority groups has not been investigated. The most accurate method of reporting the incidence and prevalence of a cleft palate is not perfected in reporting practices, according to Sayetta, Weinrich, and Coston (1989). Methodologic difficulties include varied methods of case selection (e.g., through birth or death certificates, professional reports, or hospital records); semantic confusion over incidence versus prevalence in data reports; inaccuracies in cleft classifications; and exclusion of stillbirths and aborted fetuses from incidence data. Despite these methodologic encumbrances, investigators have provided evidence of differing distributions of cleft palate occurrence across racial groupings (Vanderas, 1987). Vanderas (1987) examined the literature on epidemiologic studies of cleft lip, cleft palate, and cleft lip and palate across racial groupings and provided a picture of the incidence of a cleft palate in blacks, American Indians, Chinese, and Japanese. Some of the data were extracted from international studies, as well as from studies on the incidence in the United States. For the minority groups on which Vanderas (1987) focused, the incidence of cleft palate in the United States per 1,000 population was highest for Chinese (4.04%), second highest for American Indians (0.79–3.62%), third highest for Japanese (0.82–2.41%), and fourth highest for blacks (0.80–1.67%). Vanderas (1987) looked at one study from multiple sources to report incidence in the Chinese, whereas multiple sources were used to report incidences for other groups. Incidence reports for Filipinos and Hispanics were shared from a more limited pool of studies (Vanderas, 1987). For Filipino births in Hawaii, the incidence was 2.45% per 1,000 population. An international focus on Puerto Ricans and Mexicans showed incidence ranging from 0.42% to 2.27%, with Puerto Ricans showing slightly greater incidence than Mexicans per 100,000 population (Vanderas, 1987).

Vanderas (1987) also reported on incidence trends of the different kinds of conditions (i.e., cleft lip, cleft palate, and cleft lip and cleft palate). Among blacks, the incidence of cleft palate tended to be greater than that of cleft lip with cleft palate, which in turn was greater than that of cleft lip alone. For American Indians, the incidence of cleft lip with palate tended to be greater than the incidence of cleft lip alone or cleft palate alone. For the Chinese, the incidence of cleft lip with cleft palate tended to be greater than that of cleft lip or cleft palate alone in some studies. In other studies, the incidence of cleft lip with cleft palate tended to be equal to that of cleft palate, although the incidence of both was greater than that of cleft lip alone. For the Japanese, the incidence of cleft lip with cleft palate was greater than that of cleft lip alone, which was greater than the incidence of cleft palate alone.

The gender ratios for each racial group revealed that, for the most part, men tend to have a higher incidence of cleft palate than women. Specifically, for each group and each cleft classification the following was noted:

- Black men showed a greater incidence for all cleft types than black women.
- American Indian men showed a greater incidence for cleft lip with palate and cleft palate alone than American Indian women. Both showed an equal incidence of cleft lip alone.
- The Chinese showed an unclear ratio on gender differences for cleft lip with cleft palate, but men showed a greater incidence of cleft palate alone than women.
- Japanese men showed a greater incidence of cleft lip with palate, but women showed a greater incidence of cleft palate alone. It was unclear which gender dominated the ratio for cleft lip alone.

In summary, it appears that, except for blacks, minority groups follow the incidence trend of the general population—that is, a cleft lip with cleft palate occurs more often than a cleft palate alone (Shaw, Croen, & Curry, 1991). Among blacks, a cleft palate occurs more often. The gender ratio is less clear for minority groups and may not follow the trend found in the general population (i.e., that women are more likely to be born with a cleft palate alone than men) (Shaw et al., 1991). American Indians and the Japanese followed this trend; however, it is not followed by Chinese (women equal men in the incidence of cleft palate alone) or blacks (male incidence of cleft palate is greater than that of women).

Health Issues Related to Voice Dysfunction

To adequately address voice disorders in multicultural groups, the health-related conditions that predispose and precipitate voice disorders must be considered. This section, therefore, examines health problems that have a direct or an indirect effect on the voice production system. The database material was taken from the 1988–1992 SEER program (Miller et al., 1996). The SEER program collected data on the incidence of cancer in the general population. SEER data for 1988–1992 represented 14% of the total U.S. population. The areas that supplied the SEER database for 1988–1992 were Connecticut; Hawaii; Iowa; New Mexico; Utah; Atlanta; Detroit; Los Angeles, San Francisco, Oakland, San Jose, and Monterey, California; Seattle and Puget Sound, Washington; and areas identified by the Alaska Area Native Health Service.

Carcinomas with Direct or Indirect Effect on Voice

According to the National Cancer Institute (Miller, Kolonel, & Bernstein, 1996), overall cancer incidence rates were higher in men than women for regions included in the SEER database. SEER data showed trends that affected racial groupings. Racial groupings reported in the SEER data included black, American Indian, Alaska Native, Chinese, Filipino, Hawaiian, Hispanic (nonwhite), Hispanic (white), Japanese, Korean, non-Hispanic white, Vietnamese, and white. For men, the average annual rate of cancer per 100,000 population from highest to lowest incidence by racial and ethnic group is as follows:

Black (560)
Non-Hispanic white (481)
White (469)
Alaska native (372)
Hawaiian (340)
Hispanic (white) (336)
Vietnamese (326)
Japanese (322)
Hispanic (nonwhite) (319)
Chinese (282)
Filipino (274)
Korean (266)
American Indian (New Mexico) (196)

For women, the "average annual" rate of cancer per 100,000 population from highest to lowest incidence by racial and ethnic group is as follows:

Black (319)
Hawaiian (239)
Alaska Native (225)

Non-Hispanic white (217)
White (213)
Chinese (139)
Hispanic (white) (134)
Japanese (133)
Hispanic (nonwhite) (129)
American Indian (New Mexico) (123)
Filipino (105)
Korean (not available)
Vietnamese (not available)

Predispositions to Cancers That Affect Voice
Genetic Factors

The genetic predisposition for cancer is unclear, despite the fact that research on skin cancer tentatively shows genetic differences between blacks and whites in the development of cancer. Moreover, the genetic influence on cancers that have environmental causes is even less clear. Certain teratogens and health practices put people at risk for cancer. Known risk factors include tobacco (i.e., smokeless tobacco), alcohol, certain diet ingredients, and carcinogenic substances in the workplace and environment.

Smoking

Smoking is known to be causally related to cancer of the larynx, oral and pharyngeal cavities, lungs, and esophagus. In 1994, an estimated 48 million adults (men and women) were smokers. A 1996 Centers for Disease Control and Prevention report states that "[r]acial/ethnic group-specific prevalence was highest for American Indians/Alaskan Natives . . . and lowest for Asians/Pacific Islanders. . . . With the exception of persons with 0–8 years of education, smoking prevalence varied inversely with level of education and was highest among persons with 9–11 years of education. . . . Smoking prevalence was higher among persons living below the poverty level . . . than among those living at or above poverty" (Centers for Disease Control and Prevention, 1996). Miller et al. (1996) reported the following smoking rates for men and women in the United States:

	Men (%)	*Women (%)*
American Indians and Alaskan Natives	53.7	33.1
Blacks	33.9	21.8
Whites	28.0	24.7
Hispanics	24.3	15.2
Asian and Pacific Islanders	20.4	7.5

Alcohol

Alcohol is known to increase the risk for cancer of the oral cavity, pharynx, larynx, and esophagus. The percentage of use across minority groups is difficult to ascertain because of small sample sizes within the large national studies. However, existing data suggest that alcohol consumption patterns vary across racial groupings (Page & Asire, 1985). The occurrence of cirrhosis of the liver has been used as an indicator of alcohol consumption patterns, although caution is exercised because confounding socioeconomic variables have an impact on health care provision and can inflate incidence rates among minorities. The cirrhosis data, however, reveal that the death rate for those with cirrhosis of the liver is highest for American Indians (men, 43.7%; women, 29.9%), second highest for blacks (men, 29.4%; women, 13.5%), and lowest for Asians and Pacific Americans (Page & Asire, 1985). The death rate for Hispanics was not available.

Nutrition

Nutritional factors tend to combine with other risk factors to affect the cancers that have an impact on voice-related concerns. Exposure to teratogenic agents combined with a reduced nutritional intake probably increases the risk of cancer. Indeed, it is suggested that salt-cured, smoked, and nitrite-cured foods are linked to cancer of the esophagus. Although no data exist that implicate nutritional factors in the development of cancers that have an effect on vocal systems, it has been suggested that dietary habits influence disease incidence (Baquet, Horm, Gibbs, & Grenwald, 1991). Dietary ingredients implicated in cancer control include carotenoid (found in dark vegetables, fruits, and carrots), vitamin A (found in liver, milk, cheese, butter, and egg yolks), fiber (found in fruits, vegetables, beans, peas, and whole-grain cereals), vitamin E, and selenium. Dietary ingredients known to cause cancer include fats ingested at high levels and molds and fungi produced in foods that use curing agents. Culturally rooted dietary habits, often reinforced by conditions of poverty or low socioeconomic potential, can put minority groups at risk for cancer (Baquet et al., 1991). For example, Hargreaves, Baquet, and Gamshadzahi (1989) reviewed the nutritional habits of African Americans and found that African American food tended to be high in protein, fat, and carbohydrates and low in fiber, thiamine, riboflavin, vitamins A and C, and iron.

Environmental and Chemical Factors

Exposure to carcinogenic substances in the workplace puts individuals at risk for cancers that affect the vocal production systems

(Parnes, 1990). No studies exist that show correlations between cancer and occupational trends among minority populations. However, low-paying, high-risk jobs have historically been the employment avenues for minorities in the United States (National Center for Health Statistics, 1991). As such, these groups have been exposed to industrial processes and chemicals that increase the risk of cancer. The National Cancer Institute has identified exposure to chemicals in the workplace as an environmental risk (Page & Asire, 1985). Among the industries with a high risk of exposure are furniture manufacturing, boot and shoe manufacturing and shoe and boot repair, auramine manufacturing, rubber manufacturing, mining (with exposure to radon), isopropyl alcohol manufacturing, and nickel refining. Among the carcinogenic chemicals to which workers are exposed are 4-aminobiphenyl, arsenic and arsenic compounds, asbestos, benzene, benzidine, bis(2-chloroethyl)-2-naphthylamine (chlornaphazine), bis(chloromethyl)ether and technical-grade chloromethyl methyl ether, chromium and certain chromium compounds, 2-naphthylamine, soot, tars, oils, and vinyl chloride.

Incidence of Cancers in Minority Groups
Laryngeal Cancer
    The annual incidence of laryngeal cancer in the United States is most often reported for whites and blacks. According to SEER data for 1988–1992, black men had a higher incidence than white men and black and white women (Miller et al., 1996). Black men showed an incidence of 12.7 cases per 100,000 population, as compared with 7.5 per 100,000 for white men. Black women showed an incidence of 2.5 cases per 100,000 population, as compared with 1.5 per 100,000 for white women (Miller et al., 1996). Of all minority groups, blacks had the highest incidence of laryngeal cancer (Miller et al., 1996). Several minority groups had less than 25 cases of laryngeal cancer per 100,000 population, and calculations were not conducted for them. Groups affected by the low incidence were Alaska Native, American Indian (New Mexico), Hawaiian, Korean, and Vietnamese.

Esophageal Cancer
    SEER data for 1988–1992 on the incidence of esophageal cancer show that blacks (men and women) have a higher incidence of this cancer than whites and other minority groups (Miller et al., 1996). This report states that "the incidence rate for black men is 60% higher than that for Hawaiians and more than 2.7 times greater than the rate for non-Hispanic white men. The rates for Chinese, Japanese, and non-Hispanic white men are similar to

each other (within the range of 5.2 to 5.6 per 100,000 men) and are modestly higher than the rate for white Hispanic men." Limited data were available for women with only black, white, and Hispanic groups represented. Hispanic and non-Hispanic white women had lower incidences of esophageal cancer than black women.

Lung Cancer

SEER data for 1988–1992 on the incidence of lung and bronchus cancer show that, "among men, . . . lung cancer incidence rates (per 100,000) range from a low of approximately 14 among American Indians to a high of 117 among blacks, an eightfold difference. Between these two extremes, rates fall into two groups ranging from 42 to 53 for Hispanics, Japanese, Chinese, Filipinos, and Koreans and from 71 to 89 for Vietnamese, whites, Alaskan Natives and Hawaiians. The range among women is much narrower, from a rate of approximately 15 among Japanese to nearly 51 among Alaska Natives. . . . Rates for the remaining female populations fall roughly into two groups with low rates of 16 to 25 for Korean, Filipino, Hispanic, and Chinese women and rates of 31 to 44 among Vietnamese, white, Hawaiian, and black women" (Miller et al., 1996).

Nasopharyngeal Cancer

The Chinese are suspected to have a genetic predisposition to nasopharyngeal cancer (Hung-Dhiu Ho, 1982). Mortality rates among Chinese are as high as 11.5% for women and 13.5% for men in population-specific regions of the United States (Rice & Yu, 1982). According to SEER reports for 1988–1992, the highest incidence rates of nasopharyngeal cancer were among the Chinese (Miller et al., 1996). Rates were also high in Vietnamese and Filipino men. Black, white, and Hispanic men and white women showed low incidences compared with male and female Chinese, Filipinos, and Vietnamese.

Oral Cavity Cancer

SEER data for 1988–1992 indicate that for men, oral cavity cancer is highest in blacks, followed by whites, Vietnamese, and native Hawaiians. For women, high rates occur in non-Hispanic whites, blacks, and Filipinos (Miller et al., 1996).

Thyroid Cancer

SEER data for 1988–1992 show that thyroid cancer affects women more than men. The highest rates for thyroid cancer were among Filipino, Vietnamese, and Hawaiian women. The lowest were among black women (Miller et al., 1996).

Thyroid Disease with Direct or Indirect Effects on Voice

The incidence of endocrinologic diseases among minority populations has been researched very little. Williams (1975) identified some of the disorders among blacks based on international and national cases. Thyrotoxicosis, often symptomatic of Graves' disease, was listed among the diseases affecting blacks. It is known to produce conditions of hyperthyroidism and toxic nodular goiters. The incidence of Graves' disease among black Africans has been studied, and it is suggested that toxic nodular goiter does not often accompany the disease, although some degree of hyperthyroidism is evidenced (Kalk & Kalk, 1989). The Chinese have also shown a susceptibility to thyrotoxicosis (Blum, 1982; Gee, 1982). In a study that investigated the incidence of thyroid dysfunction in adults 55 years and older, differences in the incidence rates for blacks and whites were observed as well (Bagchi, Brown, & Parish, 1990). The incidence of hypothyroidism and hyperthyroidism was lower in blacks compared with whites. The study contained more women than men, which may have affected the results; however, both black and white women showed a greater proportional incidence than black and white men (Bagchi et al., 1990).

Respiratory Disease with Direct or Indirect Effects on Voice

Upper and lower respiratory tract bacterial and viral infections need to be researched relative to their distribution among the races. Current data-reporting and management systems do not appear to track the allergens and infectious causes of respiratory distress across racial groups. Chronic and persistent cough has been noted in the Chinese population and indicates a variety of respiratory difficulties, including postnasal drip, chronic bronchitis, bronchial asthma, and pulmonary tuberculosis (Chen, 1982). According to the Centers for Disease Control and Prevention (1996), tuberculosis showed an increase of 9.4 cases per 100,000 population between 1989 and 1990 and 2.3 cases per 100,000 population between 1990 and 1991. The incidence figures for 1990 showed that minorities account for the greatest incidence of tuberculosis. The cases per 100,000 population were 41.6 for Asian and Pacific Americans, 33.0 for blacks, 18.9 for American Indians, 21.4 for Hispanics, and 4.2 for whites (Centers for Disease Control and Prevention, 1991). It has been noted that some races have less resistance to tuberculosis, which suggests a genetic predisposition to the disease (Williams, 1975). Other reasons for the increase in tuberculosis infections may be that the virus causes acquired immunodeficiency syndrome, homelessness, drug use, and the influx of immigrants who are at high risk for tuberculosis.

Cerebrovascular Disease with Direct or Indirect Effects on Voice

It is known that conditions of neuromotor compromise often result in dysarthric conditions and can affect the system of voice production. Age-adjusted death rates for cerebrovascular disease for 1988 were higher for black men (57.8%) and women (46.6%) per 100,000 population than for white men (30.0%) and women (25.5%) (National Center for Health Statistics, 1991). Across minority groups, the 1988 death count due to cerebrovascular disease was 8,098 for black men, 10,381 for black women, 791 for Asian and Pacific-American men, 789 for Asian and Pacific-American women, 171 for American Indian men, and 200 for American Indian women (National Center for Health Statistics, 1991).

Reflux, Laryngitis, and Related Disorders

The phenomenon referred to as *laryngopharyngeal reflux* (LPR) appeared in the literature beginning in 1991. Sataloff and his colleagues (1997) reported that 265 of 583 singers who sought medical care for vocal disorders during a 12-month period had reflux-related disorders. LPR is a multisystem disorder. It involves the sphincter between the stomach and the distal esophagus, the entire length of the esophagus, the upper esophageal sphincter, the structures of the larynx, pharynx, oral cavity, trachea, and the lungs. Because it is a multisystem disorder, a team, including a laryngologist, gastroenterologist, pulmonologist, speech-language pathologist, and voice specialist, must manage the treatment. The team should also include cooperation and consultation from a psychologist and nutritionist.

Typical symptoms of LPR include morning hoarseness, prolonged voice warm-up time, halitosis, excessive phlegm, frequent throat clearing, dry mouth, coated tongue, sensation of a lump in the throat, throat tickle, dysphagia, regurgitation of gastric contents, chronic sore throat, nocturnal cough, recurrent cough, difficulty breathing, aspiration, asthma-related characteristics, and heartburn.

The treatment team may recommend pharmacologic and surgical management of LPR. However, lifestyle changes may also be recommended. This may involve alteration in foods and eating habits and patterns. Recent popular movies such as *Chocolat, Soul Food, Big Night,* and *Like Water for Chocolate* show the importance of food on health and lifestyle. Changes in lifestyle and foods may be particularly challenging for persons from cultural groups who prefer foods that aggravate LPR. Avoiding foods such as high fat and fried foods, tomato products, spicy foods, and caffeine-containing beverages such as coffees and colas may be more of a challenge for many African Americans and Latinos than those who prefer a blander diet such as rice and wheat products preferred by many Asians and Europeans (Kittler & Sucher, 1998). This may be particularly difficult during cultural celebrations and holidays in which special foods are prepared and considerable cultural value may be placed on participating in family celebrations with feasts. For example, in the Mexican American community, *Cinco de Mayo* (May fifth) is a special event that is celebrated with festivals and feasting on traditional Mexican foods such as tamales and enchiladas that contain spicy tomato sauces, which may aggravate the LPR.

Racial and Ethnographic Factors Related to Voice

Current knowledge about the anatomic, physiologic, acoustic, and perceptual parameters related to the normal voice of minority populations in the United States is almost nonexistent. The few existing studies focus on the voice characteristics of African Americans, and these are shared in this section. Specifically, this section mentions literature that suggests anatomic, physiologic, acoustical, and perceptual differences between African Americans and the majority population. At the end of this section is a discussion of how the voice is used in the cultural-linguistic patterns of African American English to perpetuate the oral tradition of the culture. It is probable that other minority groups use parameters of voice to maintain cultural connection as well; however, existing literature has best identified this phenomenon in African Americans.

Anatomic Factors

In examining the larynges of blacks in South Africa, Boshoff (1945) found that the larynges of black cadavers were larger than those of white cadavers. It has been suggested that blacks have shorter trunks and longer limbs, which contributes to respiratory differences (Williams, 1975). Cole (1980) reviewed the orofacial characteristics of blacks that must be considered in the health and professional service to cleft palate patients.

Among the structural traits were a short columella, obtuse nasal arch, wide nasal tripod, septal cartilage producing a rounded nasal tip relative to the bridge of the nose, fullness of the vermilion border of the lips, propensity to develop keloids, and depigmentation or hypopigmentation when scarring of the skin occurs.

Physiologic Factors

Williams (1975) reviewed research of pulmonary function in blacks. This research suggested that black men of all ages have smaller vital capacities than those of whites of the same age, height, and weight. Black women also demonstrated smaller vital capacities than white women. Additionally, total lung capacity and residual volume were found to be smaller in blacks compared with whites.

Acoustic Factors Across Age Groups

The fundamental frequency characteristics of African American children, preadolescents, adolescents, young adults, and elderly have undergone some investigation. For all age groups, the fundamental frequency of African Americans is reportedly lower than that of whites, even when this lower frequency level does not appear to be statistically significant (Awan & Mueller, 1996; Ducote 1983; Hollien & Malcik, 1962; Hudson & Holbrook, 1981; Wheat & Hudson, 1988). The following review of the literature moves chronologically across the age span to illuminate racial differences that may be present and observable through acoustical analysis.

Awan and Mueller (1996) compared speaking fundamentals of African American, Hispanic, and white kindergartners (ages 5–6 years and 3 months). Visual inspection of the mean speaking fundamental measures taken from this study revealed that the fundamental frequencies of white and Hispanic women and men were closer in range to each other than were the fundamental frequencies of female and male African American children. The mean values for girls and boys, respectively, were 243.35 Hz and 240.07 Hz for whites, 248.04 Hz and 248.99 Hz for Hispanics, and 231.48 Hz and 241.31 Hz for African Americans. The mean speaking fundamental for African American girls was lower than any other group (boys and girls). African American girls' standard deviation (14.99 Hz) was near to the lowest noted in the study, with deviation ranging from 14.45 (Hispanic girls) to 22.17 Hz (white girls). Despite this observable gender difference in the data, statistical analysis suggested that there was no significant difference between the groups for gender. Moreover,

Awan and Mueller (1996) found no statistically significant difference in fundamental frequency variability (i.e., pitch sigma for gender or across racial grouping). One statistically significant finding in this study was that male and female African American kindergarten children exhibited a lower mean speaking fundamental frequency compared with Hispanics (236.40 Hz and 248.51 Hz, respectively). No statistically significant difference was found between the mean speaking fundamental frequencies of white kindergarten children (241.71 Hz) and African American (236.40 Hz) or Hispanic (248.51 Hz) groups. A finding in the study was that the speaking range (in semitones) was more reduced for the Hispanic kindergartners than for either the black or white groups. Awan and Mueller (1996) interpreted their findings to suggest that applying normative mean speaking fundamental frequency measures from one racial grouping to another may not be appropriate.

Studies that precede that of Awan and Mueller (1996) also indicate that, for young children, racial differences can be traced in the acoustic properties of voice output. Wheat and Hudson (1988) conducted a study with children ranging in age from 6 years to 6 years and 11 months. The fundamental frequencies were 219.5 Hz for African American boys and 211.3 Hz for African American girls. These pitch levels are lower than those determined for whites, who had a range of 280–365 Hz for boys and 270–395 Hz for girls (Wilson, 1979). No significant difference was found for gender in the fundamental frequencies of 6-year-old African Americans (Wheat & Hudson, 1988).

Racial differences can be detected acoustically in preadolescent and adolescent youths. Hollien and Malcik (1962) measured the fundamental frequency of preadolescent and adolescent African American boys. Mean fundamental frequency values were 210 Hz at 10 years old, 158 Hz at 14 years old, and 121 Hz at 18 years old (Hollien & Malcik, 1962), as compared with the majority norms of 235 Hz, 190 Hz, and 125 Hz for the respective ages (Wilson, 1979).

Hudson and Holbrook (1981) measured the fundamental frequency of young adult African American men and women from 18 to 29 years of age and compared their findings with data gathered for young adult white men and women (Fitch & Holbrook, 1970). African American men and women showed mean fundamental frequency ranges that were greater than those of their white counterparts. The mean modal fundamental frequency for African American men was 110.15 Hz (Hudson & Holbrook, 1981), as compared with 116.65 Hz for white men (Fitch & Holbrook, 1970). The fundamental frequency for African American women was 193.10 Hz (Hudson & Holbrook, 1981), as compared with 217.00 Hz for white women (Fitch & Holbrook, 1970).

A more recent study by Mayo, Watkins, and Richmond (2001) compared the reading fundamental frequency of 30 normal African American, Caucasian American, and Native American women. The results also showed that the African American women have the lowest reading fundamental frequency (201.2 Hz), followed by the Native American women (209.0 Hz). The white American women had the highest mean values (220.2 Hz); however, a 3 × 5 factorial analysis revealed that there was no significant difference between the reading fundamental frequencies of the three groups of speakers.

Hudson and Holbrook (1981) noted that the variability of frequency in African Americans was double that of white Americans and that African Americans tended to have greater flexibility above their mean modal frequencies. Findings for whites were just the opposite. The white Americans showed a greater range below their mean modal frequency. Hudson and Holbrook (1981) suggested that the lower modal frequency and degree of change above the modal frequency are factors that lead to racial identification through the voice.

However, a more recent study by Mayo et al. (2001) studied the speaking pitch range of African American, white American, and Native American women. Analysis showed that whereas the African American and Native American women differed statistically, no statistical differences were found in the measures between the African American (374.9 Hz) and white American (338.3 Hz) women, nor the Native American (284.8 Hz) and white American women (338.3 Hz). Mayo et al. (2001) suggested that the difference between their findings and those of Hudson and Holbrook (1981) may be due to the similarity in geolinguistic dialect used by their speakers as opposed to the disparate geolinguistic dialects of the speakers in the Hudson and Holbrook study.

Ducote (1983) measured the fundamental frequency of black men and women ages 50–79 years. This study examined fundamental frequencies while the subjects were reading and speaking. The reading fundamentals showed significant differences between the younger male speakers (50–60 years) and the older group; female speakers showed no differences. For black men, the mean fundamental frequencies for speaking across the age groups were 118.13 Hz (50–60 years), 113.33 Hz (60–70 years), and 116.33 (70–79 years). These measures are below the fundamental frequency as reported for the majority male population within this age span, which is 162 Hz (Hon & Isshiki, 1980). For black women, the mean fundamental frequencies for speaking across the age groups were 168.22 Hz (50–60 years), 163.26 (60–70 years), and 150.46 Hz (70–79 years) (Ducote, 1983). These measures are below the fundamental frequency as reported for the majority female population within this age span, which is 177 Hz (Hon & Isshiki, 1980).

As these data suggest, the fundamental frequencies for black men and women tend to be lower than those of white men and women. In some instances, the differences between fundamental frequency in blacks and whites appear to be significant (e.g., for 6-, 10-, 14-, and 50- to 79-year-old men and for 6-, 18- to 29-, and 60- to 79-year-old women). In all instances, the actual measures are different and must be taken into account as levels of normal production are considered. It appears that the fundamental frequency for speaking for aged black men falls close to the range for the 18- to 29-year-old group (Hudson & Holbrook, 1981). If this holds true with additional research, the general population trend, which indicates an increase in fundamental frequency as men age, should be revisited as data on minority groups are added to the reference tables for norms.

To further support the need for revised norms to reflect racial variation, research of voice onset time differences across races is emerging. In a preliminary study of differences in voice onset time between blacks and whites, Ryalls, Zipper, and Baldauff (1997) found that there is significantly more prevoicing during voiced consonant production in blacks than in whites.

Perceptual Variables

Since 1962, perceptual studies of the speech and voice of blacks have been conducted (Baker, 1982; Dickens & Sawyer, 1962; Irwin, 1977; Larimer, Beatty, and Broadus, 1988; Lass, Mertz, and Kimmel, 1978; Lass et al., 1979, 1982; Saniga, Carlin, & Farrell, 1984; Walton & Orlikoff, 1994; Wright, Motley, & Phelan, 1976). Paradigms have included panelist judgment of (1) unaltered recorded samples of black speakers (Baker, 1982; Dickens & Sawyer, 1962; Irwin, 1977; Lass et al., 1979; Saniga et al., 1984; Walton & Orlikoff, 1994); (2) altered recorded samples to determine whether temporal features affect perception of race in the speech and voice (Lass et al., 1978; Wright et al., 1976); and (3) samples of vocally disguised speech wherein white speakers disguise their speech and voices to feign black native production (Lass et al., 1982).

Under the unaltered-recorded-samples paradigm, judges correctly identified the speaker's race or racial attributes, which implies a differentiation between the races (speakers were black or white). This occurred regardless of whether the judges were black or white. One attribute noted in a study of the use of vocal fry register in black and white speech was that black speakers were perceived to use vocal fry vocalization more often than white speakers (Saniga et al., 1984). A second attribute alluding to racial differentiation is the tendency for older blacks to be perceived as younger than their age more frequently than whites (Baker, 1982). Although studies using the unaltered-speech paradigm suggest that racial differences are perceivable in the speech and voice, factors often affect perception, particularly when the judge is not a member of the racial group targeted for study.

In a study of personality as portrayed through speech and voice (Larimer et al., 1988), social class status affected the judgment of white panelists. White judges tended to rate low-income blacks lower on the scaled items than they rated middle-class black and white speakers. White judges did not rate middle-class black and white speakers with significant difference. On the other hand, black judges rated black speakers equally regardless of social class.

Under the altered-recorded-samples paradigm, judges tended to have difficulty and performed at the chance level in identifying the race of the speaker. One study reported a bit greater than chance performance among judges who identified white and black male speakers based on prolonged vowel productions (Walton & Orlikoff, 1984). When the unaltered recorded sample and the altered sample appeared in the same study, however, judges clearly identified race with significant degrees of accuracy under the unaltered speech or voice condition (Wright et al., 1976). The distortions used to alter the speech and voice parameters appear to interfere with listener judgment. Indeed, these paradigms attempt to determine the aspects of the speech and voice as perceptual clues to racial identity. Thus far the examination of timing alterations seems to suggest that timing is a critical parameter for perception of racial differences. That is, listeners lose their capability to identify the speaker's race when timing is distorted or when timing is isolated as the only cue to the speaker's racial identity (Lass et al., 1978; Wright et al., 1976). In addition to timing, judges appear to note a characteristic of noise in the voice of black speakers as compared with white speakers (Walton & Orlikoff, 1994).

Under the vocal-disguise paradigm, judges were able to distinguish race when speakers used their native speech characteristics and when they attempted to disguise the speech to sound like black speakers. Because only white speakers and white judges were the subjects of the disguise study, it is difficult to determine the veracity of the paradigm in identifying racial perceptions (Lass et al., 1982).

Cultural and Linguistic Variables

It is known that speech and voice interact in the production of linguistic suprasegmentals, and speakers are recognized by their pitch contours (Atal, 1968; Atkinson, 1973; van Dommelen, 1987). These features of the voice appear to play a pivotal role in speaker identification (Pittam, 1987; Pittam & Gallois, 1986; van Dommelen, 1987); ethnic background (Baker, 1982; Larimer et al., 1988; Lass et al., 1978, 1979, 1982; Saniga et al., 1984; Wright et al., 1976); and cultural-linguistic heritage (Pitts, 1989; Smitherman, 1975; Tarone, 1973; Vandepitte, 1989). The oral traditions of blacks are used to illustrate the point that cultural-linguistic inheritance is portrayed in the speaker's use of voice.

Discourse analysis of communication and of miscommunication in speaker-listener dyads has suggested that intonation and the use of tone serve pragmatic functions (Vandepitte, 1989). The use of intonation contours and tone is said to indicate the speaker's assumptions about the background knowledge of the listener, as well as to suggest the speaker's illocutionary force or commitment to the relevance of information being shared (Tarone, 1973; Vandepitte, 1989). Tarone (1973) provided the following anecdotal account of how voice can be misinterpreted by those outside the relevant cultural sphere and experience: A white police officer arrested several African American youths when he mistook their lively verbal jousts to be indications of hostility and threats of violence. The African American youths were demonstrating their commitment to the verbal game, but their illocutionary force was misinterpreted by the officer who did not share their background and was not aware of the intent of the verbal exchange (Tarone, 1973).

Acquired oral traditions of cultures probably bespeak the function of the voice and speech production systems as much as do genetically inherited racial, anatomic, or physiologic traits. As noted earlier, acoustic findings have suggested that African American speakers have low fundamental frequencies and flexible ranges and tend to use the higher end of the range more flexibly than the lower end (Ducote, 1983; Hollien & Malcik, 1962; Hudson & Holbrook, 1981; Wheat & Hudson, 1988). These findings seem to be corroborated by studies of the oral traditions used by African American speakers (Pitts, 1989; Smitherman, 1975; Tarone, 1973). Intonation features of speakers of African American English include (1) the use of a wide range of pitches that frequently shift to falsetto register when points of emphasis are being made, (2) frequent use of level and rising final pitch contours on all sentence types, (3) use of falling pitch contours (demanding format) in formal and threatening contexts to express yes and no questions (which in Standard English requires a rising intonation), and (4) use of nonfinal intonation contours to express conditionality in a sentence (Tarone, 1973).

The oral traditions that affect the use of voice in African American English have been identified in the linguistic literature (Pitts, 1989; Smitherman, 1975). Smitherman (1975) discussed sacred and secular discourse modes used in African American English. Both types of discourse capture the vocal habits of speakers of African American English and are vestiges of African cultural-linguistic styles. The speech patterns that are found in secular and sacred discourse have accompanying vocal traits. Among them are the low moaning and groaning (*mm . . . hmm*) vocal postures that are used in the call and response pattern and the loud whispered and raspy affirmation (*yessuh*) in the same pattern. Other examples are the rhythmic, loud, and sometimes shrieking falsetto that is used in the "songified" pattern and vocal strain from the loud, rapid, and quickly varying vocal tones in the more secular styles of the playing the dozens, signifyin', or the toast (Smitherman, 1975).

Pitts (1989) verifies these vocal traits in his observations of West African poetics in the style of preaching used by African American ministers. He suggests that the voice as used by African American preachers has a West African heritage. The preacher's style includes use of vocal harshness; varying speech rate, from rapid to slowed and chanting; use of loud falsetto shrieks; rushing many syllables into a single breath group; loud gasping inhalations; and inhalatory stridors (Pitts, 1989). Secular and sacred oral traditions of African Americans preserve the cultural-linguistic heritage. The examination of African American English suggests that the voice is used as a cultural-linguistic device, and the voice plays a role in cultural transmission.

Obviously, the oral traditions of other minority groups should be examined as well. For instance, it is interesting to observe the vestiges of tonality in Asian groups and how this affects the use of the voice and voice production.

Research Needs

The literature reviewed in this chapter indicates that anatomic, acoustic, physiologic, and perceptible differences exist for the speech and voice of blacks and whites. It is unclear exactly which parameters within each of these studies make the differences and whether a combination of these parameters is critical to racial or ethnic identification in speech and voice. It is clear that laryngeal dynamics are affected by the subglottic and supraglottic systems (Zajac, 1990), and these systems work synergistically to produce a voice that is unique to individuals and their group affinity. Research of the anatomic support for racial differences should review more than the weight of the larynges. It should also consider the body type configurations that affect voice, including weight, height, thoracic cavity, and oropharyngeal and nasopharyngeal cavity construction. These areas of study indicate how the vocal source is structured to coordinate with the subglottal and supraglottal systems. Physiologic research needs to examine the pulmonary functions to determine how racial differences in volumes and capacities affect the voice production system. Additionally, physiologic studies of the supralaryngeal systems as they couple with the subglottic and glottic systems should be conducted to determine any differences between the races. Research of the acoustic support for racial differences needs to examine fundamental frequency across all age groups to determine which ranges fall within or outside the norm. Moreover, acoustic research needs to examine the concept of pitch contouring, as habitually used by differing racial and ethnic groups. Such examination would provide insight to the source and filter characteristics that coordinate to make the voice identifiable to a racial or ethnic group. Research of the perceptual support for racial differences needs to examine intraracial and interracial factors (e.g., cultural-linguistic biases) that affect the listener's perception of speech and voice. Moreover, perceptual research needs to examine how perceptions of rate, rhythm, stress, prosody, and intonation influence judgment of racial or ethnic affinity of a speaker. Obviously, all these research efforts need to be conducted across all minority groups in the United States and internationally.

Role of the Speech-Language Pathologist in Prevention and Assessment

Prevention

The projected changes in the composition of the American population in the next few decades require that speech-language pathologists join other health care professionals in rethinking their assumptions about the consumers of health services. To assist in this effort, the literature reviewed in this chapter attempts to identify evidence of real and probable service needs of minority populations in the United States as related to voice and its disorders. The incidence, mortality, and survival information suggests that disease and hereditary conditions that affect the voice and its functioning are variously found among the minority groups. Moreover, it appears that disease susceptibility may have a racial basis, which is evidenced by the incidence of nasopharyngeal cancer among certain groups in the Asian population. The ethnographic information suggests that different ethnic groups may have anatomic, physiologic, and acquired cultural traits that work singularly or interactively to affect the use of the voice. It is the speech-language pathologist's task to be knowledgeable about the predisposition to voice disorders for these groups. Furthermore, the speech-language pathologist must be prepared to join other health care professionals in prevention programs for racially, ethnically, and culturally diverse populations. Marge (1984) discusses three levels of prevention and defines them as follows:

1. "Primary prevention is the elimination or inhibition of the onset and development of a communicative disorder by altering susceptibility or reducing exposure for susceptible persons."

2. "Secondary prevention is the early detection and treatment of communicative disorders. Early detection may lead to the elimination of the disorder or the retardation of the disorder's progress."

3. "Tertiary prevention is the reduction of a disability by attempting to restore effective functioning. The major approach is rehabilitation of the disabled individual who has realized some residual problem as a result of the disorder."

These prevention roles have been adopted by the American Speech-Language-Hearing Association as best practice procedures for professionals (Marge, 1984). Moreover, the American Speech-Language-Hearing Association indicated that taking on the professional role of preventionist means (1) playing a "significant role in the development and application of prevention strategies . . . [,] (2) expand[ing] research into the causes of communication disorders and variables which influence the development and maintenance of communication abilities . . . [, and] (3) educating colleagues and the general public relative to personal wellness strategies as they relate to prevention" (ASHA, 1988).

Predisposers and precipitants of voice pathology that are preventable include vocal abuse; upper respiratory infections; allergies; airborne irritants; smoking; trauma and injury; faulty respiration (due to allergies, infections, and emphysema); substance abuse; and some genetic disorders (Marge, 1984). Clearly, a need exists for additional epidemiologic data to determine whether certain minority groups are more susceptible than others to predisposing and precipitating conditions affecting voice. Moreover, a need exists for information on the incidence (rate of new occurrences) and prevalence (total proportion of cases in the population at any one time) of vocal pathologies within the minority groups.

Despite the need for additional research, the speech-language pathologist must use the information that is currently available to develop prevention strategies that are culturally sensitive and relevant. Several prevention strategies are already used by health professionals and can be adapted for multicultural groups presenting voice-related disorders (Marge, 1984). They include the following:

- Prenatal care (as related to cleft palate especially)
- Genetic counseling (as related to cleft palate)
- Mass screenings and early identification (across the ages for any voice-related concern)
- Early intervention (as related to vocal abuse)
- Public education about vocal hygiene and voice-related disorders (across the ages)

- Advocacy and political action on all issues related to health care that affect the voice and its functioning (including environmental quality control and government programs to ensure that minority groups have the resources to effectively prevent and reduce debilitating conditions that lead to voice disorders)

Critical to the success of these prevention strategies is their use in a culturally sensitive manner. It must be remembered that each cultural minority group is heterogeneous and that subgroupings exist within each basic group. Thus, it behooves the speech-language pathologist to be always cognizant that the clientele within these groups do not "look alike" nor are they "all the same." The speech-language pathologist needs to engage in community-based prevention programs, which means distributing materials to targeted groups through community organizations (e.g., churches, public and private community schools, and social groups). The language used in all public awareness programs must be appropriate to the targeted population (ASHA, 1985). The speech-language pathologist must be sensitive to the cultural traits (e.g., thoughts, beliefs, traditions, mores, teachings) that affect the interactions of the various groups with the health professional.

The Secretary's Report on Black and Minority Health attempted to identify "social characteristics" of the minority groups (U.S. Department of Health and Human Services, 1985). A recurrent theme across all groups was the strength of family ties. Health beliefs and comfort with health professionals varied among the groups. To some degree, all groups showed underuse of health-related services. This underuse appears to have been caused by a preference for non-Western medical treatments and lack of economic access. The preferences for non-Western health care included folk medicine for African Americans; the healing force of family for Hispanics; herbalists, acupuncturists, and traditional non-Western medicine for Asians and Pacific Americans; and medicine men for American Indians. These traditional patterns of health care affect beliefs about the usefulness of health professionals in meeting health care needs.

In addition to beliefs and levels of comfort with health professionals, some members of ethnic or racial minority groups have reduced economic capability, which also acts as a deterrent to health care use. The Institute of Medicine (1989), in its study of allied health professions, noted the following:

- Minorities are more likely than whites to lack health care insurance, and they consistently report greater difficulty than whites in gaining access to medical care.

- Twenty-six percent of Hispanics have no medical coverage compared with 9% of whites and 18% of blacks.

These differences between whites and minorities in access to health care are reflected in health care use rates. Twenty percent of blacks and 19% of Hispanics indicate that they have no usual source of medical care, compared with 13% of whites. Between 1978 and 1980, the percentage of people 4–16 years old who had never received dental care was higher among Mexican Americans (30.7%) than among blacks (22.3%) or whites (9.7%). Similarly, the percentage of individuals with no physician contact was higher among Mexican Americans (33.1%) than among other Hispanics (3.9%), blacks (23.8%), or whites (20.4%).

The roles and responsibilities of prevention, in light of addressing the needs of minority groups, present opportunity and challenge to the profession of speech-language pathology. Speech-language pathologists are encouraged to familiarize themselves with the voice-related health problems of multicultural populations and with the cultural deterrents to health care use. These vital pieces of knowledge make the work of prevention easier.

Assessment

It is important for the speech-language pathologist to understand *normal voice* functioning before embarking on assessment techniques of the abnormal voice. The voice of humans has often been likened to musical instruments. The organs of the voice are similar to wind instruments. To make pitch adjustments the larynx follows patterns found in string instruments. In many cultures the melodic patterns of voice may be considered music to the ear (e.g., the songified pattern of African American English or the chant of the African American preacher). No one definition of what constitutes a normal voice is accepted by all. In this chapter, voice is considered as unique as a person's eyebrow pattern, fingerprint, or smile. It is influenced by race, gender, age, socioeconomic standing, emotional swings, and situational moments. Normal voice is also defined as that which is accepted by the listener and the native speaking environment. Physiologically, the normal voice can be affected by viral infections, benign or malignant tumors, neurologic impairments, and psychological factors. Currently, we have little guidance from research to direct our efforts to address the factors that affect normalcy judgments as made by various racial or ethnic groups (DeJarnette, 1996). The speech-language pathologist must therefore interview the patient to determine what is aesthetically pleasing. In doing so, he or she should use questions such as the following (DeJarnette, 1996):

- What voice pitch do you believe would best represent you to family, everyday community, religious community, and work community?

- What loudness level (soft or loud) do you believe would work best for your voice with family, everyday community, religious community, and work community?
- What vocal tone (smooth, breathy, or harsh and rough) do you believe would work best for your voice with family, everyday community, religious community, and work community?
- What degree of versatility do you believe would work best for your voice with family, everyday community, religious community, and work community?

Responses to these questions allow the speech-language pathologist to search for a culturally appropriate voice that fits with the client's best voice production capability. Moreover, these questions can provide important insight as the speech-language pathologist tries to identify and decrease abuse and misuse vocal behaviors. Having the client identify cultural models of voice can enhance the clinical relationship and provide a sense of ownership and commitment to the therapeutic process.

When assessing voice disorders among multicultural populations, the speech-language pathologist should first consider the patient's point of view. Many minority groups, if they accept professional intervention at all, approach clinical diagnosis and intervention cautiously. Some are hesitant to trust professionals who have a cultural perspective that differs from their own; this may be based on past experience or the perception that mainstream cultural values are used to judge capability and progress. Others may trust only certain professionals, such as doctors, believing that all others are pseudoprofessionals. Therefore, the speech-language pathologist should be prepared for the patient who approaches the diagnostic appointment with reticence. If the patient is a child, the speech-language pathologist should consider the anxiety level of the child and parents. In all cases, the speech-language pathologist must be aware that the patient's attitudes can be influenced by age, source of the referral, family status, occupation, and understanding of his or her own voice. The clinician should remember that, before clinical intervention begins, medical clearance is warranted. Achieving medical clearance can be affected by the client's experience or lack of experience in negotiating medical systems, the client's belief system regarding Euro-American medicine, or both. The speech-language pathologist, therefore, may need to assist the client with negotiating medical systems.

General Outline of Diagnostic Procedures

Before the diagnostic session, the speech-language pathologist needs to get a sense of the client's cultural point of view to know what clinical procedures the client sees as taboo (e.g., physical contact, direct eye contact). The speech-language pathologist uses perceptual and acoustic measures, when possible, to determine the patient's voice characteristics, the severity of the disorder, and the benefit that can be derived from therapy. Much of the data for making these determinations are based on findings from a monocultural source—that is, from mainstream speakers and voices. As noted earlier, there is a sparse database to inform the speech-language pathologist of multicultural factors to use in determining normal versus deviant voice in multicultural populations. However, a more client-centered approach can fill that knowledge gap at the present time.

A client-centered approach allows the speech pathologist to consider the notion that racial, ethnic, and cultural groups can present more risk for specific types of organic voice disorders (e.g., laryngeal, esophageal, and lung cancer in blacks and nasopharyngeal cancer in Asian populations). Moreover, a client-centered approach allows the speech pathologist to be informed by the patient regarding the cultural influences that affect voice production and voice intervention. Indeed, the diagnostic intake and interview provide opportunities for the speech-language pathologist to be client-centered. Much like the questions listed in Assessment, above (DeJarnette, 1996), the client should be asked to inform the speech-language pathologist of cultural beliefs or practices that might affect evaluation and intervention.

Good clinical practice should be informed by a client-centered approach. An assessment protocol should include at least (1) a description of the patient, including culturally relevant biographic information and observation of the client's physical presentation at the time of the diagnostic session; (2) the history of the disorder, including events in the patient's life that appear to be related to the problem; (3) a description of the speech mechanism and the characteristics of the voice (e.g., measures of fundamental frequency, optimum and habitual pitch, vocal range); (4) an audio or video recording during the interview and spontaneous voice sampling procedures; (5) the results of an indirect examination of the vocal cords; (6) a video fluoroscopic study (when appropriate); and (7) the patient's self-assessment of voice.

Although medical clearance must be ensured before intervention is initiated, the speech-language pathologist must not hesitate to inspect the patient's medical status for voice-related concerns. The speech-language pathologist should explain all procedures thoroughly. He or she must secure the client's permission to touch the patient and conduct any physical examination. It is imperative that the speech-language pathologist conducts an examination of the vocal tract (i.e., respiratory tract, larynx, oro- and nasopharynx, and oral peripheral cavity), keeping in mind possible health and environmental conditions that affect various racial and ethnic groups. Knowledge of the vocal tract improves the speech-language pathologist's ability to communicate effectively with medical staff and to understand the patient's physical limitations and conditions. If the client's ethnic or cultural beliefs prohibit such an examination or physical contact, the speech-language pathologist should explain the need and invite suggestions from the client about how to conduct the examination. For instance, significant others can be trained to position a client for clinical observation by the speech-language pathologist; this should be accepted as a way to conduct the examination.

The diagnostician should exercise caution when using norms that are based on measures of predominantly white subjects, because differences between majority and minority populations exist for anatomic, physiologic, acoustic, and perceptual parameters related to voice. As data accrue on these parameters in multicultural populations, these differences will be clarified, and norms will be generated that are more racially or culturally appropriate. It is exceedingly important for speech-language pathologists to keep this in mind as they prepare to provide services to minority populations. Care should be taken to investigate what is considered normal for each group and subgroup.

Examination of the External Vocal Tract

The speech-language pathologist's examination follows the audio or video recording of the patient. It should start with the external observation of the neck area and include palpation of the larynx and neck muscles. Notation should be made of the patient's breathing pattern and the resting position of the lips. The mobility of facial muscles, puckered lips, and protruded tongue should be noted. These procedures reveal general control and symmetry of the face. Clearly, facial muscles are not involved at the glottal level of voice production; however, their asymmetry can signal neurologic concerns. The speech-language pathologist must consider the research on the anatomic differences between races as such observations are made.

Examination of the Oral Pharynx

Attention should next be directed to the oropharynx. The symmetry, color, and condition of teeth should be observed. The protruded tongue and its mobility must be examined. Again, abnormal function could be indicative of neurologic concerns. Standard oral cancer assessment techniques should be followed that include palpation of the oral cavity. Note the coloration of mucosal lining and any edema, as these are important for future medical referrals. Note the movement of the velum when the patient produces the sound /a/ (*ah*) or /e/ (*eh*). The soft palate should move upward and backward quickly and symmetrically bilaterally; if not, paralysis is suspected. If scars or any abnormality are observed in this structure, then exploratory questions and medical consultation should be sought. The examination continues with viewing the faucial and pharyngeal regions. Scars are observed if tonsils have been removed. If the posterior wall of the pharynx slides laterally when an attempt is made to close the velopharyngeal valve, then unilateral paralysis of the pharyngeal constrictor muscle is indicated.

Nasal passages should be observed during the production of a prolonged hum by occluding one ala of the nostril at a time. If partial or complete stoppages are present, then attention to denasal voice quality should be noted. The patient should be questioned regarding allergies, colds, and injuries.

Examination of the Interior Larynx

The final phase of the examination is the interior larynx. The authors suggest that experience be gained in using the laryngeal mirror or the telescopic laryngeal scope. Medical staff normally completes fiberoptic, stroboscopic techniques. If the speech-language pathologist is not experienced in these techniques, he or she should at least be present during the medical examination. The function of the vocal cords during examination is pertinent to planning therapeutic techniques.

Observation of vocal cord color and size; movements in adduction and abduction; and the presence of symmetry, nodules, edema, and papillomas should all be noted. Photographs or video recordings can contribute to the rehabilitation plan.

Assessment of and Intervention in Voice Disorders

The speech-language pathologist should be sensitive to the fear factor when approaching the assessment of and intervention plan for a culturally diverse client with organic voice disorders. In addition, a thorough educational approach must be followed to ensure that the patient clearly understands the medical implications of the disorder.

It is not uncommon for an African American laryngectomee not to ask the doctor about his or her chances for survival, quality of life, or body hygiene techniques. This is why it is imperative that the speech-language pathologist be knowledgeable about the patient's disorder and be able to disseminate this knowledge at the patient's level of understanding.

The following steps are suggested for assessing vocal disorders such as nodules, polyps, paralysis, and alaryngeal voice:

1. Review all medical records—that is, operative reports, radiologic reports (including viewing of x-rays), pathology reports, and discharge summaries. It is imperative that the speech-language pathologist thoroughly understands all medical interventions. For example, the speech-language pathologist must recognize when a gastric pull-up procedure has been performed in addition to removal of the larynx.
2. Educate the patient about the disorder using graphs and video presentation. Verbal instructions should be accompanied by visual imagery.
3. Time is a critical factor in patient education, counseling, and therapeutic success. Often, the fact that the speech-language pathologist can offer extended time for discussion with the patient allows rapport and trust to develop, thus ensuring a positive therapeutic relationship.

An additional consideration that must be kept in mind is the patient's perception of what constitutes an aesthetically normal voice for his or her cultural community. As a way of determining what the client thinks is the ideal voice, he or she might be asked to provide models or recordings of voices from the cultural community that he or she would like to emulate. Additionally, the speech-language pathologist can develop a library of voice recordings from various cultural backgrounds and allow the client to choose among them.

In terms of intervention strategies, the speech-language pathologist must be cognizant that a number of the voice-facilitating techniques can seem awkward, if not culturally inappropriate, to clients from various racial or ethnic backgrounds. For example, "chant talk," with its monotone presentation, may be awkward for the African American speaker who uses pitch and intonation shifts to express meaning and commitment, and it may be equally difficult for speakers of tonal-based languages (Asian American speakers). Other techniques, such as head positioning, open-mouth approach, tongue protrusion, yawn and sigh, use of artificial laryngeal devices, and so on, can be perceived as obtrusive to cultural styles. Thus, the speech-language pathologist must explain the technique, determine the client's cultural comfort level with using the technique, and be prepared to make adaptations to the technique so that it fits the client's cultural style. Again, the speech-language pathologist should check with the client about the usefulness of any intervention strategy in the client's cultural milieu. Moreover, the speech-language pathologist must be open to suggestions from the client about how to adapt a technique for greater usefulness.

Conclusion

This chapter discusses the incidence of voice-related pathologies in minority groups in the United States; health issues related to voice dysfunction; ethnographic and racial factors related to voice; and the role of the speech-language pathologist in prevention, assessment, and intervention. A review of the literature concerning the epidemiology of voice-related pathologies in minority groups illuminates the need for increased research of the incidence and prevalence of causal factors leading to voice disorders and the types of voice disorders found among the minority populations in the United States. The available literature suggests that health risk factors are variously distributed among the minority groups in terms of their incidence and prevalence rates and their gender ratios. Among these risk factors are access to health care (Institute of Medicine, 1989), occupational and daily living exposure to teratogens, substance abuse, and possible predispositions to certain disease processes that are the combined effect of biological inheritance and environmental conditions (Baquet et al., 1991; Blum, 1982; Gee, 1982; Hargreaves et al., 1989; Hung-Dhiu Ho, 1982; Kalk & Kalk, 1989; National Center for Health Statistics, 1991; Parnes, 1990; Rice & Yu, 1982; U.S. Department of Health and Human Services, 1985, 1986; Williams, 1975). As in the case of carcinoma, the health risks tend to affect the entire vocal tract system and include respiratory and laryngeal and supralaryngeal resonatory systems. Moreover, health risks include disease and trauma effects on the endocrinologic system and on cerebrovascular functioning insofar as these affect voice production (Blum, 1982; Gee, 1982; Kalk & Kalk, 1989; National Center for Health Statistics, 1991; Williams, 1975). Vocal pathologies can also have different patterns of distribution in terms of proportions and gender ratios across multicultural groups (Dobres et al., 1990; Sayetta et al., 1989; Shaw et al., 1991; Vanderas, 1987). Thus, speech-language pathologists need to ascertain the magnitude of the health risks and the incidence and prevalence rates of voice disorders among the various minority groups so that prevention, identification, diagnosis, and intervention can be effectively provided for these groups.

The delivery of appropriate, relevant, and quality voice care to multicultural groups is affected by the speech-language pathologist's knowledge of the racial, ethnographic, and cultural factors that affect voice production and use. This chapter makes the case that ethnographic implications exist for all parameters of study that provide a knowledge base of what voice is across the spectrum of the human continuum (Awan & Mueller, 1996; Baker, 1982; Boshoff, 1945; Cole, 1980; Dickens & Sawyer,

1962; Ducote, 1983; Fitch & Holbrook, 1970; Hollien & Malcik, 1962; Hon Jo & Isshiki, 1980; Hudson & Holbrook, 1981; Irwin, 1977; Lass et al., 1978, 1979; Saniga et al., 1984; Walton & Orlikoff, 1994; Wheat & Hudson, 1988; Williams, 1975). These parameters include anatomic, physiologic, acoustic, perceptual, cultural, and linguistic realms of study. It is suggested that each avenue of study has the potential to expose knowledge about the "differences that make a difference" in the production and perception of voice in racially, ethnically, and culturally differing groups. For the speech-language pathologist, the acquisition of knowledge about the ethnocultural differences between groups is as critical to quality care as is knowledge of the health risks. Developing culturally sensitive, client-centered, and relevant approaches to voice service delivery permits speech-language pathologists to fulfill their roles and responsibilities as preventionists, diagnosticians, and interventionists in working with multicultural groups.

References

American Cancer Society. (1998). *Cancer facts and figures, 1998–1999*. Atlanta: American Cancer Society.

ASHA Committee on Prevention of Speech, Language and Hearing Disorders. (1988). Prevention of communication disorders. Position statement. *ASHA, 30*(3), 90.

ASHA Committee on the Status of Racial Minorities. (1985). Clinical management of communicatively handicapped minority language populations. *ASHA, 27*(6), 29–32.

Atal, D. S. (1968). *Automatic speaker recognition based on pitch contours*. Doctoral dissertation, Polytechnic University, Brooklyn, NY.

Atkinson, J. E. (1973). *Aspects of intonation in speech: Implications from an experimental study of fundamental frequency*. Doctoral dissertation, University of Connecticut, Farmington, CT.

Awan, S. N., & Mueller, P. B. (1996). Speaking fundamental frequency characteristics of white, African American, and Hispanic kindergartners. *Journal of Speech and Hearing Research, 39*, 573–577.

Bagchi, N., Brown, T. R., & Parish, R. F. (1990). Thyroid dysfunction in adults over age 55 years: A study in an urban U.S. community. *Archives of Internal Medicine, 150*(4), 785–787.

Baker, L. L. (1982). *Speech and voice characteristics of aging Afro-American female and male speakers based on listener perceived age estimates*. Doctoral dissertation, Wichita State University, Wichita, KS.

Baquet, C. R., Horm, J. W., Gibbs, T., & Grenwald, P. (1991). Socioeconomic factors and cancer incidence among African Americans and whites. *Journal of the National Cancer Institute, 83*(8), 551–557.

Blum, A. S. (1982, May). *Thyrotoxicosis among the Chinese.* Paper presented at the Conference on Health Problems Related to Chinese in America, San Francisco.

Boshoff, P. (1945). The anatomy of the South African Negro larynges. *South African Journal of Medical Sciences, 10,* 35–50.

Centers for Disease Control and Prevention. (1991). Surveillance summaries. *Morbidity and Mortality Weekly Report, 40,* 3.

Centers for Disease Control and Prevention. (1996). Cigarette smoking among adults—United States, 1994. *Morbidity and Mortality Weekly Report, 45,* 588–591.

Chen, H. (1982, May). *Chronic persistent cough in Chinese in America.* Paper presented at the Conference on Health Problems Related to Chinese in America, San Francisco.

Cole, L. (1980). Blacks with orofacial clefts: The state of the dilemma. *ASHA, 22,* 557–560.

DeJarnette, G. (1996, December). *Multicultural issues in voice care: Focus on the African American voice.* Paper presented at the meeting of the American Speech-Language-Hearing Association, Seattle.

Dickens, M., & Sawyer, G. M. (1962). An experimental comparison of vocal quality among mixed groups of whites and Negroes. *Southern Speech Journal, 18,* 178–185.

Dobres, R., Lee, L., Stemple, J. C., et al. (1990). Description of laryngeal pathologies in children evaluated by otolaryngologists. *Journal of Speech and Hearing Disorders, 55*(3), 526–532.

Ducote, C. A. (1983). *A study of the reading and speaking fundamental frequency of aging black adults.* Doctoral dissertation, Louisiana State University, Baton Rouge, LA.

Fitch, J. L., & Holbrook, A. (1970). Modal vocal fundamental frequency of young adults. *Archives of Otolaryngology, 92,* 379–382.

Gee, P. (1982, May). *Thyrotoxic periodic paralysis: An unusual presentation of thyrotoxicosis in Oriental men.* Paper presented at the Conference on Health Problems Related to Chinese in America, San Francisco.

Hargreaves, M. K., Baquet, C., & Gamshadzahi, A. (1989). Diet, nutritional status and cancer risk in American African Americans. *Nutrition and Cancer, 12*(1), 1–28.

Hollien, H., & Malcik, E. (1962). Adolescent voice change in southern Negro males. *Speech Monographs, 29*(1), 53–58.

Hon Jo, I., & Isshiki, N. (1980). Laryngoscopic and voice characteristics of aged persons. *Archives of Otolaryngology, 106,* 149–150.

Hudson, A. I., & Holbrook, A. (1981). A study of the reading fundamental vocal frequency of young African American adults. *Journal of Speech and Hearing Research, 24,* 197–201.

Hung-Dhiu Ho, J. (1982, May). *Etiology and control of nasopharyngeal carcinoma (NPC).* Paper presented at the Conference on Health Problems Related to the Chinese in America, San Francisco.

Institute of Medicine Committee to Study the Role of Allied Health Personnel. (1989). *Allied health services avoiding crises.* Washington, DC: National Academy Press.

Irwin, R. B. (1977). Judgments of vocal quality, speech fluency and confidence of African American and white speakers. *Language and Speech, 20* (3), 261–266.

Kalk, W. J., & Kalk, J. (1989). Incidence and causes of hyperthyroidism in African Americans. *South African Medical Journal, 75*(3), 114–117.

Kittler, P. A., & Sucher, K. P. (1998). *Food and culture in America* (2nd ed.). Belmont, CA: West Wadsworth.

Landis, S. H., Murray, T., Bolden, S., & Wingo, P. A. (1998). *Cancer statistics 1998.* Atlanta: American Cancer Society.

Larimer, G. S., Beatty, E., & Broadus, A. C. (1988). Indirect assessment of interracial prejudices. *Journal of Black Psychology, 14*(2), 47–56.

Lass, N. J., Mertz, P. J., & Kimmel, K. L. (1978). The effect of temporal speech alterations on speaker race and sex identifications. *Language and Speech, 21,* 279–290.

Lass, N. J., Tecca, J. E., Mancuso, R. A., & Black, W. I. (1979). The effect of phonetic complexity on speaker race and sex identifications. *Journal of Phonetics, 7,* 105–118.

Lass, N. J., Trapp, D. S., Baldwin, M. K., et al. (1982). Effect of vocal disguise on judgments of speakers' sex and race. *Perceptual and Motor Skills, 54*(3), 1235–1240.

Marge, M. (1984). The prevention of communication disorders. *ASHA, 26,* 35–38.

Mayo, R., Watkins, T. R., & Richmond, A. A. (2001). RF_0 characteristics in three groups of females: Cross-linguistic analysis. *Communication Disorders and Sciences in Culturally and Linguistically Diverse Populations, 7*(2), 3–7.

Miller, B. A., Kolonel, L. N., Bernstein, L., et al. (1996). *Racial/ethnic patterns of cancer in the United States, 1988–1992.* Washington, DC: National Institutes of Health, National Cancer Institute (NIH Pub. No. 96-4104).

National Center for Health Statistics. (1991). *Health United States, 1990.* Washington, DC: U.S. Government Printing Office (Department of Health and Human Services Pub. No. PH591-1232).

Page, H. S., & Asire, A. J. (1985). *Cancer rates and risks* (3rd ed.). Washington, DC: National Institute of Health (DHHS Pub. No. 85-691).

Parnes, S. M. (1990). Asbestos and cancer of the larynx: Is there a relationship? *Laryngoscope, 100*(3), 254–261.

Pittam, J. (1987). The long-term spectral measurement of voice quality as a social and personality marker: A review. *Language and Speech, 30,* 1–12.

Pittam, J., & Gallois, C. (1986). Predicting impressions of speakers from voice quality: Acoustic and perceptual measures. *Journal of Language and Social Psychology, 5*(4), 233–237.

Pitts, W. (1989). West African poetics in the African American preaching style. *American Speech, 64*(2), 137–149.

Rice, D. P., & Yu, E. (1982, May). *Health of the Chinese in America.* Paper presented at the Conference on Health Problems Related to the Chinese in America, San Francisco.

Ryalls, J., Zipper, A., & Baldauff, P. (1997). A preliminary investigation of the effects of gender and race on voice onset time. *Journal of Speech, Language, and Hearing Research, 40,* 642.

Saniga, R. D., Carlin, M. F., & Farrell, S. C. (1984). Perception of fry register in African American dialect and standard dialect English speakers. *Perceptual and Motor Skills, 59*(3), 885–886.

Sataloff, D. M., Pursnani, K., Hoyo, S., Zayass, F., et al. (1997). An objective assessment of laparoscopic antireflux surgery. *American Journal of Surgery 174,* 63–67.

Sayetta, R. B., Weinrich, M. C., & Coston, G. N. (1989). Incidence and prevalence of cleft lip and palate: What we think we know. *Cleft Palate Journal, 26*(3), 242–247.

Shaw, G. M., Croen, L. A., & Curry, C. J. (1991). Isolated oral cleft malformations: Associations with maternal and infant characteristics in a California population. *Teratology, 43*(3), 225–228.

Smitherman, G. (1975). *Black language and culture: Sounds of soul.* New York: Harper & Row.

Tarone, E. E. (1973). Aspects of intonation in Black English. *American Speech, 48*(1–2), 29–36.

U.S. Department of Health and Human Services. (1985). *Report of the Secretary's Task Force on Black and Minority Health (Vol. 1): Executive summary.* Washington, DC: Government Printing Office (Department of Health and Human Services, Pub. No. 491-313/44706).

U.S. Department of Health and Human Services. (1986). *Report of the Secretary's Task Force on Black and Minority Health (Vol. 2): Cancer.* Washington, DC: Government Printing Office (Department of Health and Human Services, Pub. No. 621-605:00171).

van Dommelen, W. A. (1987). The contribution of speech, rhythm and pitch to speaker recognition. *Language and Speech, 30*(4), 325–338.

Vandepitte, S. (1989). A pragmatic function of intonation: Tone and cognitive environment. *Lingua, 79*(4), 265–297.

Vanderas, A. P. (1987). Incidence of cleft lip, cleft palate, and cleft lip and palate among races: A review. *Cleft Palate Journal, 24*(3), 216–225.

Walton, J. H., & Orlikoff, R. F. (1994). Speaker race identification from acoustic cues in the vocal signal. *Journal of Speech and Hearing Research, 37*(4), 738–745.

Wheat, M. C., & Hudson, A. I. (1988). Spontaneous speaking fundamental of 6-year-old African American children. *Journal of Speech and Hearing Research, 31*, 723–725.

Williams, R. A. (1975). *Textbook of black-related diseases.* New York: McGraw-Hill.

Wilson, D. K. (1979). *Voice problems of children* (2nd ed.). Baltimore: Williams & Wilkins.

Wright, C. R., Motley, M. T., & Phelan, J. G. (1976). Discrimination of dialect from temporal patterns of the speech signal. *Psychology Report, 38*(2), 1059–1067.

Yang, P. C., Thomas, D. B., & Davis, S. (1989). Differences in the sex ratio of laryngeal cancer incidence rates by anatomic subsite. *Journal of Clinical Epidemiology, 42*(8), 755–758.

Zajac, D. J. (1990). *Effects of respiratory effort and induced oronasal coupling on laryngeal aerodynamics and oscillatory behaviors.* Doctoral dissertation, University of Pittsburgh, Pittsburgh.

11 ⬜⬜⬜ ⬜⬜⬜ ⬜⬜⬜

Multicultural Aspects of Hearing Disorders and Audiology

Diane M. Scott

What does it mean to be an audiologist in today's culturally diverse society? In 1990, 61 million people, or approximately 24% of the U.S. population, were members of racially or ethnically diverse populations (U.S. Bureau of the Census, 1990). The U.S. Census 2000 ethnicity reports were issued in March 2001. If the Hispanic ethnic classification is excluded from the population estimates, then 75.1% of the population is white, 12.3% is African American, 0.9% is American Indian, Eskimo, and Aleut, 3.6% is Asian, 0.1% is Native Hawaiian or Other Pacific Islander, 5.5% is some other race, and 2.4% is two or more races. More than 47 million people are from racial minority groups. When the Hispanic ethnic classification is included among the racial or ethnic designations, 69.1% of the population is white; 12.1% is African American; 0.7% is American Indian, Eskimo, and Aleut; 3.6% is Asian; 0.1% is Native Hawaiian or Other Pacific Islander; 0.7% is some other race; 1.6% is two or more races; and 12.5% is Hispanic (U.S. Bureau of the Census, 2001). Therefore, over 30% of the U.S. population of more than 280 million people are members of racially and ethnically diverse groups.

According to the National Institute on Deafness and Other Communication Disorders (NIDCD), approximately 46 million individuals in the United States of both genders and all races have some type of communication disorder (NIDCD, 1995). Among these individuals, more than 28 million have a hearing disorder (NIDCD, 1999). The number of children with disabilities between the ages of 6 and 21 years served in the public schools under the implementa-

Table 11-1 Percent of U.S. Population with Hearing Impairment by Age

Age (yrs)	Percent (of general population)
Under 18	1.5
18–44	4.6
45–64	14.3
65–74	23.3
Over 75	31.0

Source: Benson, V., & Marano, M. A. (1994). Current estimates from the National Health Interview Survey, 1992. *Vital and Health Statistics Series 10(189)*. Hyattsville, MD: National Center for Health Statistics.

tion of the Individuals with Disabilities Education Act Part B in the 1996–1997 school year was 5,235,952. Of these children, 68,766 (1.3%) received services for hearing impairment (U.S. Department of Education, 1998).

It should be noted that, although racially and ethnically diverse groups have the same types of communication disorders, other contributing factors affect the distribution of the types of disorders across racial and ethnic groups. This can be seen in the distribution of Americans with hearing impairment from different racial and ethnic populations shown in Tables 11-1, 11-2, and 11-3. Table 11-3 illustrates the shift in race and ethnicity of children with hearing impairment from 1973–1994. According to the Gallaudet Research Institute (1999), 45.2% of deaf and hard of hearing children are racial and ethnic minorities. Hispanics constitute 20.4% of the children. Seventeen percent of the children are African American, 4.2% Asian and Pacific Islander, 0.8% American Indian, and approximately 3% are other or multiethnic.

In a culturally diverse community, audiologists and the clients and families they serve may not share a common language or worldview. Lack of a common language can lead to difficulties in establishing rapport between cli-

Table 11-2 Prevalence of Hearing Impairment in the United States by Age Group and Race

Age (yrs)	African American (%)	White (%)
3–17	1.2	1.9
18–44	2.1	4.9
45–64	7.2	13.4
65 and older	18.7	30.1
Total	**4.2**	**9.4**

Source: Data from the National Center for Health Statistics. (1994). *National Health Interview Survey*. Series 10, No. 188, Table 2. Hyattsville, MD: National Center for Health Statistics.

Table 11-3   Annual Surveys of Deaf and Hard of Hearing Children and Youth by Race and Ethnicity, 1973–1974 and 1993–1994

	1973–1974 (%) (n = 41,070)	1993–1994 (%) (n = 46,099)
African American	16	17
Asian and Pacific Islander	<1	4
Hispanic	7	16
Other	<1	3
White	76	60
Total	**100**	**100**

Source: Schildroth, A. N., & Hotto, S. A. (1995). Race and ethnic background in the Annual Survey of Deaf and Hard of Hearing Children and Youth. *American Annals of the Deaf, 140* (2), 96–99.

ent and audiologist and in finding language-appropriate test materials. Seeing the world from the family's view is not always easy or reinforcing for an audiologist. The audiologist's values may not be so highly appreciated by others, yet the audiologist must be culturally sensitive. Anderson and Fenichel (1989) define cultural sensitivity as follows:

> Cultural sensitivity cannot mean knowing everything there is to know about every culture that is represented in a population to be served. At its most basic level, cultural sensitivity implies rather a knowledge that cultural differences as well as similarities exist. . . . [Cultural] sensitivity further means being aware of the cultures represented in one's state or region, learning some of the general parameters of those cultures, and realizing that cultural diversity will affect families' participation in intervention programs. Cultural knowledge helps a professional to be aware of possibilities and to be ready to respond appropriately. (pp. 8–9)

Audiologists and other professionals in hearing clinics must strive to become culturally competent. Roberts (1990) asserts that cultural competence refers to the ability to honor and respect those beliefs, interpersonal styles, attitudes, and behaviors of the families who are clients and of the professional staff. Cultural competence incorporates these values at the levels of policy, administration, and practice. Clinical programs that provide culturally competent services do not become that way by accident. There is commitment at all levels of the organization. The organization reaches out to the community it serves and involves the community in establishing short- and long-range objectives and in determining policy. The program hires staff that mirrors the community it serves and continually educates itself regarding cultural issues.

Cultural Issues in the Practice of Audiology

Case History Information

Cultural sensitivity begins with methods used to obtain case history information. The usual audiologic case history form may not contain all of the questions an audiologist should ask to obtain culturally relevant information (e.g., race and ethnicity; place of birth, as well as year of birth; designation of same-gender parents; natural healing methods, as well as medications prescribed and taken; and language in the home).

Race and ethnicity are important because "Hispanic" is an ethnic classification and not a racial one. For example, a person can be Hispanic and African American. Place of birth is important in possible identification of the cause of a hearing disorder. For example, if a person was born in a refugee camp, then exposure to certain contagious diseases may have occurred, or, if a person was born outside of the United States and had a serious illness, then the country of birth may have used ototoxic drugs in treating the illness. Most case history forms request the name of the mother and the father. Case history forms do not request names and identifying information about the parents without gender specification. Lack of gender specification allows for the possibility of same-gender couples. Knowledge of language use in the home is necessary in determining the need for an interpreter during the evaluation and choosing tests for speech audiometric testing. Knowledge of any natural healing methods used by a family can be vital in determining how a medically treatable auditory disorder was treated. As an example, a family from South America would regularly burn candles as treatment for the son's otitis media. (For more information on modifying the case history form to make it culturally appropriate, see Orque, Block, & Monrroy [1983].)

As shown in Chapter 1, at least 31.8 million or one in every seven U.S. residents speaks a language other than English at home (U.S. Bureau of the Census, 1993). Spanish is the most common language, other than English, spoken in American homes (U.S. Bureau of the Census, 1993). The number of homes in which Spanish was the primary language spoken increased 50% between the 1980 and 1990 Census. The hiring of cultural and linguistic interpreters may be needed if the audiologist serves a large non-English–speaking population.

As audiologists collect case history information, they need to know whether certain auditory disorders (e.g., genetic disorders, otitis media, presbycusis, and noise-induced hearing loss) are more common in certain racially and ethnically diverse populations than in others. They then can be on heightened alert for the symptoms associated with a given auditory disorder.

Cross-Racial Factors in Assessment

Cultural knowledge is needed at the next step in the audiologic evaluation: the assessment. Research studies have indicated that there are differences in auditory sensitivity between male and female populations and between African American and white populations, particularly in those older than 30 years (Berger, Royster, & Thomas, 1977; Bunch & Raiford, 1931; Jerger et al., 1993; Post, 1964; Royster et al., 1980; Royster & Thomas, 1979). The differences noted between male and female auditory sensitivity include the following:

- Hearing threshold levels for women show almost no age effects, such as increases in the threshold level due to aging, before age 30 years, which is not true for men.
- In general, women have larger age effects in the lower frequencies with advancing age, whereas men have larger age effects in the higher frequencies (Royster & Thomas, 1979).
- The same pattern of gender differences holds true for African American and white populations. Studies also indicate better auditory sensitivity for African American men across all frequencies compared to white men. African American women have better auditory sensitivity than white women (Royster et al., 1980; Royster & Royster, 1982) (Table 11-4).

Audiologic norms, therefore, actually may vary as a function of gender and race. Jerger, Chmiel, Stach, and Spretnjak (1993) examined hearing survey data covering more than 50 years from several countries including the United States, Jamaica, Finland, Scotland, and Sudan. The data again show a consistent gender difference in pure tone thresholds. Men show more hearing loss than women at frequencies higher than 1,000 Hz, whereas women show more loss than men below 1,000 Hz. At 1,000 Hz, there is typically no gender difference. The effect increases with age and hearing threshold. The gender effect remains after individuals with a history of noise exposure are factored out of the data (Jerger et al., 1993). Data still need to be collected from other racial groups in the United States (i.e., other than African Americans and whites).

Table 11-4   Mean Hearing Threshold Levels at 4,000 Hz for White and African American Women and Men Not Exposed to Industrial Noise in the United States as a Function of Age

	Age (yrs)				
	20–29	30–39	40–49	50–59	60–69
White men (Royster & Thomas, 1979)	10.8	19.3	27.7	37.4	37.7
White women (Royster & Thomas, 1979)	4.5	8.7	12.4	17.4	30.5
African American men (Royster et al., 1980)	4.0	8.3	14.6	17.6	31.9
African American women (Royster et al., 1980)	3.8	8.4	8.6	12.7	13.2

Linguistic Factors in Assessment

Providing testing instructions in the client's native language can be very important. Pantomime is not appropriate, because it shows a lack of respect for the client when the audiologist does not make use of the services of an interpreter. Children especially need to establish rapport with the audiologist and a common language helps that process.

Use of English-language speech test materials with individuals who do not speak English with native or near-native proficiency is inappropriate. Materials in Spanish and a few other languages are available (Cokely & Yager, 1993; Comstock & Martin, 1984). Audiologists should not use these materials unless they are qualified to provide services in the dialect and language of the client or unless they are able to work with a dialect- and language-appropriate interpreter. The languages (or dialects) of the audiologist and the client should match or test results could be altered by differences in vocabulary and pronunciation. Furthermore, audiologists must remember to look at the norming of any non-English tests used and determine the country of origin, language, and dialect of the speaker, if using recorded materials. Picture tasks have been developed for children. The pictures are probably reflective of vocabulary from mainstream American culture, which may not be familiar to children who have not lived in the United States for a long period of time and are learning English as a second language.

Miller, Heise, and Lichten (1951) evaluated the use of alternative speech materials for testing the hearing of adults. They recommended the use of numbers for testing purposes. Rudmin (1987) found that numbers are among the 500 most frequently used words in English. In a series of studies,

Ramkissoon and her colleagues (Ramkissoon, in press, 2000; Ramkissoon, Bilger, & Proctor, 2000) used numbers to develop a digit-speech reception test for individuals acquiring English as a second language. Results revealed that adults who were nonnative English speakers displayed improved performance on the digit-speech reception test, as compared to the traditional spondee word list.

There are also individuals who use other forms of communication besides oral language, such as cued speech and sign language. The Internet and computer software can provide resources for audiologists and other professionals wishing to improve their skills with these forms of communication.

Cued speech resources include

- *Gaining Cued Speech Efficiency: A Manual for Parents, Teachers, and Clinicians* by Walter J. Beaupre is an online book with extensive information about cued speech (http://www.uri.edu/comm_service/cued_speech).
- *Cue that Word!, Cue Reading 1,* and *Computer Fingers* provide practice sessions in receptive and expressive cueing for beginners, adults, and children. They can be obtained from Soundbytes at http://www.sound-bytes.com.

Finger spelling and sign language resources include

- Sign the Alphabet (http://www.funbrain.com/signs/index.html).
- Downloadable finger spelling fonts for Macintosh and Windows computers can be found at http://babel.uoregon.edu/yamada/fonts/asl.html.
- American Sign Language Browser (http://commtechlab.msu.edu/sites/aslweb/browser.htm) from Michigan State University's Communication Technology Laboratory provides "video of thousands of ASL signs."
- HandSpeak (http://www.handspeak.com) hosts a sign language dictionary containing more than 2,800 signs. This site contains stories in sign and categories of signs such as "animals," "colors," and so on.
- Steinberg's *The American Sign Language Dictionary* on CD-ROM New Version 2.0 can be found at http://www.soundbytes.com. The CD-ROM video simulates 2,400 signs as well as finger spelling and games. The user can also find signs by typing in English, Spanish, German, French, or Italian.

Cultural Factors in Assessment

The amount and type of physical contact permissible between individuals are highly influenced by culture. Examples of "don't touch," "middle ground" (i.e., touching is appropriate in some situations but not in others), and "touch" cultures are indicated below (Axtell, 1991).

Don't Touch	Middle Ground	Touch
Japan	France	Middle Eastern countries
United States	China	Latin countries
Canada	Ireland	Italy
England	India	Greece
Scandinavia		Spain
Other Northern European countries		Portugal
Australia		Some Asian countries
Estonia		Russia
Korea		

Audiologists must be careful in generalizing, because differences across cultures are also influenced by differences in age, gender, religion, and personal preference.

For example, in the United States, it is not unusual to see members of the opposite gender holding hands or kissing in public. In other parts of the world, such public displays of affection between men and women are not tolerated; however, it is commonplace to see members of the same gender holding hands as a sign of friendship. Among many Chinese and Asian groups, hugging, backslapping, and handshaking are not typical and should be avoided by the audiologist. In cases in which there is a language difference between audiologist and client, appropriate gestures and tone of voice can help establish rapport.

Touching the client around the head may be an important factor to consider in hearing assessment. Many Asians believe the head is the residence of the soul, and, among East Indians, there is the belief the head is so fragile that it should not be touched (Devine & Braganti, 1986). Touching may be a factor in immittance, auditory brain stem response, or electro-nystagmography testing, as well as in general interactions as the audiologist places electrodes or earphones on the client.

Cross-Racial Variables in Hearing Disorders

Etiology of Hearing Impairments

For more than 30 years, the Gallaudet Research Institute has conducted an Annual Survey of Deaf and Hard-of-Hearing Children and

Youth. The survey represents the largest data base of information on deaf and hard-of-hearing children in the United States (Holden-Pitt & Diaz, 1998).

The Annual Survey collects different kinds of data, including etiology of hearing loss. For more than 10 years, heredity, meningitis, and prematurity have been identified as the three primary causes of hearing loss across all racial and ethnic groups. Recent advances in genetic research have increased the frequency with which genetic syndromes are reported to the Annual Survey. In addition, the number of instances of cytomegalovirus reported to the Annual Survey has climbed steadily since the mid-1980s (Holden-Pitt & Diaz, 1998).

Over the years, African American and Hispanic or Latino children have been disproportionately represented in the categories of prematurity and meningitis. African American children have also been disproportionately represented among cases of cytomegalovirus. A study conducted by Van Naarden and Decoufle (1999) examined the prevalence and relative risks for congenital bilateral sensorineural hearing impairment in lower birth-weight infants. The study produced some noteworthy results. Van Naarden and Decoufle (1999) examined 169 children living in the metropolitan Atlanta area. Lower birth weight was directly related to a higher prevalence of bilateral sensorineural hearing loss, which was expected. The study also found that African American children weighing less than 2,500 g had much higher rates of hearing impairment than their white peers. The prevalence rates of hearing impairment for normal birth weight and borderline normal birth weight African American males were consistently higher than those for white children of both genders and African American females. Although etiologic data were limited, for 12 of the normal birth-weight African American males with known etiology for the hearing impairment, seven were the result of meningitis. Research is needed to identify risk factors that may explain the high prevalence of hearing loss among normal birth-weight African American males, including the association between meningitis and hearing impairment (Van Naarden & Decoufle, 1999).

Genetics

For half of all infants born with severe-to-profound hearing loss, the hearing loss is due to hereditary factors, or it is genetic. A breakdown of the etiology of severe-to-profound hearing loss reveals that 25% are nongenetic, 25% are unknown, 38% are recessively inherited, 11% are dominantly inherited, and 1% are X-linked or mitochondrial inherited (Gorlin, Toriello, & Cohen, 1995).

In dominant inheritance, one parent exhibits the inherited trait, in this case the hearing loss. There is a 50% chance of a child's inheriting the gene with each pregnancy. If a child inherits the gene, then she will present with the hearing loss. In recessive inheritance, both parents are clinically normal. For the child to manifest the hearing loss, she must inherit two abnormal genes, one from each parent. If a child inherits only one abnormal gene, she is a carrier. There is a 25% chance of a child's inheriting both genes with each pregnancy. For X-linked inheritance, the gene is located on the X chromosome, meaning girls are carriers of the trait, whereas boys are the ones affected by the trait.

Genetic mapping of hearing loss has occurred for many years. As of September 2000, the Hereditary Hearing Loss Homepage (http://dnalab-www.uia.ac.be/dnalab/hhh) lists the chromosome location for numerous inherited hearing disorders, including those that are associated with syndromes, such as Usher syndrome (Van Camp & Smith, 2000). The homepage provides links to the original published research that was used in determining the loci of the genetic disorders.

One of the more common recessive hearing losses is the gene labeled *DFNB1*. It accounts for approximately 50% of recessive nonsyndromic hearing losses. The hearing loss is a bilateral severe-to-profound sensorineural loss. The *DFNB1* gene encodes a protein called connexin 26 (Cx26). Cx26 is an essential component of the potassium pathway, a flow loop facilitating potassium circulation to maintain the high potassium concentration in scala media within the cochlea (McGuirt & Smith, 1999).

Although more than 22 different deafness-causing mutations of Cx26 have been described, in many populations it appears that a single mutation predominates. Different single mutations have been shown to exist in different populations. The carrier rate for one such mutation, 35delG, in the Midwestern U.S. is approximately 2.5%. However, in the Ashkenazi Jewish population another Cx26 mutation predominates, the 167delT mutation. It has a carrier rate of 4.03%, compared to a carrier rate of 0.73% for the 35delG mutation (Green et al., 1999). In the Japanese population, the 35delG mutation also is not a common cause of Cx26-related deafness (Usami et al., 1999).

Otitis Media

Differences have been found in the incidence of otitis media among racial groups (National Center for Health Statistics, 1986). American Indians, Alaskan Eskimos, and Aborigines have the highest incidence rates, and African Americans have the lowest incidence among racial groups. The differences in the incidence of otitis media may be caused in part by differences in the structure and function of the eustachian tube among racial groups. Evidence exists in support of this hypothesis (Beery et al., 1980;

Doyle, 1977). Doyle (1977) reported anatomic differences in the eustachian tubes of the Alaskan Eskimo, American Indian, white, and African American adult populations. The shorter, straighter eustachian tube of American Indians is associated with a higher incidence of chronic middle-ear disease (Beery et al., 1980; Doyle, 1977). In addition, differences in eustachian tube function have been found between White Mountain Apache Indians with a history of otitis media and whites also with a history of otitis media (Beery et al., 1980). Spivey and Hirschhorn (1977) studied a group of Apache Indian children adopted into middle-class homes outside the reservation and a group of Apache children living with their families on the reservation. They reported that, although the incidence of most infectious diseases decreased among the adopted Apache children, the incidence of otitis media remained comparable to the incidence for Apache children on the reservation (Spivey & Hirschhorn, 1977).

Intraracial differences in the incidence of otitis media also exist. Not all American Indian tribes have the same incidence rates of otitis media nor do all peoples of African descent (e.g., Nigerians, black South Africans, and African Americans). Individual variability must be taken into account in examining incidence or prevalence rates of otitis media, as well as familial or genetic factors, climate, and exposure to antibiotics.

Sickle Cell Disease and Hearing Loss

Sickle Cell Disease: Definition and Incidence

Sickle cell disease (SCD) is recognized as a world health problem predominantly affecting people of African descent in the United States, Africa, and the Caribbean. It also affects Israeli Arabs, Saudis, Turks, Greeks, Sicilians, Cypriots, and other races from areas adjacent to the Mediterranean Sea and Indian Ocean. Within the United States, there is regional variability in the incidence of SCD. There is a higher incidence of SCD in the Southern states than in the Northern states, probably due to the greater numbers of African Americans who live in the South.

SCD is a genetically inherited abnormality of the hemoglobin molecule, which is responsible for carrying oxygen in red blood cells (RBCs). SCD is a term used to refer to sickle cell anemia, sickle cell trait, and sickle cell variants, which are combinations of the sickle cell gene and another gene responsible for hemoglobin production. More than 50,000 African Americans have SCD.

One in 375 Americans of African ancestry is born with sickle cell anemia, whereas 1 in 12 carries one copy of the sickle cell gene, called *sickle cell trait*. Approximately 1 in 835 African Americans is born with the sickle cell gene and a gene for hemoglobin C, referred to as *sickle cell–hemoglobin C disease*. Sickle cell–hemoglobin C disease is milder than sickle cell anemia. Approximately 1 in 1,667 African Americans is born with the sickle cell gene and a beta thalassemia gene, referred to as *sickle cell–beta thalassemia disease*. This disease is variable, ranging from being indistinguishable from ordinary sickle cell anemia to being almost symptom free, depending on the nature of the thalassemia mutation (Bloom, 1995).

Normal RBCs are always soft, flexible, and rounded. They are able to easily squeeze through even the smallest blood vessels. In normal RBCs, hemoglobin is dissolved in a watery solution and remains dissolved under all conditions. In the RBC of a person with SCD, hemoglobin is dissolved under some conditions and is not dissolved under others. Instead of remaining liquid, hemoglobin forms crystals that twist the RBC out of shape. The RBC is no longer soft and flexible but, rather, becomes formed like a crescent-shaped sickle.

One of the clinical manifestations of the disease is that sickle-shaped cells form clumps that occlude smaller veins and capillaries, possibly including those supplying blood to the cochlea. In addition, central nervous system (including the auditory pathways) manifestations are frequent in SCD. It is postulated that central nervous system involvement could be due to small-vessel obstruction, although angiographic studies have revealed people with SCD who have partial or complete occlusion of such major intracranial vessels as the internal carotid, middle, and anterior cerebral arteries. The exact incidence of central nervous system involvement in SCD is unknown; however, a review of the literature reveals incidence figures of 4–40% (Sarniak et al., 1979).

Forty states, Puerto Rico, and the Virgin Islands have sickle cell screening programs for newborn infants. As of 1994, universal screening (all infants are screened regardless of race) was provided in 34 states. People with SCD now live longer, more comfortable lives. In 1973, the average lifespan was 14 years. Now, it is 48 years for women and 42 years for men. For persons with sickle cell–hemoglobin C disease, the lifespan is 68 years for women and 60 years for men (Bloom, 1995).

Auditory Involvement in Sickle Cell Disease

Considering the vaso-occlusive nature of SCD, the potential for auditory involvement is not unexpected. Some individuals with SCD have severe to profound sensorineural hearing losses, with partial or complete recovery of their hearing in some cases. These reactions in the auditory system are similar to vasospasm of the internal auditory artery.

Crawford et al. (1995) conducted a longitudinal study at Howard University to assess auditory function in a group of pediatric clients with SCD (ages

Table 11-5 Crawford et al.'s and Gould et al.'s Studies of the Prevalence of Hearing Impairments in Adults with Sickle Cell Disease*

Hemoglobin Type	Number	Number with Sensorineural Hearing Loss	Percent of Hearing Loss by Hemoglobin Type
Sickle cell anemia (HbSS)	50	18	36
Sickle cell-C disease (HbSC)	13	9	69
Sickle cell-beta thalassemia (HbS$_{b+}$–thal)	8	4	50
Sickle cell–beta thalassemia (HbS$_{b0}$–thal)	4	0	0
Total	**75**	**31**	**41**

*Central auditory system abnormalities were found, but there was no consistent pattern of abnormality.
Source: Adapted from Crawford, M. R., Gould, H. J., Smith, W. R., et al. (1991). Prevalence of hearing loss in adults with sickle cell disease. *Ear and Hearing, 12*, 349; Gould, H. J., Crawford, M. R., Smith, W. R., et al. (1991). Hearing disorders in sickle cell disease: Cochlear and retrocochlear findings. *Ear and Hearing, 12*, 352.

5 months to 16 years). Twenty-four subjects received a comprehensive audiologic evaluation that included pure tone and speech audiometry and immittance measurements. Eight subjects also received electrophysiologic testing. Six children exhibited a mild bilateral conductive hearing impairment, one exhibited a slight high-frequency sensorineural hearing impairment, and one exhibited a mild conductive impairment in the low frequencies and a slight sensorineural impairment in the high frequencies. Some children also exhibited abnormalities on acoustic reflexes and acoustic reflex decay and auditory brain stem response waveforms and latencies. Tables 11-5 and 11-6 compare the results of the Howard University study to other studies involving children and adults with SCD as subjects.

There is evidence of peripheral and central auditory dysfunction in children with SCD. Permanent peripheral dysfunction is most likely to manifest itself as a high-frequency sensorineural hearing impairment. Central auditory dysfunction is not uncommon but shows no consistent pattern. There appear to be differences in the prevalence of sensorineural hearing impairment in children versus adults with SCD (with a greater prevalence in adults) but not in the presence and variability of central auditory dysfunction. If damage due to SCD occurs mainly in the cochlea and is associated with crisis episodes, then greater hearing impairment over time would be expected, resulting in higher prevalence rates of hearing loss in adults.

Table 11-6 Audiologic Studies of Children with Sickle Cell Disease

Researcher(s)	Number	Age	Number and Percentage of Sensorineural Hearing Loss	Number and Percentage of Conductive Hearing Loss
Friedma et al. (1980)[a]	43	7–18 yrs	5 (12.0%)	0 (0.0%)
Forman-Franco et al. (1982)[b]	54	Mean = 12 yrs	2 (3.7%)	4 (7.4%)
Scott (1986)[c]	24	5 mo to 16 yrs	2 (8.0%)	7 (29.0%)
MacDonald et al. (1999)[d]	84	Mean = 7.8 yrs	3 (3.5%)	19 (22.6%)

[a]All of the children had sickle cell anemia (HbSS). Three of the five subjects with sensorineural hearing loss had history of cerebrovascular accidents of varying severity.

[b]All of the children had sickle cell anemia (HbSS). Thirteen of 28 children tested showed evidence of mild central auditory dysfunction.

[c]Seventeen children had sickle cell anemia (HbSS), four had sickle cell–C disease (HbSC), two had sickle cell–beta thalassemia (HbS$_b$–thal), and one had sickle cell–D disease (HbSD).

[d]All of the children had sickle cell anemia (HbSS).

Future study of the impact of SCD should include more longitudinal studies, the use of otoacoustic emissions to examine cochlear function, and the use of magnetic resonance imaging to examine central auditory anatomy.

Human Immunodeficiency Virus and Acquired Immunodeficiency Syndrome

Definition and Incidence of Human Immunodeficiency Virus and Acquired Immunodeficiency Syndrome

The human immunodeficiency virus (HIV) causes acquired immunodeficiency syndrome (AIDS). HIV is a ribonucleic acid retrovirus that infects white blood cells, the brain, the bowel, the skin, and other tissues. The most severe manifestation of HIV infection is AIDS (Simonds & Rogers, 1992). The immune system of the AIDS-infected individual is significantly compromised.

Through December 1999, the Centers for Disease Control and Prevention (2001a) reported 733,374 AIDS cases, with 272,881 of those cases occurring among African Americans. Although representing only 12% of the total U.S. population, African Americans make up almost 37% of all AIDS cases reported. AIDS cases are increasing among Hispanics in the United States. They accounted for 19% of the new cases reported in 1999. The 1999 rate of reported AIDS cases among African Americans was 66 per 100,000 population, whereas the rate for Hispanics was 25.6 and 7.6 for whites (Centers for Disease Control and Prevention, 2001a, 2001b, 2001c).

In the past, 6,000 infants were born to HIV-positive women each year, with 25–35% of the infants becoming HIV-positive (Ellerbrock, Bush, Chamberland, & Oxtoby, 1991). HIV infects children from all cultural groups, socioeconomic levels, family structures, and regions of the country. The majority of children with HIV infection are born to mothers who were intravenous drug users or who were sexual partners of intravenous drug users. A disproportionate number of these women and their children are African Americans, Hispanics, and members of lower socioeconomic groups. In 1998, African American children comprised 61% and Hispanic children 11% of all children reported with HIV. Twenty-six percent of children with HIV in the United States were white (Centers for Disease Control and Prevention, 1998).

The rate of HIV infection among children is changing. Audiologists may be less likely to evaluate children with hearing loss related to HIV or AIDS. The reason is that the number of children in the United States contracting AIDS from their mothers at birth dropped 43% between 1992 and 1996, because women are getting tested earlier and beginning drug treatment (Centers for Disease Control and Prevention, 1997).

Physicians believe most mothers who pass HIV to their babies do so during delivery, when the infant is exposed to the mother's blood and other fluids. Across the United States, the antiviral drug AZT has been given regularly during pregnancy since a successful 1994 experiment (Centers for Disease Control and Prevention 1997). As stated previously, without treatment, more than 25% of HIV-positive mothers will pass the virus to their newborns. With AZT, the rate drops to approximately 8% (Centers for Disease Control and Prevention, 1997).

Auditory Function in Human Immunodeficiency Virus and Acquired Immunodeficiency Syndrome

A large portion of clients with HIV has head and neck symptoms. The most common otologic and audiologic manifestations of HIV and AIDS include Kaposi's sarcoma of the ear, otitis caused by *Pneumocystis carinii*, eustachian tube obstruction caused by nasopharyngeal mass, serous otitis media, abnormal auditory response in the brain stem, sensorineural hearing loss, and facial palsy (Lalwani & Sooy, 1992).

A hearing impairment associated with HIV and AIDS is generally viewed as a secondary disorder arising from at least three primary etiologies: (1) effects of immunosuppression caused by HIV and direct infection of the hearing mechanism by HIV itself, (2) other opportunistic infections that attack the hearing mechanism, and (3) damage to the hearing mechanism due to toxic side effects of medications prescribed to treat the HIV or any associated opportunistic infections (Lalwani & Sooy, 1992; Madriz & Herrera, 1995). The hearing impairment can be manifested as a conductive, sensorineural, or central auditory disorder. In addition, a high prevalence of tinnitus has been reported in people with HIV and AIDS (Lalwani & Sooy, 1992).

Estimates of the prevalence of hearing loss in this population vary widely. Lalwani and Sooy (1992) estimated that sensorineural hearing loss in HIV-positive and AIDS clients ranged from 20.9–49.0%. The NIDCD, on the other hand, estimated that "75% of adult AIDS clients and 50% of ARC [AIDS-related complex] clients show clinical auditory system abnormalities" (NIDCD, 1989).

Recurrent infection, including upper respiratory infections and otitis media, are the most frequently reported medical problems of school-age children who are HIV positive (Papola, Alvarez, & Cohen, 1994). In addition, the density of recurrent otitis media has been reported to correlate with disease progression and immunologic suppression (Chen, Ohlms, Stewart, & Kline, 1996). Hearing losses have been reported for 7% of HIV-positive children (Chen et al., 1996). Whenever a psychological or language impairment is identified in a child who is HIV positive, the possibility of a hearing disorder should be investigated as a possible cause, especially for children having a history of recurrent otitis media (Mintz, 1998).

Noise-Induced Hearing Loss

Exposure to loud sounds can result in temporary or permanent hearing loss. Whether a hearing loss actually results from exposure to the loud sound depends on many factors, including the length of exposure, the intensity and frequency of the sound, and the susceptibility of the individual.

Differences in rates of hearing loss based on gender and race have been found in industrial noise-exposed populations. The differences are similar to the differences found in nonindustrial noise-exposed populations, as discussed in Cross-Racial Factors in Assessment. African American women show the least effects of noise on auditory thresholds, followed by white women and African American men, and then white men (Jerger, Jerger, Pepe, & Miller, 1986). African American women, therefore, show the least standard threshold shift on audiologic tests, and white men show the most (Royster & Royster, 1982). Audiologists must be aware of these differences in judging the effectiveness of hearing conservation programs.

It has been postulated that inner-ear melanin (a biological polymer responsible for pigmentation) may serve to protect the ear from excessive noise (Barrenäs & Lindgren, 1990). In addition to having more melanin content in the skin and eyes, individuals with darker skin have more melanin in the inner ear (La Ferriere, Kaufman-Arenberg, Hawkins, & Johnson, 1974). Some studies (Hood, Poole, & Freedman, 1976; Tota & Bocci, 1967) have found that, when exposed to noise, brown-eyed individuals have less temporary threshold shift (TTS) than blue-eyed individuals; Karlovich (1975) did not. Barrenäs and Lindgren (1990) conducted an experiment using 44 white male Swedish subjects with three different skin types. They found that TTS was inversely related to pigmentation. The least pigmented subjects showed the greatest TTS and the most pigmented subjects showed the least TTS.

Presbycusis

Hearing acuity declines with advancing age; the speed of decline is affected by gender and race. Women hear better than men, and African Americans hear better than white individuals. The median hearing threshold levels of an unscreened African American nonindustrial noise–exposed population (NINEP) were compared to the median threshold levels of four previously established presbycusis databases. The databases were all normalized relative to age 18 years. Comparisons were made between the African American NINEP and the presbycusis databases for different gender and age groupings. The African American NINEP exhibited hearing thresholds similar to the presbycusis databases for ages under 35–45 years. For ages older than 35–45 years, the hearing thresholds of the African American NINEP were generally lower (indicating better hearing) than those of the presbycusis databases, even though the NINEP exhibited significant nonindustrial noise exposures and medical and pathologic problems, which were not screened out of the population (Driscoll & Royster, 1984). Although it will be difficult, if not impossible, to separate the various factors contributing to changes in auditory sensitivity over time, more research is needed. As a start, population audiologic studies are needed for all racial groups. Several factors, including physiologic aging, diet, stress, noise exposure, disease processes, and racial and genetic factors, should be studied (Scott, 1993).

It is interesting to note that the U.S. Census 2000 reports on gender and median age of the various racial and ethnic populations. Women outnumber men within the white, African American, and Asian and Pacific Islander populations. For American Indians, women are almost equal in number to men, whereas, for Hispanics, men slightly outnumber women.

The median age of the racial and ethnic minority groups is significantly younger than the median age of whites. The median age for Hispanics is 26.6 years, for African Americans 30.6 years, for American Indians 28.5 years, and for Asian and Pacific Islanders 32.4 years. The median age for whites is 38.6. Based on these numbers, white men are the group most likely to be seen for hearing loss due to presbycusis.

Intervention for Hearing Disorders

An individual's culture is not a diagnostic category. Cultural heritage does not wholly explain how an individual thinks and acts, but it can help audiologists anticipate and understand how and why individuals and families make certain decisions. Audiologists must keep in mind an individual's and family's view of the disability. Three almost universal issues have been identified concerning the social implications of chronic illness and disability (Groce & Zola, 1993). The audiologist must consider the culturally perceived cause of chronic illness or disability and how this relates to the client's and family's view of the cause of the hearing loss. The audiologist must also determine the cultural expectation of survival or response to intervention. Finally, the audiologist must consider the resources in the home and community to assist with the rehabilitation of the hearing impairment.

Some examples of the influence of culture on intervention follow:

- A 3-year-old Hmong child was identified as having a bilateral sensorineural hearing impairment. Rehabilitation services were being offered through the public schools, but the parents first needed to have their son examined by a physician. They had been very slow in complying with that requirement. The parents were very willing to be responsible for taking care of their son at home; they were unsure that the public schools could do anything useful for their son. The solution was to have the parents meet with a Hmong adult with a hearing loss who had received intervention services.
- An African American mother whose son had a unilateral conductive hearing loss would not work with the audiologist in requiring her son to wear his hearing aid. Some of the children in his class did tease him about the hearing aid; however, the principal reason the mother was uncooperative was that she blamed herself for her son's hearing loss. She was sure she had done something during her pregnancy to cause the loss. She felt very guilty, because she believed that the hearing loss was evidence of a transgression. The conductive loss was actually

attributed to a congenital malformation of the ossicles. The mother remained uncooperative.

Part of the audiologic intervention process usually involves the selection and use of hearing aids and assistive listening devices. The following are examples of cultural influences that audiologists should keep in mind during this process:

- The color of hearing aids and ear molds is important. Hearing aids and ear molds will be more acceptable to people of color if the aids and ear molds more closely match their skin color. The audiologist must consider that there is considerable heterogeneity in skin tones.
- Some families may consider that the boys need hearing aids more than the girls.
- The deaf do not view the use of cochlear implants as appropriate for young deaf children. They do not believe a deaf child's hearing needs to be "fixed."

Other forms of aural rehabilitation also must be culturally appropriate. The family and significant family members need to be involved in the assessment and intervention as much as possible and according to their expectation of their role in the intervention process. The family structure may include single parents, gay and lesbian parents, and nuclear families or large extended families. The choice of language for (re)habilitation needs to be made with full consideration of the language used by the family. This will allow the client to develop and use language with those most significant in their daily life.

Hearing disability among racial and ethnic minority groups has received little attention. Hanyak (1992) conducted a study to determine the use of a modified Hearing Handicap Inventory for the Elderly–Screening Version (HHIE-S) for the assessment of hearing handicap and the incidence of self-reported hearing handicap in Hispanic adults. The Spanish version of the HHIE-S was shown to be a useful screening tool with Hispanic adults. In his conclusions, Hanyak (1992) recommended that the HHIE-S Spanish version be administered by bilingual interpreters. The reading level should be considered when administering the test to the elderly.

Access to hearing services in low-income racially and ethnically diverse communities is an important issue. In a survey of hearing health care needs among racial and ethnic minorities, Jones and Richardson-Jones (1987) found that only 9% of 230 respondents knew that they should seek an audiologist for hearing health care, and none knew where they could find an audiologist in their communities. They also found that 73% of the respondents rated hearing health care as a low priority. In 1986, Jones had found that African American populations were using hearing aids at a rate that was only one-fifth that of the majority population in the United States (Jones, 1986). Jones and Richardson-Jones (1987) stated that there are a number of reasons for the underuse of hearing health care services, including the need for more effective hearing health education in racial and ethnic minority communities, the costs of hearing services, and the nonpromotion of hearing services by hearing aid manufacturers in racial and ethnic minority communities.

Experience has shown that many elderly African Americans identified with hearing impairment do not ultimately purchase hearing aids or assistive listening devices. The cost of hearing aids is a factor, but many elderly do not believe that their lifestyles warrant the need for a hearing aid.

A study conducted by Lavizzo-Mourey, Smith, Sims, and Taylor (1994) tested the effectiveness of culturally sensitive education material and hearing screenings on evaluating the prevalence of hearing impairment among urban African American and Hispanic seniors.

Informational booklets on hearing loss were mailed to households and senior centers in 45 census tracts with high concentrations of racial and ethnic minority elderly. The elderly were then invited to have their hearing screened. Subjects with possible hearing impairments were referred for more testing and later telephoned to determine whether they received subsequent care. Four hundred thirty-three persons responded to three mailings by presenting themselves for a hearing evaluation. Of the 296 individuals screened for hearing loss, 174 (59%) had abnormal hearing thresholds, but only 26% obtained further testing.

Conclusion

Cultural competence is often described as consisting of three areas—knowledge, affect, and skills. A person who is culturally competent possesses a willingness and capability to draw on community-based values and customs and to work with others in developing focused interventions, communications, and other supports. Cultural incompetence is manifested by having no knowledge of cultural issues and having apathy in caring about cultural issues. Audiologists may physically or otherwise harm the client by being culturally incompetent. For example, the failure to detect a life-threatening auditory disease, such as cancer or a tumor along the auditory pathway, might result in death or, in other cases, result in a reduced quality of life. Kittrell and Arjmand (1997) found that white children were diagnosed with sensorineural hearing loss significantly earlier than African American or Hispanic children, regardless of socioeconomic status.

References

Anderson, P. P., & Fenichel, E. S. (1989). *Serving culturally diverse families of infants and toddlers with disabilities.* Washington, DC: National Center for Clinical Infant Programs.

Axtell, R. E. (1991). *Gestures: The do's and taboos of body language around the world.* New York: Wiley.

Barrenäs, M. L., & Lindgren, F. (1990). The influence of inner ear melanin on susceptibility to TTS in humans. *Scandinavian Audiology, 19,* 97–102.

Beery, Q. C., Doyle, W. J., Cantekin, E. I., et al. (1980). Eustachian tube function in an American Indian population. *Annals of Otology, Rhinology, and Laryngology, 89*(Suppl 68), 28–33.

Benson, V., & Marano, M. A. (1994). Current estimates from the National Health Interview Survey, 1992. *Vital and Health Statistics Series 10(189).* Hyattsville, MD: National Center for Health Statistics.

Berger, E. H., Royster, L. H., & Thomas, W. G. (1977). Hearing levels of nonindustrial noise exposed subjects. *Journal of Occupational Medicine, 19,* 664–670.

Bloom, M. (1995). *Understanding sickle cell disease.* Jackson, MS: University Press of Mississippi.

Bunch, C. C., & Raiford, T. S. (1931). Race and sex variations in auditory acuity. *Archives of Otolaryngology, 13,* 423–434.

Centers for Disease Control and Prevention. (1997, November 21). CDC: Rate of babies born with HIV down 43 percent in 4 years. *News & Record* (Greensboro, NC), A6.

Centers for Disease Control and Prevention. (1998). *HIV/AIDS surveillance report,* Vol. 10. Atlanta: Centers for Disease Control and Prevention.

Centers for Disease Control and Prevention. (2001a). *HIV/AIDS among African Americans* [On-line]. Available: http://www.cdc.gov/hiv/pubs/facts/afam.htm.

Centers for Disease Control and Prevention. (2001b). *HIV/AIDS among Hispanics in the United States* [On-line]. Available: http://www.cdc.gov/hiv/pubs/facts/hispanic.htm.

Centers for Disease Control and Prevention. (2001c). *HIV/AIDS among U.S. women: Minority and young women at continuing risk* [On-line]. Available: http://www.cdc.gov/hiv/pubs/facts/women.htm.

Chen, A. Y., Ohlms, L. A., Stewart, M. G., & Kline, M. W. (1996). Otolaryngologic disease progression in children with human immunodeficiency virus infection. *Archives of Otolaryngological Head and Neck Surgery, 122,* 1360–1363.

Cokely, J. A., & Yager, C. R. (1993). Scoring Spanish word-recognition measures. *Ear and Hearing, 14,* 395–400.

Comstock, C. L., & Martin, F. N. (1984). A children's Spanish word discrimination test for non-Spanish speaking clinicians. *Ear and Hearing, 5,* 166–170.

Crawford, M. R., Gould, H. J., Smith, W. R., et al. (1991). Prevalence of hearing loss in adults with sickle cell disease. *Ear and Hearing, 12,* 349–351.

Crawford, M. R., Burch-Sims, G. P., Scott, D. M., et al. (1995, April). *Audiologic considerations in sickle cell disease.* Paper presented at the annual convention of the American Academy of Audiology, Dallas.

Devine, E., & Braganti, N. L. (1986). *The traveler's guide to Asian customs and manners.* New York: St. Martin's Press.

Doyle, W. J. (1977). *A functiono-anatomic description of eustachian tube vector relations in four ethnic populations—an osteologic study.* Doctoral dissertation, University of Pittsburgh.

Driscoll, D. P., & Royster, L. H. (1984). Comparisons between the median hearing threshold levels for an unscreened black nonindustrial noise exposed population (NINEP) and four presbycusis data bases. *American Industrial Hygiene Association Journal, 45*(9), 577–593.

Ellerbrock, T., Bush, T., Chamberland, M., & Oxtoby, M. (1991). Epidemiology of women with AIDS in the U.S., 1981–1990. *Journal of the National Medical Association, 265,* 2971.

Forman-Franco, B., Karayalcin, G., Mandel, D. D., & Abramson, A. L. (1982). The evaluation of auditory function in homozygous sickle cell disease. *Otolaryngology—Head and Neck Surgery, 89,* 850–856.

Friedman, E. M., Luban, N. L. C., Herer, G. R., & Williams, I. (1980). Sickle cell anemia and hearing. *Annals of Otology, Rhinology, and Laryngology, 89,* 342–349.

Gallaudet Research Institute. (1999). Regional and national summary report of data from 1998–1999. *Annual Survey of Deaf and Hard-of-Hearing Children and Youth.* Washington, DC: Gallaudet University.

Gorlin, R. J., Toriello, H. V., & Cohen, M. M. (1995). *Hereditary hearing loss and its syndromes.* Oxford, UK: Oxford University Press.

Gould, H. J., Crawford, M. R., Smith W. R., et al. (1991). Hearing disorders in sickle cell disease: Cochlear and retrocochlear findings. *Ear and Hearing, 12,* 352–354.

Green, G. E., Scott, D. A., McDonald, J. M., et al. (1999). Carrier rates in the midwestern United States for GJB2 mutations causing inherited deafness. *Journal of the American Medical Association, 281*(23), 2211–2216.

Groce, N. E., & Zola, I. K. (1993). Multiculturalism, chronic illness, and disability. *Pediatrics, 91*(Suppl), 1048–1055.

Hanyak, R. E. (1992, November). *Perdida de audicion en los adultos Hispanos (Hearing handicap in Hispanic adults).* Paper presented at the annual convention of the American Speech-Language-Hearing Association, San Antonio.

Holden-Pitt, L., & Diaz, A. (1998). Thirty years of the Annual Survey of Deaf and Hard-of-Hearing Children & Youth: A glance over the decades. *American Annals of the Deaf, 143*(2), 72–76.

Hood, J. D., Poole, J. P., & Freedman, L. (1976). The influence of eye color upon temporary threshold shift. *Audiology, 15,* 449–464.

Jerger, J., Jerger, S., Pepe, D., & Miller, R. (1986). Race difference in susceptibility to noise-induced hearing loss. *American Journal of Otology, 7,* 425–429.

Jerger, J., Chmiel, R., Stach, B., & Spretnjak, M. (1993). Gender affects audiometric shape in presbycusis. *Journal of the American Academy of Audiology, 4,* 42–49.

Jones, R. C. (1986). *Does the hearing aid industry discriminate against minorities?* Unpublished report.

Jones, R. C., & Richardson-Jones, J. T. (1987). Strategies for marketing hearing healthcare services to minority populations. *Hearing Journal, 40*(1), 13–16.

Karlovich, R. S. (1975). Comments on the relation between auditory fatigue and iris pigmentation. *Audiology, 14,* 238–243.

Kittrell, A. P., & Arjmand, E. M. (1997). The age of diagnosis of sensorineural hearing impairment in children. *International Journal of Pediatric Otorhinolaryngology, 40*(2–3), 97–106.

La Ferriere, K. A., Kaufman-Arenberg, I., Hawkins, J. E., & Johnson, L. G. (1974). Melanocytes of the vestibular labyrinth and their relationship to microvasculature. *Annals of Otology, Rhinology, and Laryngology, 83,* 685–694.

Lalwani, A., & Sooy, D. (1992). Manifestaciones otológicas y neuro-otológicas del SIDA. *Clínicas Otorrinolaringologicas de Norte América, 6,* 1239–1254.

Lavizzo-Mourey, R., Smith, V., Sims, R., & Taylor, L. (1994). Hearing loss: An educational and screening program for African-American and Latino elderly. *Journal of the National Medical Association, 86*(1), 53–59.

MacDonald, C. B., Bauer, P. W., Cox, L. C., & McMahon, L. (1999). Otologic findings in pediatric cohort with sickle cell disease. *International Journal of Pediatric Otorhinolaryngology, 47,* 23–28.

Madriz, J. J., & Herrera, G. (1995). Human immunodeficiency virus and acquired immune deficiency syndrome: AIDS-related hearing disorders. *Journal of the American Academy of Audiology, 6,* 358–364.

McGuirt, W. T., & Smith, R. J. H. (1999). Connexin 26 as a cause of hereditary hearing loss. *American Journal of Audiology, 8,* 93–100.

Miller, G. A., Heise, G. A., & Lichten, W. (1951). The intelligibility of speech as a function of the context of the test materials. *Journal of Experimental Psychology, 41,* 329–340.

Mintz, M. (1998). Clinical features of HIV infection in children. In H. E. Gendelman, S. A. Lipton, L. Epstein, & S. Swindells (Eds.), *The neurology of AIDS* (pp. 385–407). New York: Chapman & Hall.

National Center for Health Statistics. (1986). *Current estimates from the National Health Interview Survey, United States 1984.* (Vital and Health Statistics. Series 10, No. 156. DHHS Pub. No. [PHS] 86-1584. Public Health Service). Washington, DC: U.S. Government Printing Office.

National Center for Health Statistics. (1994). *National Health Interview Survey.* Series 10, No. 188, Table 2. Hyattsville, MD: National Center for Health Statistics.

National Institute on Deafness and Other Communication Disorders. (1989). *A Report of the Task Force on the National Strategic Research Plan.* Bethesda, MD: National Institutes of Health.

National Institute on Deafness and Other Communication Disorders. (1995). *Research in human communication.* Bethesda, MD: Author.

National Institute on Deafness and Other Communication Disorders. (1999). *Health information: Hearing and balance* [On-line]. Available: http://www.nih.gov/nidcd/health/hb.htm.

Orque, M., Block, B., & Monrroy, L. (1983). *Ethnic nursing care: A multicultural approach.* St. Louis: Mosby.

Papola, P., Alvarez, M., & Cohen, H. J. (1994). Developmental and service needs of school-age children with human immunodeficiency virus infection: A descriptive study. *Pediatrics, 94,* 914–918.

Post, R. H. (1964). Hearing acuity variation among Negroes and whites. *Eugenics Quarterly, 11,* 65–81.

Ramkissoon, I. (2000). *Digit-speech reception thresholds among non-native speakers of English.* Presented at the 2nd International Symposium on Communication Disorders in Multilingual Populations, Kwa Maritane, Republic of South Africa.

Ramkissoon, I. (in press). Speech recognition thresholds for multilingual populations. *Communication Disorders Quarterly.*

Ramkissoon, I., Bilger, R. C., & Proctor, A. (2000). Digit-speech recognition thresholds among nonnative speakers of English. *ASHA Leader, 5*(16), 72.

Roberts, R. N. (1990). *Workbook for developing culturally competent programs for children with special needs.* Washington, DC: Georgetown University Child Development Center.

Royster, L. H., & Thomas, W. G. (1979). Age effect hearing levels for a white nonindustrial noise-exposed population (NINEP) and their use in evaluating industrial hearing conservation programs. *American Industrial Hygiene Association Journal, 40,* 504–511.

Royster, L. H., & Royster, J. D. (1982). Methods of evaluating hearing conservation program audiometric databases. In P. W. Alberti (Ed.), *Personal hearing protection in industry* (p. 571). New York: Raven.

Royster, L. H., Driscoll, D. P., Thomas, W. G., & Royster, J. D. (1980). Age effect hearing levels for a black nonindustrial noise-exposed population (NINEP). *American Industrial Hygiene Association Journal, 41,* 113–119.

Rudmin, F. (1987). Speech reception threshold for digits. *Journal of Auditory Research, 27,* 15–21.

Sarniak, S., Soorya, D., Kim, J., et al. (1979). Periodic transfusions for sickle cell anemia and CNS infarction. *American Journal of the Diseased Child, 133,* 1254–1257.

Schildroth, A. N., & Hotto, S. A. (1995). Race and ethnic background in the Annual Survey of Deaf and Hard of Hearing Children and Youth. *American Annals of the Deaf, 140*(2), 96–99.

Scott, D. (1986). Sickle-cell anemia and hearing loss. In F. H. Bess, B. S. Clark, & H. R. Mitchell (Eds.), *Concerns for minority groups in communication disorders* (pp. 69–73). Rockville, MD: American Speech-Language- Hearing Association (ASHA Reports 16).

Scott, D. M. (1993). Aging and hearing loss: Race and gender differences in African Americans and Euro-Americans. *Howard Journal of Communications, 4,* 369–379.

Simonds, R., & Rogers, M. (1992). Epidemiology of HIV infection in children and other populations. In A. C. Crocker, H. J. Cohen, & T. A. Kastner (Eds.), *HIV infection and developmental disabilities: A resource for service providers* (pp. 3–14). Baltimore: Brookes.

Spivey, G. H., & Hirschhorn, N. (1977). A migrant study of adopted Apache children. *Johns Hopkins Medical Journal, 140,* 43–46.

Tota, Y., & Bocci, G. (1967). The importance of the colour of the iris on the evaluation of resistance to auditory fatigue. *Rev Oto-Neuro-Ophthalmology, 42,* 183–192.

Usami, S., Abe, S., Shinkawa, H., et al. (1999). *Prevalent mutations in connexin 26 gene in sporadic and recessive non-syndromic deafness in Japanese population.* Unpublished data presented at February 1999 Association for Research in Otolaryngology, St. Petersburg, FL.

U.S. Bureau of the Census. (1990). *Statistical abstract of the United States: 1990* (110th ed.). Washington, DC: U.S. Bureau of the Census.

U.S. Bureau of the Census. (1993). *Language spoken at home and ability to speak English for United States, regions, and states: 1990, CPH-L-133.* Washington, DC: U.S. Bureau of the Census.

U.S. Bureau of the Census. (2001). *Census 2000 brief: Overview of race and Hispanic origin 2000* [On-line]. Available: http://www.census.gov/prod/cen2000/index.html.

U.S. Department of Education. (1998). *To assure the free appropriate public education of all Americans: Twentieth annual report to Congress on the implementation of the Individuals with Disabilities Education Act* (Pub No. 1998-716-372/93547). Washington, DC: U.S. Government Printing Office.

Van Camp, G., & Smith, R. J. H. (2000). *Hereditary hearing loss homepage* [On-line]. Available: http://dnalab-www.uia.ac.be/dnalab/hhh.

Van Naarden, K., & Decoufle, P. (1999). Relative and attributable risks for moderate to profound bilateral sensorineural hearing impairment associated with lower birth weight children 3 to 10 years old. *Pediatrics, 104*(4), 905–910.

12

Multicultural Aspects of Deafness

Zenobia Bagli

The Deaf community is a microcosm of the larger normal hearing community in which it resides. Its heterogeneity is apparent in its constituents who represent different cultures, ages, and genders. The members of this community have one common denominator—their inability to hear. The Deaf community in the United States shares a language, American Sign Language (ASL), and a culture, which is passed on from one generation to another. Members of this culture have values and beliefs about themselves and the hearing world around them. Usually, a language provides an individual with his or her ethnic identity. ASL does provide such an identity. However, Deaf persons who are also ethnic minorities hold membership in two or more minority groups and must participate and interact effectively with each group and with the dominant culture.

Before discussing the multicultural aspects of deafness, it is necessary to define the population under review in this chapter. The term *hearing impairment* is used generically in this chapter; it represents the whole audiologic continuum of hearing loss without regard to the degree and type of hearing loss or age of onset. The term *deaf* is used to identify those individuals who have a hearing impairment of 90 decibels of hearing loss or greater in the better, unaided ear across the speech frequencies. The term *Deaf* is used to identify the culture of those with the degree of hearing loss specified earlier.

Deafness may be caused by genetic factors or nongenetic factors, such as infections and ototoxic drugs. In a young child, deafness can impede normal development of language and speech and, subsequently, affect education. In the adult, it may result in vocational and economic difficulties and lead to social isolation and stigmatization. The increased life expectancy and the growing world population suggest that, in the future, there will be much larger numbers of persons with hearing impairment unless decisive public health action is taken to reduce and eventually eliminate avoidable hearing impairment and disability by implementing appropriate preventive measures (World Health Organization, 2001).

Although deafness can occur in persons of all races, genders, and ages, there are differences among ethnic groups depending on the etiologic factor under review. For instance, the leading cause of deafness in the Hispanic community is maternal rubella, but in the African American community, it is meningitis (Schildroth & Hotto, 1995). To some extent, health differences and this disparity appear to be related to the socioeconomic status. On average, white Americans have better access to the social and economic resources necessary for a healthy environment and lifestyle and better access to preventive medical services than minorities.

The population of the United States is becoming increasingly diverse; minority racial groups have each grown faster than the population as a whole. In 1970, together the minorities represented 16% of the population; by 1998, the minority population had increased to 27%. The U.S. Bureau of the Census (2000a) has projected that if current trends continue, by 2050 the minority groups will account for almost 50% of the U.S. population. The school-aged population is more diverse and already resembles the projected composition of this nation's population in 2010 (Council of Economic Advisors for the President's Initiative on Race, 1999). In this century, some of the greatest changes and challenges facing health care professionals will be related to ethnic diversity. Speech-language pathologists and audiologists will be providing services to more minorities, and culture will influence the way they operate. Professionals will have to become more conscious and knowledgeable of the cultures of the persons they serve, because culture may affect the way a family accepts a diagnosis of deafness, copes with the emotional impact of having a deaf child, interacts with the professional, implements treatment, allows the clinician to participate with the family in early intervention, and tolerates what may be perceived as intrusion from the clinician. To achieve successful outcomes, professionals will have to become more culture conscious, develop cultural competence, and design, develop, and implement assessment and treatment protocols that reflect the diversity of the individuals they serve.

Demographics

It is estimated that, in the United States, there are 28 million persons of all ages with hearing impairment (National Institute on Deafness and Other Communication Disorders, 1996). *Healthy People 2010* (U.S. Department of Health and Human Services, 2001), a national health promotion and disease prevention initiative, lists two primary goals for the next decade: (1) to increase the quality and years of healthy life, and (2) to eliminate health disparities. Recognizing that hearing is a defining element of the quality of life, one of the objectives of this initiative is to improve hearing health of the nation through prevention, early detection, treatment, and (re)habilitation. In the past, it was estimated that 1 in 1,000 live births had a congenital hearing impairment. However, data from states with universal newborn hearing screening programs suggest that the incidence may be higher; perhaps there are 2–3 per 1,000 live births with congenital hearing impairment. This estimate does not include those with late-onset or progressive hearing impairment. Additionally, Collins (1997) estimated that there were 1,465,000 persons aged 3 years or older who were deaf in both ears, whereas the National Institute on Aging (1996) estimated that approximately one-third of Americans between ages 65 and 74 years and one-half of those who were 85 years and older had hearing impairments.

Deafness affects individuals of all ages, gender, and ethnicity. The U.S. Department of Education (USDOE) (2000), in its *Twenty-Second Annual Report to Congress*, reported that during the 1998–1999 school year, 70,883 students aged 6–21 years (1.30% of all students with disabilities) received special education services under the "hearing impairment" category, and 1,609 students (0.03%) received special education services under the "deaf-blindness" category. The number of children with hearing impairment is probably higher because many children have multiple disabilities and may be served under other categories. According to the USDOE (2000), the percentage of children with hearing impairments grew by 22.4% between the 1989–1990 and 1998–1999 school years, whereas the percentage of children with deaf-blindness decreased by 1.5%.

According to the USDOE (2000), the number of students with disabilities served under the Individuals with Disabilities Education Act (IDEA) continues to grow at a greater rate than the resident population and school enrollment, although the increase varies by the disability category. The collection of race/ethnic data was a new component of the 1998 child count for all programs under IDEA. The ethnic breakdown of children between 6 and 21 years for the two disability categories (i.e., hearing impairments and deaf-blindness served under IDEA, Part B) between the 1987–1988 and 1998–1999 school years in the 50 states, District of Columbia, and Puerto Rico are shown in Figures 12-1 and 12-2. The race/ethnicity distribution of students served under IDEA and the distribution in the general population shows some disparity. Although Asian and Pacific Islander students represent 3.8%

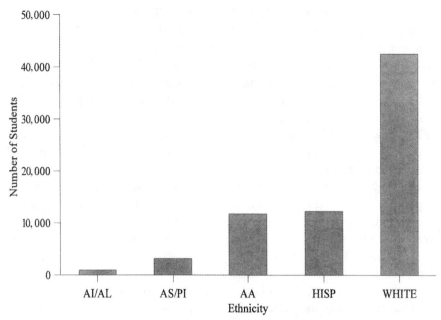

Figure 12-1   Number of students with hearing impairments by ethnicity for the 1998–1999 school year. (AA = African American; AI/AL = American Indian/Alaska Native; AS/PI = Asian/Pacific Island Native; HISP = Hispanic.) (U.S. Department of Education [2000]. *Twenty-Second Annual Report to Congress on the implementation of the Individuals with Disabilities Education Act. OSEP, Data Analysis System.* Washington, DC: U.S. Government Printing Office.)

of the general population, 4.6% are hearing impaired, and 11.3% have deaf-blindness—a significantly higher percentage than their representation in the resident population. African American students accounted for 14.8% of the general population, compared with 16.8% with hearing impairment and 11.5% with deaf-blindness. This suggests that the representation of African American children in the hearing-impaired category exceeded the resident population. The representation of Hispanic students in the hearing-impaired category was 16.3%, which is slightly higher than the 14.2% of Hispanic children in the resident population. The percentage of deaf-blindness was a lower 12.1% in the Hispanic students enrolled in special education. American Indian students represented 1.0% of the general population; however, 1.4% of the students were classified as hearing impaired, and 1.8% were categorized as deaf-blind. There were 66.0% of white children categorized as hearing impaired and 63.3% with deaf-blindness in comparison with the general population of 66.3%.

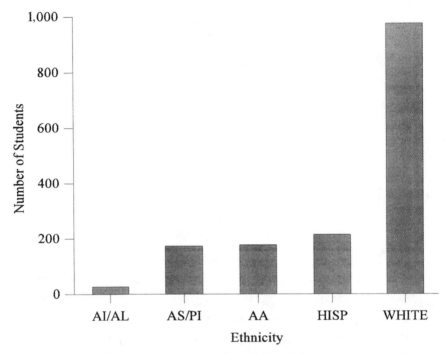

Figure 12-2 Number of students categorized as deaf-blind by ethnicity for the 1998–1999 school year. (AA = African American; AI/AL = American Indian/Alaska Native; AS/PI = Asian/Pacific Island Native; HISP = Hispanic.) (U.S. Department of Education [2000]. *Twenty-Second Annual Report to Congress on the implementation of the Individuals with Disabilities Education Act. OSEP, Data Analysis System.* Washington, DC: U.S. Government Printing Office.)

Schildroth and Hotto (1995) commented that, over the past 20 years, the demographic variable that shifted most dramatically in the *Annual Survey of Deaf and Hard of Hearing Children and Youth* was race/ethnic background. The incidence of deafness in minority children and youth increased from 24% in 1973–1974 to 40% in 1993–1994. They reported a steady increase in the number of Hispanic children with hearing impairment, as shown in Figure 12-3; specifically, this number increased from less than 3,000 in 1973–1974 to 7,500 in 1993–1994. The number of Asian and Pacific Islander children and youth reported to the Annual Survey increased by more than 500% during the same period.

Schildroth and Hotto (1995) also reported on the types of special education program settings deaf and hard of hearing children and youth from different ethnic cultures attended based on data from the 1993–1994 school year. As shown in Figure 12-4, a larger number of white students attended

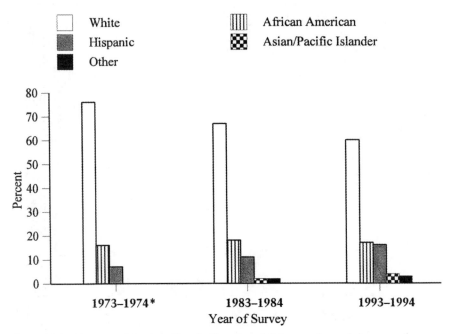

Figure 12-3 Percent of deaf and hard of hearing children and youth by year of survey. *In 1973–1974, <1% of children and youth from Asian and Pacific and other ethnic origins were reported to be deaf and hard of hearing. (Adapted from Schildroth, A. N., & Hotto, S. A. [1995]. Race and ethnic background in the Annual Survey of Deaf and Hard of Hearing Children and Youth. *American Annals of the Deaf, 140,* 96–99. Copyright 1995, Gallaudet Research Institute.)

residential and local, not integrated, programs than minorities. On the other hand, the minorities appeared to be predominantly in day school and local, integrated programs.

According to the U.S. Department of Education (2000), the majority of children with disabilities received educational services in regular classrooms, resource rooms, or separate classes in regular schools for either all or part of the day. Children with two or more disabilities were more likely to receive special education and related services in separate classes than children with one disability. The number of students with hearing impairments and those with deaf-blindness, ages 6–21 years, served under IDEA, Part B, in the 50 states, the District of Columbia, and Puerto Rico during the 1987–1988, 1997–1998, and 1998–1999 school years are shown in Figures 12-5 and 12-6, respectively.

Table 12-1 identifies states with the highest number and percentage of students (ages 6–21 years) of different race/ethnicity with hearing impair-

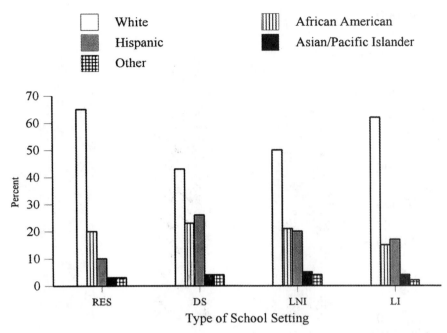

☐ White	▥ African American
▨ Hispanic	■ Asian/Pacific Islander
▦ Other	

Figure 12-4 Percent of children and youth reported to be deaf and hard of hearing by type of school setting during the 1993–1994 school year. (DS = day school; LI = local, integrated; LNI = local, not integrated; RES = residential.) (Adapted from Schildroth, A. N., & Hotto, S. A. [1995]. Race and ethnic background in the Annual Survey of Deaf and Hard of Hearing Children and Youth. *American Annals of the Deaf, 140,* 96–99. Copyright 1995, Gallaudet Research Institute.)

ment who received services under IDEA, Part B, in 1998–1999. The number and percentage of students with deaf-blindness (ages 6–21 years) from different races/ethnicities are shown in Table 12-2; these percentages should be interpreted with caution because of the small numbers of students with deaf-blindness in most states.

Data collected during the National Health Interview Survey by the U.S. Department of Health and Human Services for the years 1990, 1991, and 1992 listed "deafness" and "other hearing impairments" among the selected chronic conditions with the highest prevalence (Collins, 1997). These data showed that the largest number of persons who were deaf in both ears resided in the south (466,000), whereas the smallest number resided in the northeast (263,000). Subsequent data from the National Center for Health Statistics (2000) were reported differently, as the survey was revised to include several special topics. The data on persons with all degrees of hearing impairment were collected under the category of "hear-

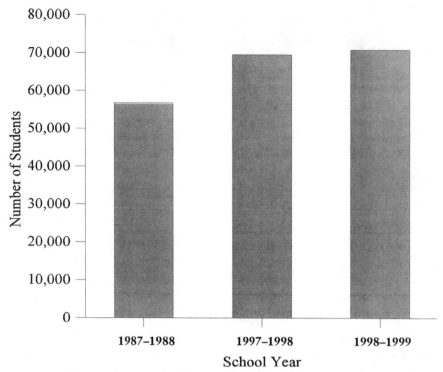

Figure 12-5 Number of students, by school year, with a hearing impairment. (U.S. Department of Education [2000]. *Twenty-Second Annual Report to Congress on the implementation of the Individuals with Disabilities Education Act. OSEP, Data Analysis System.* Washington, DC: U.S. Government Printing Office.)

ing impairment." Therefore, persons with deafness were not differentiated from persons with lesser hearing impairment. As shown in Figure 12-7, for each of the years 1993, 1994, 1995, and 1996, in which the National Health Interview Survey (National Center for Health Statistics, 2000) was conducted, a substantially greater number of men than women reported a hearing impairment. Figure 12-8 differentiates the number of persons reporting hearing impairment based on ethnicity. For each of the 4 years, white persons far exceeded the incidence of hearing impairment in the African American community. Figure 12-9 shows that more persons in the South reported having hearing impairments than in any other region in the United States for each of the 4 years that the survey was conducted, whereas the Northeast appeared to have the least number of persons with hearing impairment. When the data from the National Health Interview Survey (National Center for Health Statistics, 2000) were compared to examine the incidence of hearing impairment by age groups, it was observed that for each of

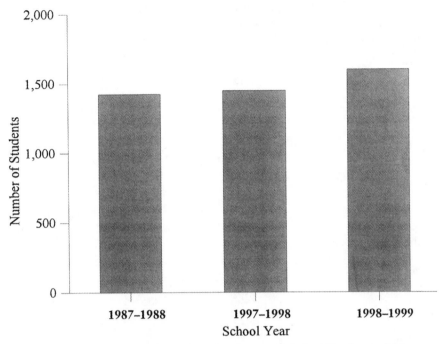

Figure 12-6 Number of students, by school year, with deaf-blindness. (U.S. Department of Education [2000]. *Twenty-Second Annual Report to Congress on the implementation of the Individuals with Disabilities Education Act. OSEP, Data Analysis System.* Washington, DC: U.S. Government Printing Office.)

the 4 years that the survey was conducted, the incidence appeared to be the highest in the 45–64-year-olds (Figure 12-10). This may suggest that the "baby boomers" are aging.

According to the National Center for Health Statistics (1997), 4.5 million persons use hearing aids, amplified telephones, closed caption television, and other assistive devices for hearing impairments. As technology has advanced, the use of assistive devices has increased dramatically over the past decade. Other factors contributing to the increased use of these devices include the aging of the population, public policy initiatives, and changes in the delivery and financing of health care. It was estimated that 69% of persons using hearing devices were older than 65 years of age.

Etiology

Deafness at birth or in early childhood can have a devastating effect on the child's language and speech development. This concern

Table 12-1   Highest Number and Percentage of Students with Hearing Impairments, Ages 6–21, by Ethnicity, Served under the Implementation of the Individuals with Disabilities Education Act during the 1998–1999 School Year

	American Indian/ Alaskan	Asian/ Pacific Islander	African American	Hispanic	White
Highest number of children with hearing impairment	Arizona (134) Alaska (76)	Colorado (1,108) New York (350)	New York (1,727) Texas (851)	California (3,941) Texas (2,297)	California (3,427) New York (2,685)
Highest percent of children with hearing impairment	Alaska (31.67%) South Dakota (18.18%)	Hawaii (86.60%) Arkansas (13.08%)	District of Columbia (83.33%) Mississippi (56.08%)	Puerto Rico (100%) New York (47.53%)	New Hampshire (97.64%) Maine (97.63%)

led to the development of the Joint Committee on Infant Hearing (1991), which has guided the early identification of hearing impairment in neonates over the past 30 years. Although risk factors associated with deafness have been known for decades, with advances in medicine, genetics, and technology, the focus has shifted over the decades from diseases such as maternal rubella, which has been controlled via immunization, to genetics and other diseases, such as cytomegalovirus (CMV). A detailed discussion of every risk factor identified by the Joint Committee on Infant Hearing (1991) is beyond the scope of this chapter. Selected etiologic factors are discussed below.

Low Birth Weight

The birth weight and gestational period are two very important predictors of a neonate's health and survival. Infants born too small or too soon have a greater risk of death, as well as short-term and long-term disabilities, than those who are born at term and who weigh 2,500 g or more. The Centers for Disease Control and Prevention (MacDorman & Atkinson, 1999) reported that in 1997, low birth weight (<2,500 g) was reported in 7.5% of the neonates; their mortality rate was six times the rate for infants weighing 2,500 g or more. The infant mortality rate for

Table 12-2   Highest Number and Percentage of Students with Deaf-Blindness, Ages 6–21, by Ethnicity, Served under the Implementation of the Individuals with Disabilities Education Act during the 1998–1999 School Year

	American Indian/ Alaskan	Asian/ Pacific Islander	African American	Hispanic	White
Highest number of children with deaf-blindness	Arizona (7) Arkansas (5)	Hawaii (132) California (17)	Pennsylvania (18) Texas (16)	California (46) Puerto Rico (28)	Utah (142) Connecticut (52)
Highest percent of children with deaf-blindness	Wyoming (50%) Alaska (40%)	Guam (100%) N. Maranas (100%) Palau (100%) Hawaii (84.08%)	District of Columbia (91.67%) Pennsylvania (78.26%)	Puerto Rico (100%) New Mexico (71.43%)	Kentucky, Maine, Montana, Nebraska, New Hampshire, South Dakota, Tennessee, Vermont, West Virginia (100%)

Source: U.S. Department of Education (2000). *Twenty-Second Annual Report to Congress on the Implementation of IDEA.* OSEP, Data Analysis System. Washington, DC: U.S. Government Printing Office.

very low birth weight (<1,500 g) was over 90 times greater than that for infants with a birth weight of 2,500 g or more. Factors associated with low birth weight in neonates include the age of the mother (e.g., teenage pregnancies), delayed or no prenatal care, mother's disadvantaged background, and tobacco use during pregnancy. Data reported by MacDorman and Atkinson (1999) indicated that the percentage of African American mothers who gave birth to neonates weighing less than 1,500 g was higher than for any other ethnic group. Additionally, the mortality rate for infants with low birth weight was higher in African Americans than for other ethnic groups. According to the Joint Committee on Infant Hearing (2000), infants weighing less than 1,500 g are at risk for hearing impairment or deafness. Therefore, it may be inferred that more African American babies are at risk for hearing impairment or deafness than other ethnic groups.

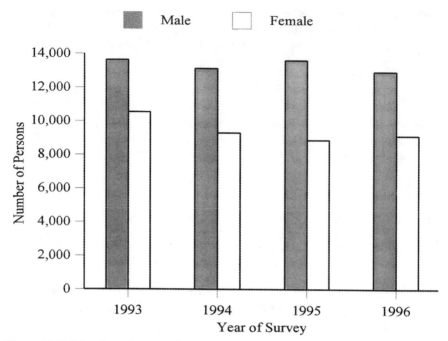

Figure 12-7 Number of men and women in thousands who reported a hearing impairment on a National Health Interview Survey conducted annually between 1993 and 1996. (Data from the National Center for Health Statistics. *Vital health statistics series.* [No. 10, 1994, 1995, 1998, 1999.] Hyattsville, MD.)

Figure 12-11 shows the percentage of very low birth weight babies born to different ethnic groups.

Genetic Hearing Loss

Epidemiologic studies in the United States have shown that approximately 1 in 1,000–2,000 children are born with or present in early childhood with severe or profound hearing impairment, of whom approximately half have a genetic cause (Parving, 1983; Newton, 1985). Recently, Marazita et al. (1993) reported that the incidence of profound early-onset deafness was present in 4–11 per 10,000 children. Of these, 37.2% of the cases were attributed to sporadic causes and 62.8% to genetic causes (47.1%, recessive; 15.7%, dominant). A genetic hearing impairment may occur in isolation (nonsyndromal) or in association with other features (syndromal). Nonsyndromal hearing impairments (70%) occur as a single gene disorder due to an autosomal dominant gene, X-linked gene, or mito-

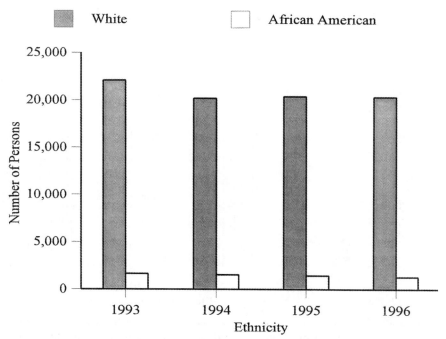

Figure 12-8 Number of individuals in thousands by ethnicity who reported a hearing impairment on the National Health Interview Survey conducted annually between 1993 and 1996. (Data from the National Center for Health Statistics. *Vital health statistics series.* [No. 10, 1994, 1995, 1998, 1999.] Hyattsville, MD.)

chondrial inheritance. For instance, adult-onset progressive hearing impairment can be caused by mutations in a single gene. Syndromal hearing impairments (30%) result from chromosomal or single gene causes. Clinical diagnosis depends on the detection of the overall pattern of anomalies. The most common mode of transmission of genetic hearing impairment was estimated to be autosomal recessive (80%), although hearing impairment may result from autosomal dominant transmission (15%) and X-linked inheritance (2–3%) also (Newton, 1985; Rose, Conneally, & Nance, 1977). More recently, Marazita et al. (1993) reported an incidence of 75% of autosomal recessive transmission. This decrease may be due to the increasing number of Deaf persons who marry and have children, which results in an increase in the frequency of cases with a dominant mode of transmission.

Parving (1996) summarized the incidence of hearing impairment in children that were attributed to genetic causes based on 14 surveys conducted internationally. The incidence of genetic hearing impairment reported in

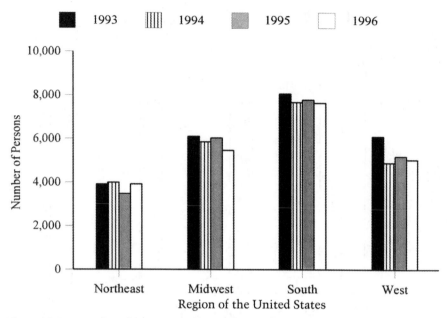

Figure 12-9 Number of persons in thousands in different geographic regions who reported a hearing impairment on the National Health Interview Survey conducted annually between 1993 and 1996. (Data from the National Center for Health Statistics. *Vital health statistics series.* [No. 10, 1994, 1995, 1998, 1999.] Hyattsville, MD.)

these surveys varied from 9–54%, whereas 16–42% of the children had hearing impairment of unknown origin. Parving (1996) suggested that it was likely that the variation in the proportion of genetic hearing impairment reflected true differences in the genetic expression in the different populations. Although, in the United States, autosomal recessive nonsyndromal hearing impairment is estimated to be 1 in 1,000 children (Morton, 1991), in England and Denmark, it is reported to be 0.7 in 1,000 children (Davis & Parving, 1994). However, in China, it is estimated that 1.1 per 1,000 are affected by profound hearing impairment (Liu, Xu, Zhang, & Xu, 1993).

The cultural practice in a community also impacts the incidence of genetic hearing impairment. In some cultures, consanguineous marriages are an accepted practice. Al-Shihabi (1994) reported that the incidence of hearing impairment was 12.9 per 1,000 in offspring in consanguineous marriages but 3.1 per 1,000 births in nonconsanguineous marriages in the same geographic area. This suggested that autosomal recessive hearing impairment was a monogenic disease.

During the last few decades, there has been rapid development of knowledge within the field of genetics concerning the structure and function of

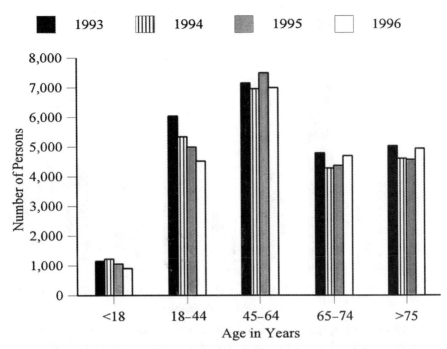

Figure 12-10 Number of persons in thousands in different age groups who reported a hearing impairment on the National Health Interview Survey conducted annually between 1993 and 1996. (Data from the National Center for Health Statistics. *Vital health statistics series.* [No. 10, 1994, 1995, 1998, 1999.] Hyattsville, MD.)

chromosomes, which has led to the localization and isolation of genes that cause hearing impairment and deafness. As mapping continues, the human genome project will be completed and will provide an invaluable resource for the diagnosis, prevention, habilitation, and rehabilitation of genetic hearing impairment and deafness (Parving, 1996).

Mueller (2000) reported that investigations of the recurrence of hearing impairment in children born to hearing-impaired or deaf couples have indicated that there are approximately 100 genes that may be responsible for nonsyndromal sensorineural hearing impairment or deafness. During the past 8 years, 28 autosomal recessive, 30 autosomal dominant, and 5 X-linked genes for nonsyndromal sensorineural hearing impairment or deafness have been cloned. The recent identification of the *connexin 26* gene allows geneticists to test for mutations in children who are sporadically affected with nonsyndromal sensorineural hearing impairment or deafness to determine whether the hearing impairment is genetic in origin and provide appropriate counseling to the parents. Connexins are proteins that are responsible for

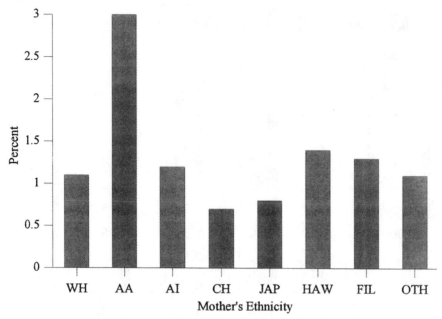

Figure 12-11 Percentage of live births of infants with a birth weight of <1,500 grams by ethnicity. (AA = African American; AI = American Indian; CH = Chinese; FIL = Filipino; HAW = Hawaiian; JAP = Japanese; OTH = other; WH = white.) (Data from MacDorman, M., & Atkinson, J. [1999]. *Infant mortality statistics from the 1997 period linked birth/infant data set.* National vital statistics reports [Vol. 47, No. 23]. Hyattsville, MD: National Center for Health Statistics.)

forming physical connections between cells. By testing for this gene, it is possible to identify the cause of deafness in 20–40% of persons with hearing impairment or deafness of unknown etiology. For instance, Morrell, Kuir, and Hood (1998) reported that the 167delT mutation had only been identified in the Ashkenazi Jewish population. On the other hand, the 35delG mutation in *connexin 26* has been shown to account for nonsyndromal sensorineural hearing impairment or deafness in Western Europe and North America (Estivill, Fortina, & Surrey, 1999; Lench et al., 1998; Zelante, Gasparini, & Estivill, 1997).

Based on data from the 1989–1990 Annual Survey of Hearing Impaired Children and Youth, Nuru (1993) reported that heredity was the primary cause of deafness among whites (15.8%), Hispanics (13.2%), and Asian Pacific Americans (6.6%). Data from the 1991–1992 Annual Survey of Hearing Impaired Children and Youth (Schildroth, 1994) indicated that heredity accounted for 17% of hearing impairment or deafness in children younger than 6 years of age. Typically, the degree of hearing impairment was substantial; 45% had profound hearing impairment, 18% had severe hearing impairment, 12% had moderately severe, and 10% reported moderate hearing impairment. Heredity as a causative factor was the highest among white (72%) children and youth when compared with peers from the Hispanic (14%), African American (10%), Asian and Pacific Islander (2%), and other (2%) communities.

Cytomegalovirus

CMV is one of the leading causes of nongenetic severe to profound hearing impairment in infants and children. CMV is a member of the herpes family. According to the Centers for Disease Control and Prevention (1999), CMV is found throughout all geographic locations and socioeconomic groups and infects between 50% and 85% of adults in the United States by 40 years of age. CMV infection is more widespread in developing countries and in areas of lower socioeconomic conditions. Healthy persons who become infected experience few symptoms and no long-term health consequences. However, persons who work with children are at risk for contacting this infection, which remains alive but usually dormant within the person's body for life. Although the virus is not highly contagious, it has been known to spread in households and among children at day care centers. For instance, Murph et al. (1998) traced some cases of congenital CMV infection to child-care environments. This virus poses a threat to the unborn baby during pregnancy and to neonates; it may be transmitted to the infant at delivery from contact with genital secretions or through breast milk. Fowler et al. (1992) observed that primary maternal CMV infection during pregnancy resulted in more serious consequences for the fetus than infection from a reactivated virus.

The Centers for Disease Control and Prevention (1999) estimated that 1–3% pregnant women get infected with CMV in the United States. Although CMV infection without symptoms is common in infants and young children, neonates who are infected prenatally may develop generalized infection with symptoms ranging from moderate enlargement of the liver and spleen to fatality. With supportive treatment, most of these infants survive. However, 80–90% develop complications such as hearing impairment, vision impairment, and varying degrees of mental retardation within the first year of life. Another 15% who are infected but symptomless at birth subsequently develop significant hearing impairment, mental retardation, and coordination problems. Williamson et al. (1992) reported that 15% of the cases developed hearing impairment over several years.

According to Dahle et al. (2000), the infection may cause latent damage to the inner ear and may result in hearing impairment months or years after birth; the hearing impairment may fluctuate and may be of the progressive type. They observed that the majority of cases showed profound hearing loss (51% in asymptomatic cases and 44.1% in symptomatic cases). Additionally, there was a consistent increase in the percentage of children with hearing impairment with increasing age, indicating the delay in onset that is characteristic of this disease. When investigators (Boppanna et al., 1992; Hanshaw, 1976; McCollister et al., 1996; Pass, Stagno, & Myers, 1980; Ramsay, Miller, & Peckham, 1991; Stagno et al., 1977) combined the incidence of CMV infection with the annual birth rate of 4.1 million, they projected that more than 6,000 children born each year experience sensorineural hearing impairment as a result of CMV infection.

Schildroth (1994) reported that the number of children with CMV as a cause of hearing impairment has increased every year since the question was first included in the Annual Survey of Hearing Impaired Children and Youth conducted by Gallaudet University during the 1985–1986 school year. Although the 1991–1992 survey data showed that CMV cases were reported in all four regions of the country, the South reported 45% of the cases. Schildroth (1994) specified that Texas, North Carolina, and California reported almost one-fourth of the CMV cases to the Annual Survey, and the large number of cases in Texas accounted for much of the survey's CMV overrepresentation in the South. This large number reported by Texas was attributed to this state's emphasis on early identification of hearing impairment. Schildroth (1994) reported that 88% of the CMV group had severe to profound hearing impairment, and 98% of the CMV children had bilateral hearing impairment. The ethnic breakdown from the survey showed that 72% of the CMV children were white, 16% were African American, 8% were of Hispanic origin, 2% were from the Asian and Pacific Islander group, and 2% were identified in the "other" category. This was consistent with USDOE's (2000) observation that in California, Texas, and New York, minority children with hearing impairments made up a large percentage of children in special education classrooms. Furthermore, according to the U.S. Bureau of the Census (2001), African American, Hispanic, and American Indian children were more likely to live in poverty and have less access to health care. At the same time, the Centers for Disease Control and Prevention (1999) has reported that CMV is more widespread in areas of lower socioeconomic conditions. Disparities in risk for the infection, access to health care, and higher incidence of poverty place minority children at a greater risk for hearing impairment.

CMV infection is not restricted to the United States. Ahlfors, Ivarsson, and Harris (1999) reported on a long-term study of maternal and congenital CMV infection in Sweden. They found 0.5% congenitally infected infants, 29.0% with transient neonatal symptoms, and 18.0% with neurologic symptoms by the age of 7 years. They observed that central nervous system disturbances in infants occurred after primary and secondary maternal infections. On the other hand, Balasubramaniam et al. (1994) reported that CMV was highly endemic in Malaysia. Congenital CMV was detected in 11.4% of infants, in comparison with congenital syphilis in 4.0%, congenital rubella in 3.7%, and congenital toxoplasma in 1.0% of infants. Furthermore, 10.4% of the infected cases had central nervous system deficits. They concluded that CMV appeared to be the most important cause of congenital infection in Malaysia.

A few studies have suggested that there may be a relationship between maternal seropositivity for CMV and the clinical features of CMV infection. The enzyme-linked immunosorbent assay is the most commonly available serologic test for measuring antibody to CMV. The result can be used to determine whether maternal antibody is present in an infant. Stagno et al. (1982) compared the prevalence of congenital CMV infection in a Chilean population with low-income and middle- and upper-class populations in Birmingham, Alabama. Although the incidence was higher in the highly seroimmune Chilean (1.7%) and low-income Birmingham (1.9%) groups than in the less immune middle- and upper-class group (0.6%), 407 autopsies did not attribute neonatal deaths to CMV in the Chilean group, whereas 1.0% of infant deaths in the Birmingham groups were attributed to CMV. The investigators concluded that in spite of an apparent lack of protection against intrauterine transmission, maternal immunity reduces the risk of severe fetal infection. Similarly, Morita et al. (1998) reported a low incidence (1.6 of 100,000 births) of symptomatic CMV disease in Japan. Major clinical manifestations were observed in 38–50% of the symptomatic neonates. Sequelae such as hearing impairment, mental retardation, and motor disability developed in 71% of survivors, whereas 35% of infected infants died or had severe disability. The investigators attributed the lower frequency of clinical findings at birth to the higher seroprevalence of pregnant women in Japan than in Europe and the United States.

Congenital Rubella Syndrome

The rubella virus causes German measles, a viral disease found throughout the world. Although it is typically harmless to the infected individual, it represents a serious threat to the fetus. When contracted during the first trimester, there is a 20% chance of spontaneous abortion; if the mother carries the baby to term, then there is an 80% chance that the baby will have congenital rubella syndrome (CRS), which includes damage to the auditory system, brain, and heart. In industrialized countries such as the United States, because of mandatory large-scale vaccination programs, CRS is almost nonexistent. According to the World Health Organization (2001), in countries in which rubella vaccination has not been introduced, low rubella activity alternates with epidemics at intervals of 4–8 years. During epidemics the incidence of CRS rises from approximately 0.1–0.2 to 1–4 per 1,000 live births. During an epidemic in the United States in the early 1960s, 12.5 million cases were reported, including 20,000 cases of CRS, which resulted in 11,000 deaf and 35,800 blind children and more than 1,800 children with mental retardation. The most recent data from the National Center for Health Statistics (2000) indicated a dramatic drop in the incidence of rubella cases over the past three decades, from 56,552 in 1970 to a substantially lower figure of 3,904 in 1980, which was reduced further to 1,125 in 1990 and a much lower number of 364 in 1998.

Schildroth (1994) reported on the *Annual Survey of Hearing Impaired Children and Youth* conducted in 1991–1992. The data indicated a higher incidence of CRS in white (53%) and Hispanic (23%) communities than among persons of African American (19%) and Asian and Pacific Islander (3%) heritage. The incidence was slightly higher in men (53%) than in women (47%), and the highest percentage of cases was reported in the South (37%). The devastating effect of CRS is reflected in the high percentage (63%) of children and youth with profound hearing impairment.

Bacterial Meningitis

Sensorineural hearing impairment is the most common complication of *bacterial meningitis*. The infection has been traced from the meninges to the labyrinth via the cochlear aqueduct. Kaplan et al. (1984) estimated the incidence to range between 2.4% and 29.0%. Typically, the hearing impairment is mild to profound and bilateral. In a few cases, some recovery of hearing has been reported. Guiscafre et al. (1984) reported that 22 of the 32 children with bacterial meningitis in Mexico recovered normal hearing. Vienny et al. (1984) examined 51 children with bacterial meningitis in Switzerland. They reported that 35 children had normal hearing, 11 children showed transient abnormalities in the auditory brain stem response, and 5 children had permanent sensorineural hearing loss. The investigators observed occurrence of deafness during the early phase of the disease with a crucial phase in the first 2 weeks, during which the hearing improved or worsened.

The Centers for Disease Control and Prevention (2000b) reported that there were 123,658 cases of meningococcal disease with 21,830 deaths in West African countries during 1996–1997. More typically, the incidence is 2% during epidemics and 0.5–5.0 per 100,000 cases worldwide for endemic disease. There is a mortality rate of 10–15%. Of patients who recover, 10% have permanent hearing impairment or other sequelae.

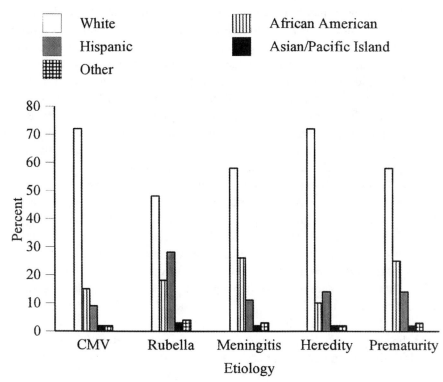

Figure 12-12 Percentage of children and youth reported to be deaf and hard of hearing by selected etiologic factors and ethnicity. (CMV = cytomegalovirus.) (Adapted from Schildroth, A. N., & Hotto, S. A. [1995]. Race and ethnic background in the Annual Survey of Deaf and Hard of Hearing Children and Youth. *American Annals of the Deaf, 140, 96–99.* Copyright 1995, Gallaudet Research Institute.)

Schildroth (1994), based on data gathered from the 1991–1992 *Annual Survey of Children and Youth,* reported that among those who developed deafness as a result of meningitis, 60% were white, 26% were African American, and 11% were Hispanic. Meningitis was the cause of deafness in more men (60%) than women (40%), and the South had the highest incidence (43%). The resulting hearing impairment was typically profound (59%). According to the National Center for Health Statistics (2000), the incidence of meningococcal disease in the United States rose until 1998; specifically, it went from 2,505 in 1970 to 2,840 in 1980, and, although the incidence was highest in 1996 (3,437), it had dropped to 2,725 in 1998.

Data from the 1991–1992 *Annual Survey of Children and Youth* provided by Schildroth (1994) are shown in Figure 12-12 to compare the incidence of CMV, rubella, meningitis, and heredity. In comparing the four etiologic factors for hearing impairment and deafness, it appears that the incidence of rubella was higher in the Hispanic community among the minorities. Limited access to health care and immunization and lack of health insurance may have contributed to the higher incidence of rubella in the Hispanic community. Data indicate that only 75% of Hispanic babies ages 19–35 months received their immunizations, and Hispanics are the most likely to be uninsured (Council of Economic Advisors for the President's Initiative on Race, 2000). Typically, children with family incomes below the poverty level have lower rates of coverage. Additionally, the data indicate that the incidence of meningitis was higher among the African Americans than in other ethnic groups. This is troubling, because meningitis is a preventable disease. Perhaps the high percentage of African American children living in poverty, lack of health insurance, and limited access to health care contributed to the higher incidence in this group. Heredity and CMV appeared to be the primary cause of hearing impairment among whites. The Asian and Pacific Islander group appeared to have a low incidence across the four etiologic factors. It should be noted that incomplete data may have played a major role in the outcome of this survey. Schildroth (1994) reported that the schools did not report a cause for 52% of the students; the question was left blank, ". . . or it was indicated that the cause of the hearing impairment could not be determined or was not available in the student's record."

Syphilis

Syphilis is a sexually transmitted disease. In the United States, 1 in 10,000 neonates is infected with congenital syphilis. Although the incidence of syphilis had declined through 1970, the incidence has gone up again in the past two decades. An infected mother may transmit the infection to the fetus in the early or late stage of the disease; however, the incidence is higher (80–90%) in the early stage. Typically, 25–30% of infected fetuses die in utero, and 25–30% die postnatally. Approximately 60% of infants with congenital syphilis are asymptomatic at birth, and 40% of neonates develop late symptomatic syphilis. Congenital syphilis may manifest as secondary syphilis in the first 2 years of life or as tertiary syphilis between 8 and 20 years. Central nervous system abnormalities and progressive sensorineural hearing impairment are common. The onset of the hearing loss is typically in early childhood. The hearing impairment is usually sudden, bilateral, and severe to profound. The National Center for Health Statistics (2000) reported a substantial decrease in the incidence of congenital syphilis, from 13,377 cases in 1950 to 4,416 cases in 1960; the incidence decreased to 1,953 cases in 1970 and 277 cases in 1980. Although the number of cases increased to

3,865 in 1990, the incidence dropped to 801 cases in 1998. In *Healthy People 2000—Statistical Notes,* the U.S. Department of Health and Human Services (2000) reported that the United States had attained the year 2000 target with a 110% reduction in the incidence of syphilis; 41 states achieved the target in 1997 and 1998, whereas 10 states in the South Atlantic, East South Central, and West South Central regions did not attain the target in 1997 or in 1998. Advanced syphilis can cause sensorineural hearing loss in adults; infection of the labyrinth or acoustic nerve may result in sudden, progressive, or bilateral sensorineural hearing impairment.

Human Immunodeficiency Virus

Human immunodeficiency virus (HIV) is a retrovirus that causes acquired immunodeficiency syndrome (AIDS). The first official report of what later came to be known as *AIDS* was published in 1981 by the Centers for Disease Control and Prevention in its *Morbidity and Mortality Weekly Report.* Initially, the proliferation of AIDS was attributed to promiscuous sexual activity among homosexuals, because the first victims were gay men. However, today it is commonly known that HIV is transmitted through sexual intercourse, use of infected needles, and use of infected blood products, as well as across the placental barrier and via infected breast milk. Some develop flu-like symptoms at the time of initial infection. Most infected persons may be asymptomatic for years after infection. When an HIV-positive person develops signs of generalized constitutional disease, opportunistic infections, neurologic disease, secondary cancers, or other systemic disease, the individual is said to have AIDS.

Matkin, Diefendorf, and Erenberg (1998) reported that pediatric AIDS patients are susceptible to infections and neurologic complications that can compromise auditory function. According to Bankaitis and Schountz (1998), ototoxicity and opportunistic infections associated with HIV and AIDS are potential causes of sensory hearing loss among HIV and AIDS cases. Ototoxicity has been associated with antiretroviral drugs, antifungal agents, antineoplastic drugs, immune modulators, and aminoglycoside antibiotics. The severity of the resulting hearing impairment varies from mild to profound depending on the patient's sensitivity, size of the dosage, and length of time the drug is taken. Besides ototoxicity, sudden-onset sensorineural hearing impairment associated with direct infection of the central nervous system, such as AIDS encephalopathy or subacute encephalitis, has also been reported. Opportunistic infections of the central nervous system such as cryptococcal meningitis and tuberculous meningitis also have been associated with deafness.

The World Health Organization (1999) reported that, since the beginning of the AIDS epidemic, 50 million individuals worldwide have been infected with HIV, of whom more than 33 million are still alive and more than 60 million have died. The Centers for Disease Control and Prevention (2000a) reported 745,103 adult and adolescent AIDS cases in the United States, of whom 620,189 were men, 124,911 were women, and an additional 8,804 were children under the age of 13. Additionally, it was reported that 438,795 persons with AIDS had died, including 433,296 adults and adolescents, 5,086 children under age 15, and 413 persons whose age at death was unknown. In a later report, the Centers for Disease Control and Prevention reported that in 1999, although there were more cumulative cases of AIDS among whites, more African Americans (37%) were reported with AIDS than any other racial or ethnic group. Specifically, 47% of the 46,400 AIDS cases reported in 1999 were among African Americans. Additionally, almost 63% of women reported with AIDS were African American, and 65% of all reported children with AIDS were African American. The 1999 rate of reported AIDS cases among African Americans was 66 per 100,000—more than twice the rate among Hispanics and eight times greater than the rate for whites. The state and metropolitan area reporting the highest number of cumulative AIDS cases were New York State and New York City. The data were interpreted to suggest that three interrelated issues played a role in the spread of this disease in communities of color: (1) continued health disparities between economic classes, (2) substance abuse, and (3) sharing needles and trading sex for drugs (Centers for Disease Control and Prevention, 2000a).

Ototoxicity

Certain drugs administered to combat life-threatening diseases have side effects, one of which is a profound hearing impairment or deafness (Gerber & Mencher, 1980). The damage is typically in the hair cells and epithelial structures of the cochlea. The severity of the damage varies; in general, the greater the dosage and longer the drug is administered, the greater the damage. Factors such as the age of the patient, nutritional status, genetic predisposition to nonsyndromic deafness renal failure, and use of more than one ototoxic drug affect the severity and morbidity (Pappas & Pappas, 1997). When ototoxic drugs are administered to pregnant women, they can cross the placental barrier and cause congenital deafness. When renal failure occurs, administration of diuretics (e.g., ethacrynic and furosemide) and a prolonged course of drug therapy may contribute to the development of fetal ototoxicity (Northern & Downs, 1991).

Deafness due to ototoxicity can occur at any age. The medical management of congenital ear disease in infants, as well as premature and low-birth-weight infants, may require the administration of ototoxic drugs such as loop diuretics and aminoglycosides. In children and adults, ototoxic drugs may be used in the treatment of endocarditis, pneumatic, tuberculosis, or meningitis. Ototoxicity has been associated with many of the drugs used to treat the HIV infection and its associated complications. Antifungal agents, antineoplastic drugs, and immune modulators have been associated with significant ototoxicity (Matkin et al., 1998). Drugs such as vinblastine, daunorubicin, and vincristine that are used in the treatment of life-threatening and opportunistic infections are known to cause deafness (Bankaitis & Schountz, 1998).

MacDorman and Atkinson (1999) reported that the incidence of babies with low birth weight (<1,500 g) is higher among African American mothers than white or other ethnic groups in the United States. Additionally, according to the Centers for Disease Control and Prevention (2000a), 63% of women and children reported with AIDS were African American. Similarly, the incidence of meningitis and tuberculosis was the highest among African Americans. Such health differences between racial and ethnic groups were noted by the Council of Economic Advisors for the President's Initiative on Race (2000), who reported that, "In general, blacks fare worse than any other group, and American Indians and Hispanics are often disadvantaged in health status relative to whites."

Cochlear Implants

A chapter on deafness would be incomplete without a discussion of cochlear implants. These neural prostheses have revolutionized the treatment of persons with deafness. Cochlear implantation improves most recipients' ability to communicate and is considered a safe and effective medical treatment for appropriately selected adults and children with bilateral severe to profound sensorineural hearing loss. The consensus panel convened by the National Institutes of Health in May of 1995 concluded that

> Cochlear implants are now firmly established as effective options in the habilitation and rehabilitation of individuals with profound hearing impairment. Worldwide, more than 12,000 people have attained some degree of sound perception with cochlear implants, and the multichannel cochlear implant has become a widely accepted prosthesis for adults and children (National Institutes of Health, 1995).

Cochlear implants are biomedical electronic devices that convert sound into electrical current that stimulates the auditory nerve, resulting in the sensation of sound. Early implants used a single electrode, which facilitated the perception of temporal cues but did not permit discrimination of auditory information across frequency ranges, and, therefore, typically did not assist in open-set speech perception. Regardless, implanted persons benefited from the temporal information, which was an excellent supplement to speech reading. More recently, substantial strides have been made in the available technology, especially in the improvement of speech processors. Newer implants use multiple electrode arrays that provide much more spectral information about the incoming auditory signal and facilitate better speech perception (Dorman et al., 1989). The latest advances in processing strategies and cochlear implant technology produce greater benefit in speech recognition. Consequently, cochlear implant users today can understand speech, and some can even converse on the telephone.

Early in the cochlear implant clinical trials, it became apparent that profoundly deaf children benefited from implantation (Osberger et al., 1991). Initially the U.S. Food and Drug Administration specified 2 years as the lower limit for implantation in children for several reasons. There was concern regarding the certainty with which one could diagnose a profound hearing loss in a very young child. Additionally, there was discomfort in implanting a young child without allowing adequate time with amplification to accurately determine its benefits. During the past decade, there have been rapid advances in technology in the areas of testing hearing in infants and in the cochlear implant device itself. Also, it is believed that 60% of skull growth is achieved by the age of 2 years, and the cochlea and the middle ear achieve adult size before term (Miyamoto, 1995). Furthermore, initial results of studies have indicated that electrical stimulation of the cochlea can partially prevent the degeneration of the spiral ganglion, and the developing brain can use the pattern of information provided by the cochlear implant, regardless of whether there have been previous audiologic experiences (Leake, 1995; Shannon, 1996). Recently, the U.S. Food and Drug Administration approved two devices—the Nucleus Mini 22-Channel (Cochlear, Ltd., Sydney, Australia) and the Clarion Multi-Strategy Cochlear Implant System (Advanced Bionics, Sylmar, California)—for children as young as 18 months of age.

Waltzman, Cohen, and Gromolin (1997) reported on the success of 38 children, 14 months to 5 years of age, who had congenital profound hearing loss and were implanted. Thirty-seven of these children were mainstreamed and used speech as their only means of communication, whereas one of the children attended a total education program in which he used speech and signed. All 38 children were functioning at age-appropriate levels.

Spencer et al. (1998) assessed linguistic performance in children with prelingual hearing impairments who used cochlear implants or hearing aids. The implanted children produced significantly more English-inflected morphemes

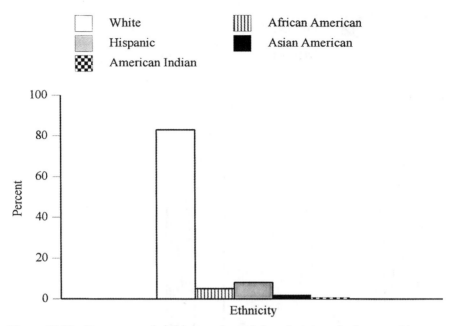

White   ▥ African American
Hispanic   ■ Asian American
American Indian

Figure 12-13 Percentage of children and youth by ethnicity who have cochlear implants. (Adapted from the Gallaudet Research Institute [1996]. *Who and where are our children with cochlear implants?* 1996 Annual Survey of Deaf and Hard of Hearing Children and Youth.)

than those with hearing aids, suggesting that cochlear implants facilitate children's ability to perceive and comprehend inflectional morphology of English. The cochlear implants offer acoustic access to sounds, and, as they begin to perceive the sounds, they incorporate them into their phonology and subsequently into their spoken morphology. Zwolan (1995) and Zwolan, Kileny, and Telian (1996) reported that prelingually deafened adults felt that they benefited from cochlear implants, although there was considerable variability among their patients in terms of their auditory skills and auditory training before implantation, postoperative speech recognition skills, as well as their perceived use and satisfaction with their devices.

The results of the 1996 *Survey of Deaf and Hard of Hearing Children and Youth* conducted by the Gallaudet Research Institute (1998) showed that, of the 48,000 survey cases, 1,344 (2.8%) children and youth between the ages of 2 and 19 years had cochlear implants, of whom 972 (72.32%) had onset of deafness before 2 years of age. The year of implantation was reported for 816 of these prelingually deaf children. Of the 816 children, 52% were female. The ethnic breakdown of these 816 children is provided in Figure 12-13. The majority (83%) of children who were implanted were white; children from all the minor-

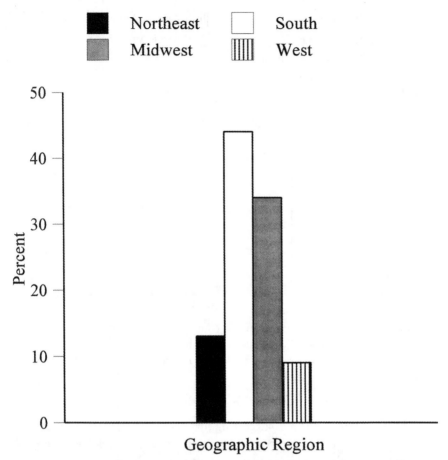

Figure 12-14 Geographic location of children and youth (percent) with cochlear implants. (Adapted from the Gallaudet Research Institute [1996]. *Who and where are our children with cochlear implants?* 1996 Annual Survey of Deaf and Hard of Hearing Children and Youth.)

ity groups combined made up less than 16% of the 816 with cochlear implants. Additionally, it was reported that the majority of the children who were implanted lived in the South and in the Midwest, as shown in Figure 12-14.

The data also showed that both parents of 99% of the 816 children were hearing, whereas 1% had one hearing and one deaf parent. Additionally, a majority of the children and youth appeared to be enrolled in regular schools, although it was possible that they could be placed in self-contained classrooms for the hard of hearing or could be mainstreamed into classrooms with children with normal hearing on a full-time or part-time basis. As shown in Figure 12-15, 63% of the children were in regular classrooms, and only 13%

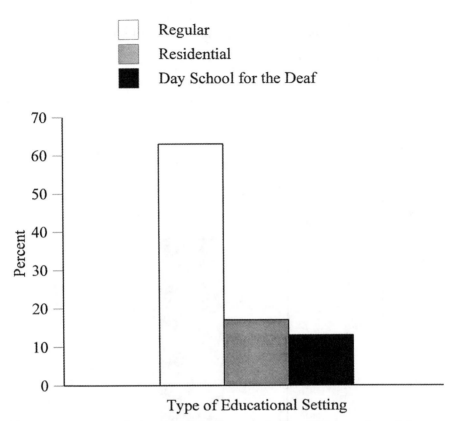

Figure 12-15 Type of educational setting attended by children and youth (percent) with cochlear implants. (Adapted from the Gallaudet Research Institute [1996]. *Who and where are our children with cochlear implants?* 1996 Annual Survey of Deaf and Hard of Hearing Children and Youth.)

attended day schools for the Deaf. Furthermore, it was reported that 58% of the children were instructed using sign language and speech, 36% used auditory or oral communication, and only 1% used only signs (Figure 12-16).

Financial Considerations

Financial counseling is an important aspect of any cochlear implant program, because cochlear implants are expensive. Koch (1996) estimated that the final cost of a cochlear implant reflects the regulatory expenses the manufacturers incur and the small size of the market. By the time the premarket approval is obtained, a manufacturer may invest $15–20 million to bring a new implant into commercial use. In 1996, Lowder esti-

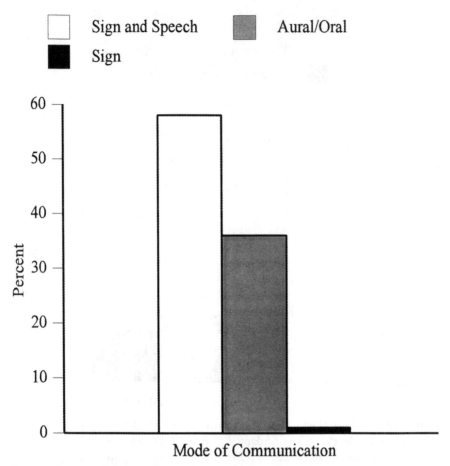

Figure 12-16   Mode of communication used by children and youth (percent) with cochlear implants. (Adapted from the Gallaudet Research Institute [1996]. *Who and where are our children with cochlear implants?* 1996 Annual Survey of Deaf and Hard of Hearing Children and Youth.)

mated that total up-front costs for unilateral cochlear implantation, including the hardware, surgery, hospital costs, surgeon's fees, and audiologic services for 1 year, were approximately $35,000. Although costs may vary from one geographic area to another, current estimates range from $40,000–50,000. Many medical insurance carriers cover cochlear implants, but often a copayment (10–20%) is required, which may pose a financial hardship for many families, especially those in the lower economic bracket. Some insurance carriers specifically exclude coverage for the implant, which poses an even greater burden on the individual.

Syrja (1999) observed that the universal focus on cost containment in the health care industry has made it more difficult for patients to obtain specialist referrals, adequate benefits for the surgical procedure, and postsurgical audiologic services. This problem is pervasive and affects families in all countries, including the United States and Canada. The lack of sufficient funding restricts patient access to cochlear implants and, in addition, does not allow adequate reimbursement for surgeons, audiologists, and hospitals. Weinick, Zurekas, and Cohen (2000) analyzed the data from the 1977 *National Medical Care Expenditure Survey*, the 1987 *National Medical Expenditure Survey*, and the 1996 *Medical Expenditure Panel Survey*, conducted in the United States to ascertain the differences, if any, in access to and use of health care services from 1977 to 1996. They found that over the 20 years, Hispanic Americans had become increasingly more likely to lack health care. Specifically, they reported that, after adjusting for health insurance, income, and other individual characteristics, in 1996, African Americans were 2.1 percentage points and Hispanic Americans were almost 10.0 percentage points more likely to lack a usual source of care than American whites. Between 1977 and 1996, this disparity for African Americans had declined by 3.2%, but the disparity for Hispanic Americans had increased by 6.5%. This change had occurred primarily between 1977 and 1987. There was no significant change in access to care for American whites between 1977 and 1996. The prohibitive cost may be one reason why the Gallaudet Research Institute (1998) reported that less than 16% of all deaf minorities combined were implanted (Figure 12-13). Among the minorities, the American Indians seemed to be the least likely to obtain cochlear implants. Federal agencies such as Veterans' Administration and the armed forces do provide coverage, as do Medicare and Medicaid; however, the level of reimbursement varies.

Cochlear Implants and the Deaf Community

The cochlear implant has been the source of much discord between the Deaf community and the hearing community, especially in the medical community. Although the position of the Deaf community has been tempered recently, the strong opposition to implanting children who are born deaf or who become deaf prelingually continues. The Deaf community's concerns regarding the cochlear implant focus around Deaf education, identity of the Deaf community, and the possibility of "cultural genocide"—the gradual and eventual elimination of Deaf culture and language (sign). The concern is that cochlear implants may eliminate the condition of deafness, which may lead to the eventual demise of Deaf culture and language (Lane, Hoffmeister, & Bahan, 1996). The Deaf community in the United States and the world subscribes to the "wellness model." The World Federation of the Deaf (2000), an international, nongovernmental, central organization of national associations of the Deaf, passed a resolution during the XIII World Congress, reaffirming the position that "Deaf people are a cultural and linguistic minority with a right to their native sign language as their mother tongue." Although acknowledging that technological and biological advances were creating changes for the Deaf community internationally, the Congress condemned genetic research ". . . which aims to eliminate Deaf people from the human race" (World Federation of the Deaf, 2000).

Tyler (1993) and Ramsey (2000) have reported that deaf persons share the conviction that deafness relates to biological and cultural characteristics, and not to a disorder or disability. Therefore, the Deaf community does not see the need for cochlear implants. Members of the Deaf community view themselves as biologically different from normal hearing persons—that is, as an ethnolinguistic group or a minority culture. Tyler (1993) reported that some deaf parents were happy when their child was born deaf, because the deafness was viewed as a family characteristic. Although a diversity of values and interests exist in the Deaf community, the feeling of family and social interactions are strong. An important characteristic of Deaf culture is sign language. The Deaf community has traditionally viewed the oral-language approach to language development and education as limiting. It is believed that the absence of visual language opportunity results in developmental delays, whereas a general education using sign language promotes cognition. Many adults in the Deaf community have attended residential schools, which have preserved the feeling of community. The Deaf community believes that when a deaf child is mainstreamed, the child does not have the advantage of deaf mentors, and this affects the child's self-image.

According to Ramsey (2000), the Deaf community views genetic research negatively, because it may lead to the elimination of certain types of deafness. Concurrently, the Deaf community considers cochlear implant surgery to be invasive and experimental and, therefore, too risky to be performed on children. A concern often expressed is the proximity of the device to the nervous system and its unknown long-term effects on the health of the child. Additionally, the extensive habilitation and rehabilitation process after surgery still leaves the individual with hearing loss. Also, there is concern about the emotional impact on the child who may grow to adolescence and adulthood without learning to sign, only to find that he or she is unable to communicate with persons who are deaf and is unable to fully participate in the hearing world and, therefore, feels isolated from both cultures. The Deaf community argues that hearing parents of a deaf child cannot know the experiences of being deaf in a hearing world and is concerned about hearing parents making surrogate decisions about implantation without fully understanding the impact on the deaf child.

In 1991, the position of the National Association of the Deaf (NAD) in the United States was in strong opposition to the cochlear implant and was critical of the U.S. Food and Drug Administration's approval of the implant and the process, which had excluded deaf persons. The NAD expressed concern about the short-term and long-term medical, social, and psychological risks of implanting children. Although the NAD's current position (2000) is more restrained, it emphasizes that before a surrogate decision is made for a deaf child, parents should understand the various options available, including all factors that might impact development. The NAD position emphasizes that the cochlear implant does not eliminate deafness; cautions that the implant may destroy residual hearing, preventing the individual from using an amplification device; and encourages parents of prelingually deaf children to research other options before making a decision. Regardless of the selected option, the NAD reminds parents to focus on the whole child, early language development, literacy, and cognitive development.

In response to the observed opposition to implanting children, the Cochlear Implant Club International developed its own position paper in 1998, which supports and endorses the rights of individuals who are deaf and parents of deaf children to choose or not to choose the cochlear implant. It opposes efforts that attempt to deny, limit, or refuse to recognize the rights of parents to choose the cochlear implant as an option for their children. The position statement includes mention of the 20,000 persons who have been implanted, of whom 8,000 are children who have reportedly shown significant improvement in their ability to hear with implants in comparison with their ability to hear with hearing aids before implantation. This group reported that 1 of 10 profoundly deaf children in the United States and Canada enjoyed the benefits of cochlear implants. The Cochlear Implant Club International has projected that within the decade one of three deaf children will be implanted. Furthermore, this organization has emphatically endorsed allowing individuals to make their own choices without intrusion from others.

A demographic reality is that only a small percentage (less than 10%) of deaf children are born to deaf parents. The majority of deaf children are born to hearing parents who seek information about educational placement, cochlear implants, or other approaches to intervention from hearing professionals. The Deaf community believes strongly that these parents should also be introduced to someone from the Deaf culture so that they can make a truly informed surrogate decision; only someone from the Deaf culture can provide hearing parents true information regarding experiences of being deaf. Holcomb (1999) indicated that the majority of deaf children are now educated in nonresidential settings (i.e., public schools in which they do not have adult deaf role models). Consequently, the process of developing a healthy self-identity as a deaf person takes a very long time. Holcomb (1999) advocates the inclusion of the Deaf community in cochlear implant programs, as is done in the Colorado early intervention program.

Educational Aspects

The education of deaf children in the United States began in the 1800s with the establishment of special schools for deaf children in New England. Deafness being a low incidence condition, the earliest schools were residential and served children from relatively wide geographic areas. The twentieth century brought about the urbanization and suburbanization of the United States, which gradually led to the spread of day schools. In the 1960s and 1970s, the Deaf joined the general movement of social unrest to voice their needs and shape their destiny. A major outcome of this rights effort was an increase in the use of manual communication in educational settings.

The passage of the Education for All Handicapped Children Act (PL 94-142) in 1975 paved the way for mainstreaming deaf children into regular classrooms. Before PL 94-142, millions of children with disabilities received inadequate or inappropriate special education services from public schools, whereas approximately 1 million children were denied a public education, because many states had laws that specifically excluded deaf children from the schools (USDOE, 1995). PL 94-142 formally recognized the right of all children with disabilities to a public education and the necessity to make educational placements on the basis of the needs of the individual child. In 1986, the law was amended by PL 99-457 to include preschoolers (3–5 years) and to assist states in developing programs for infants and toddlers. The Education of the Handicapped Act Amendment of 1990 (PL 101-476) renamed the statute the *IDEA*, and references to "handicapped children" were amended to read "children with disabilities." This change was brought about by the activism of persons with disabilities, their advocates, and their supporters. Subsequently, the IDEA Amendments of 1997 placed greater emphasis on encouraging states to provide services to infants and toddlers in their "natural environments." Each law has helped to make education available to deaf children; however, even today the educational needs of *all* deaf children are unmet. Until a learning environment is created that addresses the issues of ethnic heritage, values, and attitudes, the educational needs of all deaf children will not be met.

Historically, educational services provided to deaf persons from minority groups have been inferior to those provided to deaf persons from the majority population (Moores, 1978). An erroneous assumption that has been perpetuated in society until, approximately, the last decade was that what was known about educating deaf children in the majority culture was applicable to all deaf children without consideration for the unique cultural traits and characteristics of children from other cultures. The fallacy of this assumption has been evidenced in the frequent reports of underachievement, limited literacy, and underemployment in minorities who are deaf (Allen, 1986; Bowe, 1971).

Deaf students continue to be educated primarily in special education classes. Recent data from the 1993–1994 *Annual Survey of Children and Youth* (Schildroth & Hotto, 1995) showed that of four special educational settings, white students were primarily educated in residential schools (65%) and in local, integrated (62%) settings. Nonwhites primarily attended day schools (57%) and local, nonintegrated (50%) programs (self-contained classrooms). Among the nonwhites, more Hispanic children tended to attend day school (26%) and local, nonintegrated programs (20%), whereas more African Americans attended day schools (23%), local, nonintegrated programs (21%), and residential schools (20%). Children from Asian and Pacific communities primarily attended day schools (4%), local, nonintegrated programs (5%), and local, integrated programs (4%) (Schildroth & Hotto, 1995).

The exit rates reported on the 1993–1994 *Annual Survey of Deaf and Hard of Hearing Children and Youth* as reported by Schildroth and Hotto (1995) showed that more minorities graduated with certificates (55%) than white students (45%). There was a slightly higher percentage of Hispanic youth (25%) graduating with a certificate than African Americans (24%) and Asian and Pacific (4%) youth. Among those who graduated with a diploma, 65% were white and 35% were nonwhite, of whom 14% were African Americans, 13% were Hispanic, and 5% were Asian and Pacific Islander youth. The overall dropout rate of students aged 14 years and over reported by Schildroth and Hotto (1995) was 11–12%. Sixty percent were white and 40% were nonwhite. Hispanic (20%) students dropped out at a higher rate than African American (17%) or Asian and Pacific Islander (2%) youth.

Allen (1994) discussed data collected on deaf and hard of hearing students exiting high school and starting postsecondary education. Seventeen-year-old students leaving high schools were primarily white, 81% of whom had only one disability. Fifty percent of these students had attended public schools, whereas the remaining 50% had attended special schools. On the other hand, students exiting at the age of 20–21 years were primarily minorities, of whom 62% had one or more additional disabilities. Forty-six percent of these students had attended special schools. Of the pooled 17- to 21-year-old exiting students, only 40% demonstrated reading levels at a fourth grade equivalent or above; 52% of these students were white, 22% were African American, and 19% were Hispanic. Allen (1994) cautioned that at higher levels of achievement (i.e., at the eighth grade level of achievement), the pool of students became disproportionately white; specifically, 88% were white, 3% were African American, and 7% were Hispanic. As the minority population increases, there will be more minority deaf youth exiting schools to apply for admission to institutions of higher education where admission standards are being made more stringent. However, without adequate literacy skills, few will be admitted, and fewer still will graduate. These youth will be unable to compete for jobs and will likely settle for low-paying jobs or be unemployed and live in poverty. In fact, according to the U.S. Bureau of the Census (McNeil, 2001), the presence of a disability is associated with lower levels of income and an increased probability of living in poverty. Additionally, data on earnings collected in 1987 and 1991 by Schildroth and Hotto (1995) showed that minority deaf youth were likely to earn a lower hourly wage and work fewer hours a week and were more likely to be unemployed than white deaf youth.

Yoshinaga-Itano (2000) reported that children identified as deaf or hard of hearing before 6 months of age who receive immediate and appropriate intervention maintain age-appropriate language skills from 12 months through 3 years, regardless of the degree of hearing loss, ethnicity, socioeconomic status and mode of communication. Perhaps the chasm between the hearing-impaired person's potential and achievement level may be bridged by targeting cognitive processes so that higher-level mental processes and literacy can be enhanced (Martin, 1993). Strassman (1997) reviewed research on the link between metacognition and reading in children who are deaf. He made three observations: (1) instructional practices that emphasize school-related activities and skills, such as memorizing vocabulary, may hinder metacognitive activities in the deaf student; (2) providing students with reading material that is at a low level because it matches their assessed reading levels may, in fact, hinder metacognition by not providing the deaf student the opportunity to develop strategies to think; and (3) deaf students may benefit from instruction in metacognitive strategies.

After investigating the effectiveness of sign language in promoting spoken language development and literacy in school-aged deaf children of deaf and normal hearing parents, it has been reported that sign-supported speech facilitates child-parent and child-teacher communication but does not enhance spoken or written language abilities. Strong and Prinz (1997) reported that children educated using ASL as the primary language of communication and instruction attained higher levels of proficiency in spoken English and literacy. Findings such as these have led several countries to adopt bilingual-bicultural programs in which deaf children of hearing parents and deaf children of deaf parents are taught in the national sign language as the primary mode of communication and instruction. English or other spoken languages and their written forms are taught as second languages. Recently, based on their own study Pizzuto et al. (2000) advocated (1) the use of appropriate nonverbal tasks to assess children's cognitive skills; (2) the use of speech and sign language when evaluating language skills; and (3) consideration of the child's family, language, and educational environments when assessing the child's development.

Some have suggested that increasing the number of racially and ethnically diverse professionals and administrators will provide positive role models for deaf children and youth and encourage them to strive and achieve. It is hoped that increasing access to positive role models will help to eliminate institutional barriers for minorities who are deaf. Another solution that has been suggested is increasing state and federal funding to infuse multiculturalism and educate school administrators, teachers, and staff about multicultural issues (Akamatsu, 1993; Anderson & Grace, 1991; Cheng, 1993; Gerner de Garcia, 1993).

Allen (1986) reported that the reading comprehension scores for 12-year-old Hispanic deaf children were lower than for 8-year-old deaf white children. Investigators have attributed underachievement and poor literacy, particularly in deaf Hispanic children and other immigrant families, to the home-school mismatch. The cultural and behavioral norms of the family and school may be in conflict. For instance, in Mexican and many Asian cultures, the child is taught to be respectful to teachers and elders, be well behaved, and to work hard; these may not be typical expectations in the majority population. Additionally, the child may be subject to different expectations from deaf peers. Unless the teacher is from the same racial and cultural group, the child has to adjust between three cultures. The child may speak Spanish with the family members, English and ASL in school. Unless the family members speak English fluently or sign, or both, the child will not get much help in reading English and with homework. The problem is compounded for immigrant deaf children who may have learned the sign languages of their native countries before coming to the United States.

The African American Deaf

African American deaf children, like other minority deaf children, are faced with the problems encountered by membership in two minority cultures—Deaf and African American. This impacts their educational, personal, and social development. Although conditions have improved, the

African American Deaf continue to face discrimination in every aspect of life. They are placed in educational settings that may not promote growth and that typically ignore their culture and history. Frequently, they are maneuvered into nonacademic or vocational tracts that limit the acquisition of literacy and academic skills. Without adult African American role models to identify with and guide them to strive harder to achieve more, these students may not succeed in academics. Low academic achievement results in a high dropout rate, or large numbers leave school with certificates rather than diplomas. As a result, few go to college, and they end up with low-paying jobs or unemployment—which, in turn, results in a life of poverty. To break this cycle, a conscious effort needs to be made to upgrade the education they receive, improve access to services, establish appropriate intervention formats, and provide opportunities for postsecondary education and, subsequently, better jobs.

The Black community in the United States includes persons who are African Americans and persons from the Caribbean, Europe, Africa, and other countries. It is important to appreciate this diversity and learn about an individual's own background, cultural values, and attitudes, because these factors determine the way the deaf individual responds in society. Many educators do not understand this diversity and do not make the effort to learn about the cultural differences. For children to identify with what they are learning, the values, culture, and history of the African American community should be incorporated into their curriculum.

The deaf African American child must face and learn to deal with the prejudice associated with his or her ethnicity and with deafness. As Nuru-Holmes and Battle (1998) have eloquently observed, "The challenge of the Deaf child is to come to terms with culture of the home and culture of the school and peers and to effectively negotiate both." The deaf African American child must adapt to life in a society that is dominated by people who hear normally and possibly have attitudes, values, languages, and cultures that may be different from those of his or her family. This child must also adapt to the cultures and values of his or her peers in the school setting and use ASL. Also, in the school, this child must learn to deal with the cultures, expectations, and values of his or her teachers and administrators who may not be deaf, may not be African American, and may not understand the child's culture. At home, the child must embrace the values, attitudes, beliefs, and culture of his or her family, who typically have normal hearing and may not understand the deaf child's experiences. The deaf African American child must learn the rules of each culture, abide by them, and also develop his or her own values and self-image.

An important task for the deaf African American child is to develop a sense of self as a person who is both African American and deaf. Aramburo (1989) reported that there were differences in the socialization experiences of those who identified themselves as Deaf first, compared to those who identified themselves as African American first. The former typically attended white residential schools, had deaf parents, and were active in the Deaf community. Those who identified themselves as African American first were more familiar with the African American culture, which they had acquired from their family rather than school. They were familiar with and identified with issues related to racial discrimination and were not as active in the Deaf community. Developing a sense of the self is important, yet there is little research on how children who belong to several minority groups come to terms with this complicated issue.

Speech-language pathologists and audiologists who work with deaf African American children must understand the child's individual background, as well as his or her culture. Many children come from single-parent homes headed by the mother who probably has to work and earns just enough to support the family. African American children have a strong bond with their mothers, who tend to be firm and physical in disciplining their children. They also come from homes where self-sufficiency and toughness are promoted. Fischgrund et al. (1987) believe that this may result in cultural dissonance if teachers behave differently from the way the children expect persons of authority to behave, especially when the children display behaviors that they know are not valued in the classroom. In these situations the children may "run all over" the teachers. The need for role models the children can identify with is an issue that is frequently discussed. However, with the paucity of minority professionals, this void cannot be filled until more minority persons are recruited and trained.

Anderson and Grace (1991) observed that there were consequences to deaf African American children lacking exposure to positive adult role models from their own culture during the school years. In the absence of adult African American role models, the children may not be provided with opportunities for upward educational and occupational mobility. Without the influence of adult African American role models, there may be a failure to influence, motivate, and inspire deaf children to aspire to learn, go to college, and seek employment in a variety of professions. Another consequence may be that the absence of an adult role model may reinforce negative messages regarding their own culture and their own capabilities. Also, the potential to influence the children to understand and develop the values and attitudes of their culture may be reduced.

It is recognized that mainstreaming a deaf child with normal hearing children may have a positive or negative impact depending on the individual child. However, other environmental factors also determine the child's success in the integrated classroom. Negative teacher attitude, inhibited teacher-student interaction, limited expectations, inadequate support services, and biased educational materials and tests may impair the child's ability to perform to his or her potential. Additionally, if the deaf African American child is placed with a teacher who is unprepared, does not use ASL, does not understand deafness, and may have inappropriate expectations, the child may be doomed for failure. Cohen et al. (1990) reported that very few special programs conduct staff training activities specifically addressing the needs of minority children. Important as it is to address the needs imposed by deafness, it is equally important to attend to cultural backgrounds, home, and community.

Low socioeconomic status is associated with poor health and lack of access to health care and other services, as well as to limited educational and occupational opportunities. Many African American families live below the poverty line, which inhibits the deaf African American children's chances to lead healthy, productive, and prosperous lives.

Until the 1970s, African American and white deaf children in the South were educated in segregated schools. Although African American children learned ASL, they also developed what is called *African ASL*, which is a variation of ASL (Maxwell & Smith-Todd, 1986). The linguistic features of this sign language were perceived by some as poorly developed communication skills that served as a communication barrier and were rejected at Deaf social and cultural activities (Anderson & Bowe, 1972). Persons who use African ASL use linguistic switching—which is similar to code switching used by speakers of African American English—to communicate in formal situations (Woodward, 1982). Additionally, ASL users may demonstrate regional differences that have more colorful nonverbal expressions and body language or may be alternate versions of standard signs (Hairston & Smith, 1983).

Regrettably, racism exists in the Deaf culture. African Americans and whites in the adult Deaf community are relatively unintegrated. There is little social interaction between the two groups, although they communicate and joke with each other when the two groups attend the same social functions (Hairston & Smith, 1983).

The Asian Deaf

In 1997, 27% (6.8 million) of the United States' foreign-born population was from Asia (U.S. Bureau of the Census, 2000b). Although the Asian-born population consists of immigrants from over 40 countries, the five largest contributors in 1997 were China, India, Korea, the Philippines, and Vietnam. In view of this rapid growth of Asian-born residents, the probability is high that most speech-language pathologists and audiologists will provide services to Asian Americans. Although there are some similarities in the beliefs and values of persons of Asian origin, there are vast differences in the language, culture, and lifestyle among Asians. Therefore, it is imperative for the clinicians who work with these individuals to obtain information regarding the language(s) spoken by each family, as well as the culture, religion, values, and beliefs. Without such basic information, the clinician may not be successful in developing a positive working relationship with the individual and the family. As Cheng (2000) recommended, it is important for clinicians to have some basic information regarding the languages of the children they serve so that they understand why the children abide by or violate linguistic rules.

Based on data from the 1993–1994 *Annual Survey of Deaf and Hard of Hearing Children and Youth*, Schildroth and Hotto (1995) estimated that Asian and Pacific youth and children made up 4% of the deaf and hard of hearing population in the United States. This was an increase of 500%, compared with data from the 1973–1974 survey. One-third of these Asian and Pacific children were reported from California; 10% were from Minnesota.

In many cultures such as the Vietnamese, Chinese, Indian, and others, there is a highly disciplined extended-family system that is vertically organized and hierarchal. Respect for elders, obedience, family cohesion, harmony, and avoidance of shame are important. Parental self-sacrifice is common to ensure educational pursuits and success of children. Control, supervision, and parental emphasis on high achievement results in motivated students with high grade-point averages who seek a college education. In many Asian cultures, the group or family unit has precedence over the individual.

Attitudes toward disabilities vary and are often influenced by religious beliefs. Although some may believe that deafness is a punishment for misdeeds in the past, others may view it as a gift from God, and still others may view it as a curse. The mother of a child born with a disability may view it as a disgrace to the family and may experience guilt and shame (Wilson, 1996). Therefore, it is important to ascertain the family's views on deafness. Views on child rearing vary among the cultures and may be very different from those of the American dominant culture. Toilet training, feeding, and methods of discipline may vary widely among the cultures. If the professional does not speak the language of the family and the parents do not speak English, then interpreters trained to assist with assessment and counseling should be used. Some have suggested that professionals should team up with paraprofessionals who speak the family's language (Hamayan & Damico, 1991).

Akamastu & Cole (2000) have correctly challenged the view that ASL should be the first and natural language for all deaf children in the United States. Immigrant deaf families may use other signed languages in their homes and may know their native spoken or written language. Therefore, ASL would be a second or third language for these children. Often, immigrant parents must learn English and have the added challenge of learning ASL. Additionally, if the parents are deaf and use a sign language from the native country, then the child must use that sign language at home and ASL in school. Also, there are families with deaf members who communicate via rudimentary gestures and speech (in their native language). Speech-language pathologists and audiologists must remember that because of parents' own limited education or limited English competency or ability to sign, they may be unable to help their children. Some parents may find it difficult to participate in sign language classes because they may be taught in English or because of conflicts with work schedules (Akamatsu & Cole, 2000).

For some deaf children, education may not have been available in their native country; therefore, these children may lack the language and skills that are required in U.S. schools. The family may not have basic information regarding deafness, language communication, or the special education opportunities available to their children in the United States. They may also be unaware of their responsibilities and role as partners in their child's education (Akamatsu & Cole, 2000).

In working with Asian Americans, Akamatsu (1993) advises the clinician to remember that asking direct questions may be interpreted as prying; in such situations, parents may tell the clinician what they believe the clinician wants to hear rather than the truth. Therefore, use of indirect approaches to gather information is better, because it allows parents the choice of revealing information they feel comfortable sharing with the clinician. Reaching consensus is more productive than confrontation, because Asian parents will try not to offend the clinician if they disagree; rather than arguing, they may smile, bow their head or nod, and then do exactly what they intended to do rather than what the clinician wanted them to do.

While providing services, the clinician must remember that Asian Americans may not look directly into the clinician's eyes, which the clinician may misinterpret as an avoidance behavior. Asian Americans avoid eye contact with professionals and elders as a mark of respect and may interpret the clinician's direct eye gaze as a sign of hostility. Additionally, they value their privacy and are disinclined to discuss emotional or personal matters with individuals outside the family unit. Finally, the clinician may wish to seek the help of the appropriate ethnic organization to facilitate communication and service delivery.

The Hispanic Deaf

The number of Hispanic Deaf in the United States has more than doubled during the last two decades. Today, the Hispanic community in the United States includes persons of Mexican descent, as well as persons from Puerto Rico, Central America, Cuba, South America, and the Dominican Republic. The largest Hispanic populations are found on the coasts and southern border of the United States. Schildroth and Hotto (1995) reported that responses to the 1993–1994 *Annual Survey for Deaf and Hard of Hearing Children and Youth* showed that the states of California, Texas, and New York together made up two-thirds of all Hispanic deaf children and youth that were reported. The number of Hispanic children in these three states increased from 3,000 in 1973–1974 to 7,500 in 1993–1994. They represented 16% of deaf children and youth reported on the 1993–1994 survey.

Hispanic students have demonstrated little success in general education, as well as deaf education (Gerner de Garcia, 2000). The high school dropout rate for Hispanics continues to be high. Schildroth and Hotto (1995) reported that 20% of Hispanics dropped out of school, 25% graduated with a certificate, and 13% graduated with a diploma. This dropout rate was higher than the dropout rate for all deaf persons (11–12%) and higher than the 15% dropout rate reported in the federal statistics for all school-aged children in 1991–1992.

Hispanic deaf students in the United States, like other immigrants, are required to become trilingual and tricultural (MacNeil, 1990). The child must use Spanish at home and English and ASL at school and outside in the hearing community. This may create ambivalence and identity crises in the deaf child. Other issues such as parental education and socioeconomic level have also been reported to affect the deaf child's adjustment and success. Cohen (1993) reported that in New York City only 42% of Hispanic deaf children had parents with at least a high school diploma, and the median income of Hispanic families was lower than that of the majority population. Furthermore, 60% of Hispanic families had children under the age of 18, and 32% of these households were headed by women.

At a time when the number of Hispanic deaf children is increasing, most educators are not well prepared to meet their needs. It has been suggested that more Hispanic professionals should be hired to provide role models for Hispanic students. However, Andrews and Jordan (1993) reported that only 2% of teachers and 4% of administrators were Hispanic.

Hispanic deaf children are overrepresented in local schools with self-contained classes for the deaf, and they are underrepresented in local schools with integrated classes and in special schools. Schildroth and Hotto (1995) reported that 26% of Hispanic deaf students attended day schools and an additional 20% attended local, nonintegrated programs. Enrollment in self-contained classes has an adverse effect, because it does not allow the child the opportunity to be mainstreamed into regular classes.

Hispanic students have been reported to score lower on reading comprehension and mathematics than whites and are more likely to be placed in low-skill vocational classes. When students are placed in vocational classes rather than being provided academic instruction, the students are not likely to reach their full potential and their literacy skills are not developed. Additionally, if they leave school with certificates rather than diplomas, they are unable to enroll in postsecondary programs.

Speech-language pathologists and audiologists working with Hispanic families should be sensitive to and understand the beliefs and values of the Hispanic communities, which may differ substantially from the mainstream American culture (see Chapter 6 for information on Latino culture). The roles of the father (main authority) and mother (conducts the daily business of family) are divided. Although the mother makes the appointments and meets with professionals, a decision will require the father's approval. Female children are protected and disciplined more than male children. Furthermore, children are viewed as dependent on parents beyond the age considered appropriate by mainstream Americans. Folk beliefs regarding the causes and treatments are integral to the culture. Fatalism and an overprotective attitude toward a deaf child are likely. Parents may need guidance in assuming their role of "partner" under IDEA. They may also need guidance in understanding their role in improving their children's opportunities through representation and advocacy. Additionally, Hispanics see a person as a whole rather than qualities associated with one's professional role. Therefore, a professionals' neutral or impersonal attitude may be interpreted as lack of feeling. Hearing families with a deaf infant need early intervention. However, the family may not have transportation or child care, or both and, therefore, may be unable to attend (Gerner de Garcia, 2000).

It is necessary to determine the dominant language and language proficiency of deaf children from Spanish-speaking families. There are no standardized instruments; therefore, unless the clinician is trilingual, the help of a culturally sensitive trilingual professional is essential. Additionally, a child from an immigrant family may have acquired the Spanish language and literacy in the native country or may use gestures and homemade signs or may use a sign language used in the native land. Although difficult, it is useful to know what the child knows in each language (Gerner de Garcia, 2000).

Cheng (1987) and Christensen (1993) support the use of naturalistic assessment, which includes observation by professionals in a variety of environments the child uses, such as the classroom, school, home, and the community. This allows the evaluators to observe and document how the child uses communication in various situations and contexts and how the child uses language to learn, grow, and experience. This type of evaluation is particularly useful with culturally diverse and immigrant children who may not have experienced formal evaluations. It is also particularly useful when the immigrant child has had limited or no formal education. Most standardized tests present decontextualized or context-reduced information; therefore, this task is difficult for those culturally different children who use contextualized information to access the knowledge that they have. Additionally, evaluators who do not share the culture of the child may not be able to adequately interpret the child's performance. Finally, if the evaluator is not trilingual or bicultural, or both, or not assisted by someone who is, the results are likely to be biased (Erickson, Anderson, & Fischgrund, 1983).

Immigrant children who have not been exposed to dialects other than those used in their homes may not know the terminology used in the standardized tests. Some instruments available in English have been translated into Spanish. However, the quality of the translation varies and norms may not be available for the Spanish versions or, if available, may not apply to children who are deaf. Unless the clinician is fluent in Spanish and ASL, a trilingual person must be a part of the assessment team.

Educational outcomes for deaf Hispanic students will not improve until educators and other professionals recognize the unique needs of this population. Professionals must make the effort to learn more about the children they serve, their cultural backgrounds, and recognize diversity in the Hispanic population.

References

Ahlfors, K., Ivarsson S. A., & Harris, S. (1999). Report on a long-term study of material and congenital cytomegalovirus infection in Sweden. Review of prospective studies available in the literature. *Scandinavian Journal of Infectious Diseases, 31*(5), 443–457.

Akamatsu, C. W. (1993). Teaching deaf Asian and Pacific Island American children. In K. M. Christensen & G. L. Delgado (Eds.). *Multicultural issues in deafness* (pp. 127–142). White Plains, NY: Longman.

Akamatsu, C., & Cole, E. (2000). Immigrant and refugee children who are deaf: Crisis equals danger plus opportunity. In K. Christensen (Ed.). *Deaf plus—a multicultural perspective* (pp. 93–120). San Diego: Dawn Sign Press.

Allen, T. (1986). Patterns of academic achievement among hearing impaired students: 1974–1983. In A. Schildroth & M. Karchmer (Eds.). *Deaf children in America* (pp. 161–206). San Diego: College-Hill Press.

Allen, T. (1994). *Who are the deaf and hard-of-hearing students leaving high school and entering post secondary education?* [On-line]. Washington,

DC: Gallaudet University. Available: http://gri.gallaudet.edu/AnnualSurvey/whodeaf.html.

Al-Shihabi, B. A. (1994). Childhood sensorineural hearing loss in consanguineous marriages. *Journal of Audiological Medicine 3*, 151–159.

Anderson, G., & Bowe, F. (1972). Racism within the deaf community. *American Annals of the Deaf, 111*, 617–619.

Anderson, G., & Grace, C. (1991). Black deaf adolescents: A diverse and underserved population. *Volta Review, 93*, 73–86.

Andrews, J., & Jordan, D. (1993). Minority and minority-deaf professionals. *American Annals of the Deaf, 138*, 388–396.

Aramburo, A. (1989). Sociolinguistic aspects of the black deaf community. In C. Lucas (Ed.). *The sociolinguistics of the deaf community* (pp. 103–119). San Diego: Academic Press.

Balasubramaniam, V., Sinniah, M., Tan, D. S., et al. (1994). The role of cytomegalovirus (CMV) infection in congenital disease in Malaysia. *Medical Journal of Malaysia, 49*(2), 113–116.

Bankaitis, A., & Schountz, T. (1998). HIV-related ototoxicity. *Seminars in Hearing, 19*, 155–163.

Boppana, S., Pass, R., Britt, W., et al. (1992). Symptomatic congenital cytomegalovirus infection: Neonatal morbidity and mortality. *Pediatric Infectious Disease Journal, 11*, 93–99.

Bowe, F. (1971). Non-white deaf persons: Educational, psychological and occupational considerations. *American Annals of the Deaf, 116*, 357–361.

Centers for Disease Control and Prevention. (1981). Kaposi's sarcoma and pneumocystis pneumonia among homosexual men—New York City and California. *Morbidity and Mortality Weekly Report, 30*, 305–308.

Centers for Disease Control and Prevention. (1999). *Cytomegalovirus (CMV) infection.* Atlanta: Author.

Centers for Disease Control and Prevention. (2000a). *HIV/AIDS among African Americans.* Atlanta: Author.

Centers for Disease Control and Prevention. (2000b). *Meningococcal disease.* Atlanta: Author.

Cheng, L. (1987). Assessing Asian language performance: Guidelines for evaluating limited English proficient students. Rockville, MD: Aspen.

Cheng, L. (1993). Deafness: An Asian/Pacific Island perspective. In K. M. Christiansen & G. L. Delgado (Eds.), *Multicultural issues in deafness* (pp. 113–126). White Plains, NY: Longman.

Cheng, L. (2000). An Asian/Pacific perspective. In K. Christensen (Ed.). *Deaf plus—a multicultural perspective* (pp. 58–92). San Diego: Dawn Sign Press.

Christensen, K. (1993). Looking forward to a multicultural commitment. In K. M. Christensen & G. L. Delgado (Eds.), *Multicultural issues in deafness* (pp. 179–183). White Plains, NY: Longman.

Cochlear Implant Club International, Inc. (1998). CICI position statement— cochlear implants: The rights of children and parents acting on their behalf. *CICI CONTACT, 1st Quarter,* 40–41.

Cohen, O. (1993). Multicultural education and the deaf community: A conversation about survival. *Deaf American Monograph, 43,* 23–26.

Cohen, O., Fischgrund, J., & Redding, R. (1990). Deaf children from ethnic, linguistic and racial minority backgrounds: An overview. *American Annals of the Deaf, 135,* 67–73.

Collins, J. (1997). *Prevalence of selected chronic conditions: United States 1990–1992.* Hyattsville, MD: National Center for Health Statistics. *Vital Health Statistics, 10*(194), 1–89.

Council of Economic Advisors for the President's Initiative on Race. (1999). *Changing America—indicators of social and economic well-being by race and Hispanic origin.* Washington, DC: U.S. Government Printing Office.

Council of Economic Advisors for the President's Initiative on Race. (2000). *Changing America* [On-line]. Available: http://w3.access.gpo.gov/eop/ca/index.html.

Dahle, A. J., Fowler, K. B., Wright, J. D., et al. (2000). Longitudinal investigation of hearing disorders in children with congenital cytomegalovirus. *Journal of the American Academy of Audiology, 11,* 283–290.

Davis, A., & Parving, A. (1994). Towards appropriate epidemiology data on childhood hearing disability: A comparative European study of birthcohorts 1982–1988. *Journal of Audiological Medicine, 3,* 35–47.

Dorman, M., Hannley, M., Dankowski, K., et al. (1989). Word recognition by 50 patients fitted with the Symbion multichannel cochlear implant. *Ear and Hearing, 10,* 44–49.

Erickson, J., Anderson, M., & Fischgrund, J. (1983). General considerations in assessment. In J. Gelatt & M. P. Anderson (Eds.). *Bilingual language learning system.* Rockville, MD: American Speech and Language Association.

Estivill, X., Fortina, P., Surrey, S. (1999). Connexin-26 mutations in sporadic and inherited sensorineural hearing deafness. *Lancet, 387,* 394–398.

Fischgrund, J., Cohen, O., & Clarkson, R. (1987). Hearing-impaired children in black and Hispanic families. *Volta Review, 86,* 59–67.

Fowler, K., Stagno, S., Pass, R., et al. (1992). The outcome of congenital cytomegalovirus infection in relation to maternal antibody status. *New England Journal of Medicine, 326,* 663–667.

Gallaudet Research Institute. (1998). *Who and where are our children with cochlear implants?* [On-line]. Available: http://gri.gallaudet.edu/Cochlear/ASHA.1997/.

Gerber, S., & Mencher, G. (1980). *Auditory dysfunction* (pp. 133–147). Houston: College-Hill Press.

Gerner de Garcia, B. (1993). Addressing the needs of Hispanic deaf children. In K. M. Christensen & G. L. Delgado (Eds.), *Multicultural issues in deafness* (pp. 69–90). White Plains, NY: Longman.

Gerner de Garcia, B. (2000). Meeting the needs of Hispanic/Latino deaf students. In K. Christensen (Ed.). *Deaf plus—a multicultural perspective* (pp. 149–198). White Plains, NY: Longman.

Guiscafre, H., Benitex-Diaz, L., Martinez, M., & Munoz, O. (1984). Reversible hearing loss after meningitis. *Annals of Otology, Rhinology and Laryngology, 93,* 229–232.

Hairston, E., & Smith, L. (1983). *Black and deaf in America: Are we that different?* Silver Spring, MD: TJ Publishers.

Hamayan, E., & Damico, J. (1991). *Limiting bias in the assessment of bilingual students.* Austin, TX: PRO-ED.

Hanshaw, J. B., Scheiner, A. P., Moxley, A. W., et al. (1976). School failure and deafness after silent congenital cytomegalovirus infection. *New England Journal of Medicine, 295,* 468–470.

Holcomb, T. (1999). Early intervention/late results: The need to "depathologize" the service model. *Seminars in Hearing, 20,* 269–276.

Joint Committee on Infant Hearing (1991). Position statement. *Audiology Today, 3,* 14–17.

Joint Committee on Infant Hearing (2000). Year 2000 position statement: Principles and guidelines for early hearing detection and intervention programs. *American Journal of Audiology, 9,* 9–29.

Kaplan, S., Catlin, F., Weaver, T., & Feigin, R. (1984). Onset of hearing loss in children with bacterial meningitis. *Pediatrics, 73,* 575–579.

Koch, D. (1996). Commercial cochlear implants. *Seminars in Hearing, 17,* 317–325.

Lane, H., Hoffmeister, R., & Bahan, B. (1996). *A journey into the deaf-world.* San Diego: Dawn Sign Press.

Leake, P. A. (1995). *Long-term effects of electrical stimulation.* Paper presented at the 100th NIH Consensus Development Conference on Cochlear Implants in Adults and Children. Bethesda, MD: National Institutes of Health.

Lench, N., Houseman, M., & Newton, V., et al. (1998). Connexin-26 mutations in sporadic nonsyndromal sensorineural deafness. *Lancet, 351,* 415.

Liu, X., Xu, L., Zhang, S., & Xu, Y. (1993). Prevalence and aetiology of profound deafness in the general population of Sichuan, China. *Journal of Laryngology and Otology 107*, 990–993.

Lowder, M. (1996). Management of the adult cochlear implant patient. *Seminars in Hearing, 17*, 327–335.

MacDorman, M., & Atkinson, J. (1999). *Infant mortality statistics from the 1997 period linked birth/infant data set.* National vital statistics reports (Vol. 47, No. 23). Hyattsville, MD: National Center for Health Statistics.

MacNeil, B. (1990). Educational needs for multicultural hearing-impaired students in the public school system. *American Annals of the Deaf, 135*, 75–82.

Marazita, M., Ploughman, L., Rawlings, B., et al. (1993). Genetic epidemiological studies of early-onset deafness in the U.S. school-age population. *American Journal of Medical Genetics, 46*, 489–491.

Martin, D. (1993). Reasoning skills: A key to literacy for deaf learners. *American Annals of the Deaf, 138*, 82–86.

Matkin, N., Diefendorf, A., & Erenberg, A. (1998). Children: HIV/AIDS and hearing loss. *Seminars in Hearing, 19*, 143–153.

Maxwell, M., & Smith-Todd, S. (1986). Black sign language and school integration in Texas. *Language in Society, 15*, 81–94.

McCollister, F., Simpson, L., Dahle, A., et al. (1996). Hearing loss and congenital symptomatic cytomegalovirus infection: A case report of multidisciplinary longitudinal assessment and intervention. *Journal of American Audiology, 7*, 57–62.

McNeil, J. (2001). *Disability.* U.S. Census Bureau, Population Division and Housing and Household Economic Statistics Division [On-line]. Available: http://www.census.gov/population/www/pop-profile/disabil.html.

Miyamoto, R. (1995). Timing of implantation in children. Paper presented at the 100th NIH Consensus Development Conference on Cochlear Implants in Adults and Children. Bethesda, MD: National Institutes of Health.

Moores, D. (1978). *Educating the deaf—psychology, principles, and practices* (pp. 19–26). Boston: Houghton Mifflin Company.

Morell, R., Kuir, H., & Hood, L. (1998). Mutations in the connexin 26 (GJB2) among Ashkenazi Jews with nonsyndromic recessive deafness. *New England Journal of Medicine, 339*, 1500–1505.

Morita, M., Morishima, T., Yamazaki, T., et al. (1998). Clinical survey of congenital cytomegalovirus infection in Japan. *Acta Paediatrica Japan, 40*(5), 2–6.

Morton, N. E. (1991). Genetic epidemiology of hearing loss. *Annals of the New York Academy of Sciences, 630*, 16–31.

Mueller, R. (2000). Genetics of hearing loss. *Seminars in Hearing, 21*(4), 399–408.

Murph, J., Souza, I., Dawson, J., et al. (1998). Epidemiology of congenital cytomegalovirus infection: Maternal risk factors and molecular analysis of
cytomegalovirus strains. *American Journal of Epidemiology, 147*, 940–947.

National Association of the Deaf. (1991). Report of the task force on childhood cochlear implants. *Broadcaster, 13.*

National Association of the Deaf. (2000). [On-line]. Available: http://
www.nad.org/infocenter/newsroom/papers/CochlearImplants.html.

National Center for Health Statistics. (1997). *Trends and differential use of
assistive technology devices: United States, 1994.* (No. 292, PHS 98-
1250). Hyattsville, MD: Author.

National Center for Health Statistics. (2000). *Health, United States, 2000 with
adolescents health chartbook.* Hyattsville, MD: Author.

National Institute on Aging. (1996). *Hearing and older people* [On-line].
Available: http://www.nih.gov/nia/health/agepages/hearing.htm.

National Institute on Deafness and Other Communication Disorders. (1996).
National strategic research plan: Hearing and hearing impairment.
Bethesda, MD: U.S. Department of Health and Human Services, National
Institutes of Health.

National Institutes of Health. (1995). Cochlear implants in adults and children. *NIH Consensus Statement, 13*(2), 1–30.

Newton, V. E. (1985). Aetiology of bilateral sensorineural hearing loss in
young children. *Journal of Laryngology and Otology Supplement, 10*, 1–57.

Northern, J., & Downs, M. (1991). *Hearing in children.* 4th edition (pp.
73–74). Baltimore: Williams and Wilkins.

Nuru, N. (1993). Multicultural aspects of deafness. In D. Battle (Ed.). *Communication disorders in multicultural populations* (pp. 291–292). Boston:
Butterworth–Heinemann.

Nuru-Holmes, N., & Battle, D. E. (1998). Multicultural aspects of deafness.
In D. E. Battle (Ed.). *Communication disorders in multicultural populations* (pp. 255–277). Boston: Butterworth–Heinemann.

Osberger, M., Robbins, A., Miyamoto, R., et al. (1991). Speech perception
abilities of children with cochlear implants, tactile aids, or hearing aids.
American Journal of Otolaryngology, 12(Suppl.), 105–115.

Pappas, D., & Pappas, D., Jr. (1997). Medication and characteristics of drugs
causing ototoxicity. *The Volta Review, 99*, 195–203.

Parving, A. (1983). Epidemiology of hearing loss and aetiological diagnosis of
hearing impairment in childhood. *International Journal of Pediatric
Otorhinolaryngology, 5*, 151–165.

Parving, A. (1996). Epidemiology of genetic hearing impairment. In A. Mar-
tini, A. Read, & D. Stephens (Eds.). *Genetics and hearing impairment*
(pp. 73–81). San Diego: Singular Publishing Group.

Pass, R. F., Stagno, S., & Myers, G. J. (1980). Outcome of symptomatic congenital cytomegalic infection: Results of long-term longitudinal follow-up. *Pediatrics, 66,* 758–762.

Pizzuto, E., Caselli, M., & Volterra, V. (2000). Language, cognition and deafness. *Seminars in Hearing, 21,* 343–357.

Ramsey, C. (2000). Ethics and culture in the Deaf community: Response to cochlear implants. *Seminars in Hearing, 21,* 75–86.

Ramsay, M. E., Miller, E., & Peckham, C. S. (1991). Outcome of configured symptomatic congenital cytomegalovirus infection. *Archives of Disease in Childhood, 66,* 1068–1069.

Rose, S., Conneally, P., & Nance, W. (1977). Genetic analysis of childhood deafness. In F. Bess (Ed.). *Childhood deafness* (pp. 19–36). New York: Grune and Stratton.

Schildroth, A. N. (1994). Congenital cytomegalovirus and deafness. *American Journal of Audiology, 3,* 27–38.

Schildroth, A., & Hotto, S. (1995). Race and ethnic background in the Annual Survey of Deaf and Hard of Hearing Children and Youth. *American Annuals of the Deaf, 140,* 96–99.

Shannon, R. V. (1996). Cochlear implants: What have we learned and where are we going? *Seminars in Hearing, 17,* 403–414.

Spencer, L., Tye-Murray, N., & Tomblin, J. (1998). The production of English inflectional morphology, speech production and listening performance in children with cochlear implants. *Ear and Hearing, 19,* 310–318.

Stagno, S., Reynolds, D. W., Amost, C. S., et al. (1977). Auditory and visual defects resulting from symptomatic and subclinical congenital cytomegalovirus and toxoplasma infections. *Pediatrics, 59,* 669–678.

Strassman, B. (1997). Metacognition and reading in children who are deaf: A review of the research. *Journal of Deaf Studies and Deaf Education, 2,* 140–149.

Strong, M., & Prinz, P. (1997). A study of the relationship between American Sign Language and English literacy. *Journal of Deaf Studies and Deaf Education, 2,* 37–46.

Syrja, J. (1999). Cochlear implants and medical benefits in a competitive world. *Contact, 13,* 4–5.

Tyler, R. (1993). Cochlear implants and the Deaf culture. *American Journal of Audiology, 2,* 26–32.

U.S. Bureau of the Census. (2000a). *Projections of the total resident population by 5-year age groups, race, and Hispanic origin with special age categories* [On-line]. Available: http://www.census.gov/population/projections/nation/summary/np-t4-g.pdf.

U.S. Bureau of the Census. (2000b). *Census brief—from the Mideast to the Pacific: A profile of the nation's Asian foreign-born population. Based on findings from the* Profile of the Foreign-Born Population in the United States: 1997. Current Population Reports, Special Studies P23-195.

U.S. Bureau of the Census (2001). *Current population survey, March 2000, Racial Statistics Population Division* [On-line]. Available: http://www.census.gov.

U.S. Department of Education (1995). *Seventeenth annual report to Congress in the implementation of the Individuals with Disabilities Education Act (IDEA)*. Washington, DC: U.S. Government Printing Office.

U.S. Department of Education (2000). *Twenty-Second Annual Report to Congress on the Interpretation of the Individuals with Disabilities Education Act*. Washington, DC: U.S. Government Printing Office.

U.S. Department of Health and Human Services. (2000). *Healthy People 2000: An assessment based on the health status indicators for the United States and each state*. Hyattsville, MD: Author.

U.S. Department of Health and Human Services (2001). *Healthy People 2010*. Hyattsville, MD: Author.

Vienny, H., Despland, P., Lutschg, J., et al. (1984). Early diagnosis and evolution of deafness in childhood bacterial meningitis: A study using brain stem auditory evoked potentials. *Pediatrics, 73,* 579–586.

Waltzman, S. B., Cohen, N. L., & Gromolin, R. H. (1997). Open-set speech perception in congenitally deaf children using cochlear implants. *American Journal of Otology 18,* 342–349.

Weinick, R., Zurekas, S., & Cohen, J. (2000). Racial and ethnic differences in access to and use of health care services, 1977 to 1996. *Medical Care Research and Review, 57*(Suppl. 1), 36–54.

Williamson, W., Demmler, G., Percy, A., & Catlin, F. (1992) Progressive hearing loss in infants with asymptomatic congenital cytomegalovirus infection. *Pediatrics, 90,* 862–866.

Wilson, M. (1996). Arabic speakers: Language and culture, here and abroad. *Topics in Language Disorders, 16,* 65–80.

Woodward, J. (1982). *How are you gonna get to heaven if you can't talk with Jesus?* Silver Springs, MD: T. J. Publishers.

World Federation of the Deaf. (2000). *Resolution of the XIII World Congress of the World Federation of the Deaf* [On-line]. Available: http://www.wfd-news.org/news/news3.asp.

World Health Organization. (1999). *Press release: AIDS not losing momentum—HIV has infected 50 million, killed 16 million, since epidemic began* [On-line]. Available: http://www.who.int.

World Health Organization. (2001). *Prevention of deafness and hearing impairment* [On-line]. Available: http://www.who.int.

Yoshinaga-Itano, C. (2000). Successful outcomes for deaf and hard-of-hearing children. *Seminars in Hearing, 21,* 309–326.

Zelante, L., Gasparini, P., & Estivill, X. (1997). Connexin 26 mutations associated with the most common form of non-syndromic neurosensory and autosomal recessive deafness (DFNB1) in Mediterraneans. *Human Molecular Genetics, 6,* 1608–1609.

Zwolan, T. (1995). *Factors affecting auditory performance with a cochlear implant by prelingually deafened adults.* Paper presented at the 100th NIH Consensus Development Conference on Cochlear Implants in Adults and Children. Bethesda, MD: National Institutes of Health.

Zwolan, T., Kileny, P., & Telian, S. (1996). Self-report of cochlear implant use and satisfaction by prelingually deafened adults. *Ear and Hearing, 17,* 198–210.

Additional Resources

Alexander Graham Bell Association: http://www.agbell.org.

Centers for Disease Control and Prevention. (2001). *Basic statistics—cumulative AIDS cases.* Atlanta: Author.

Children of Deaf Adults (CODA): http://www.coda-international.org/.

Cochlear Implant Association, Inc.: http://www.cici.org.

Council on Education of the Deaf: http://educ.kent.edu/deafed.

Deafness Research Foundation: http://www.drf.org.

French, M. (1999). *Starting with assessment—a developmental approach to deaf children's literacy.* Washington, DC: Gallaudet University.

Gallaudet Research Institute: http://gri.gallaudet.edu.

Hairston, E., & Bachman, J. (1967). *A study of a segment of the Negro deaf population in the Los Angeles area.* Los Angeles: Leadership Training Program in the Area of the Deaf.

Kluwin, T. (1994). The interaction of race, gender and social class effects in the education of deaf students. *American Annals of the Deaf, 139,* 465–471.

Lewis, L., Farris, E., & Greene, B. (1994). *Deaf and hard of hearing students in postsecondary education (NCES 94-394).* Washington, DC: U.S. Government Printing Office.

Mahshie, S. (1995). *Educating deaf children bilingually.* Washington, DC: Gallaudet University.

National Association of the Deaf: http://www.nad.org/.

National Institute on Deafness and Other Communication Disorders. (1993). *National Institute of Health consensus statement. Early identification of hearing impairment in infants and young children*. Bethesda, MD: Author.

Osberger, M. J. (1995). *Effect of age at onset of deafness on cochlear implant performance*. Paper presented at the 100th NIH Consensus Development Conference on Cochlear Implants in Adults and Children. Bethesda, MD: National Institutes of Health.

Paul, P. (2001). *Language and deafness*, 3rd ed. San Diego: Singular Thomson.

Rodriguez, O., & Santiviago, M. (1991). Hispanic deaf adolescent. A multicultural minority. *Volta Review, 93*, 89–97.

Schirmer, B. (2000). *Language and literacy development in children who are deaf*. Boston: Allyn & Bacon.

Stagno, S., Dworsky, M. E., Torres, J., et al. (1982). Prevalence and importance of congenital cytomegalovirus infection in three different populations. *Journal of Pediatrics, 101*(6), 897–900.

Wolk, P., & Allen, D. (1984). A five-year follow-up study of reading comprehension achievement in a national sample of hearing impaired students. *Journal of Special Education, 18*, 161–176.

World Federation of the Deaf: http://www.wfdnews.org/.

Wrasnick, B., & Jacobson, J. 1995. Teratogenic hearing loss. *Journal of the American Academy of Audiology, 6*, 23–28.

Wright, M. H. (1999). *Sounds like home: Growing up black and deaf in the South*. Washington, DC: Gallaudet University Press.

13

Assessing the Communicative Abilities of Clients from Diverse Cultural and Language Backgrounds

Toya A. Wyatt

When working with multicultural populations, it is important to provide services that are culturally sensitive and appropriate. To accomplish this goal, speech-language pathologists and audiologists must understand how cross-cultural differences in communication styles; views toward health, illness, and disability; the nature and prevalence of communication disorders; and language differences affect the diagnostic evaluation process. This applies to every aspect of the assessment process, including obtaining the case history, test administration, interpretation, diagnosis, and report writing. This chapter discusses how some of the cross-cultural variables addressed in this text affect each of these components of the speech-language-hearing assessment process.

Case History Interview

The case history interview is a very important part of the diagnostic evaluation process, particularly when working with clients from culturally and linguistically different backgrounds. It provides an opportunity to identify possible at-risk medical, developmental, and health concerns that may help to validate a suspected communication disorder. It also provides clinicians with an opportunity to obtain important information about a client's language history, typical language use patterns, communicative difficulties, and course of communication development in English, as well as any other languages spoken.

When interviewing clients from differing cultural and language backgrounds, clinicians must recognize that there are a number of cross-cultural factors that may impact a client's willingness to disclose sensitive information. These factors include but are not limited to (1) differences in communication style; (2) differences in beliefs toward health, disability, and disorder; (3) experience and familiarity with traditional clinical service delivery models; (4) the client or family's level of English language proficiency; and (5) degree of cultural trust or mistrust.

Cross-Cultural Factors Impacting on the Case History Interview

When clinicians and families from differing cultural backgrounds and socialization experiences meet, the two parties may bring differing forms of verbal and nonverbal communication styles, values, expectations, and beliefs.

Greetings and Terms of Address

Clinicians should be familiar with the forms of greetings in the community they serve. As discussed by Cheng in Chapter 3, in traditional Asian communities, it is important to first know the social status of individuals so that appropriate forms of address can be used. The clinician must know, for example, whether the person to be addressed is of higher, equal, or lower status than the clinician (Matsuda, 1989). Clinicians should use formal third party introductions to help establish the appropriate degree of formality and respect and the clinician's credibility (Matsuda, 1989). When meeting clients and families from traditional Asian backgrounds, the clinician should introduce all members of the diagnostic team by name, title, professional role, and clinical responsibilities. The introductions are best carried out by the member of the team who has had the most contact with the family or client before the session or by the person with the highest professional status on the team.

Clinicians should also consider the terms of address used with clients and family members. In many culturally and linguistically diverse communities, addressing clients by their first name may be viewed as socially inappropriate and, in some cases, disrespectful. This is of particular concern when the client is older and has had more life experience than the clinician. Clinicians should always greet clients formally and address them using traditional titles (e.g., "Mr." or "Mrs.") and last names. When working with Spanish-speaking clients, it is also important for clinicians to use the more proper form of *you* (*usted* vs. *tu*) when addressing parents, adults, or older clients (Langdon, 1992).

Nonverbal Communication Differences

Cultural communities differ in the use of nonverbal communication behaviors such as eye gaze during conversation, touch, physical distance from listeners while speaking, gestures, and facial expressions. For example, sustained and directed eye gaze serves as a signal of active listening and attentiveness in some cultural communities (e.g., Westernized, mainstream American communities and Arab or Middle Eastern communities). It can, however, be viewed as a form of disrespect in other communities (e.g., African American, Latino, and Asian cultures) in which diverted eye gaze is used to convey active listening and respect. Similarly, although head nodding in some cultural communities may serve as a sign of verbal agreement among some communicators, it may simply serve as a sign of verbal acknowledgment in others. Failure to correctly interpret and understand nonverbal behaviors can lead to misunderstandings. This becomes important during counseling in which recommendations are shared and the client's understanding is essential.

The use and interpretation of facial expressions can also vary cross-culturally. For example, when interacting with individuals from cultural communities in which emotional restraint is valued, the excessive use of smiling could be viewed as an expression of insincerity. Emmons (1998) compared American and Japanese subjects' interpretations of various facial emotions. He observed that 98% of Americans interpreted the picture of a smiling face as an expression of happiness; however, only 70% of the Japanese interpreted it as such. Instead, 10% of the Japanese subjects interpreted the smiling face as "disgust," 9% interpreted it as "sadness," and 7% interpreted the expression as a form of "contempt." Differing interpretations of a facial expression can potentially impact on the degree to which some clients trust or disclose, or both, sensitive information to clinicians.

Conversational Turn-Taking

Communicators from different cultural backgrounds may also vary in their views of turn-taking. In some communities, it is appropriate to allow longer periods of silence and pausing between turns than observed in Standard American interactions. For example, some Asian speakers provide listeners with time to reflect on what has been said before responding (Matsuda, 1989; Roseberry-McKibbin, 1995). The opposite, however, is true in interactions between African American communicators. According to Kochman (1981), Schieffelin and Eisenberg (1984), and van Kleeck (1994), African American communicators are more likely to engage in rapid turn-taking sequences, characterized by less pause and greater overlap than observed in exchanges between communicators from Euro-American backgrounds.

Clinicians must also be aware of the ways in which communicators from diverse backgrounds initiate, sustain, and terminate conversations. For example, in Latino communities, conversations always begin with discussion of family and other personal issues (Langdon, 1992). In some American Indian communities, the client may remain silent at the beginning of initial social encounters (Saville-Troike, 1986). Clinicians may, therefore, need to plan at least two meetings for diagnostic evaluations with American Indian clients displaying this social discourse style. The first meeting should be used to establish rapport, and the subsequent sessions should be used to obtain necessary information.

In the African American community, listener attentiveness is frequently signaled through the use of call and response (Terrell, Battle, & Grantham, 1998). Call and response involves the ongoing use of phrases and statements such as "Mm-hm," "um-um-um," "You know that's right," "Tell me about it," and ". . . I know what you talkin' 'bout," during another speaker's turn. It is a means for confirming or acknowledging what the speaker is sharing. It is a very important conversational tool for sustaining the flow of conversation and signaling active listening. Clinicians who are unfamiliar with this pattern of responding may inappropriately perceive African American listeners as being interruptive and respond accordingly. To do so, however, could have a negative impact on the establishment of rapport.

Conversational Style

Cultural communities can also differ in how they value and interpret direct and indirect styles of communication. Mainstream American communicators generally prefer a more direct communication style; however, an indirect communication style is more highly valued in the Asian community (Matsuda, 1989). Communicators who use a direct communication style may be viewed as critical or prying by traditional Asian communicators. Clinicians should use an indirect manner of asking questions of traditional Asian clients, particularly when asking questions dealing with sensitive topics and information. Using more pausing between turns and allowing more time for reflection after questions may also help to enhance information sharing and disclosure.

The preservation of harmony during group discourse is also important in Asian communities (Matsuda, 1989). Some Asian communicators may say "yes" or "okay" even when they are not in agreement with statements or suggestions.

Perceived Appropriateness of Topics and Requests for Information

The establishment of rapport during the information-sharing process can also be affected by the types of topics addressed, questions asked, and the manner in which questions are asked. Questions about birth history, place of residence, and nature of communication difficulties may be perceived by some clients as being too personal, intrusive, inappropriate, or irrelevant to the speech evaluation process. In some American Indian communities, for example, the mere mention or discussion of an individual's disability can be viewed as putting that person at risk for greater difficulties (Harris, 1998). Fairly neutral questions such as "Where do you live?" may be viewed with suspicion by clients with a high level of cultural mistrust. Some clients may interpret requests for this type of information as an attempt to obtain personal information about their socioeconomic or immigration status. This may have a negative have a impact on their willingness to disclose important information. To minimize potential barriers, clinicians should preface questions with an explanation of the use of the information in clinical service. Introductory statements such as "Some of the questions I will need to ask you may be a little personal, but they are important for helping me to understand your speech and language needs" may help the client understand the intent of the questions and thus minimize any suspicions or concerns. Clinicians may also want to have a cultural informant—who is knowledgeable about the client's cultural community—review case history questions and the process to be used before the interview to determine their cultural appropriateness.

Beliefs about Health, Disability, and Disorder

Cultural communities can also differ in the ways in which disorders and disabilities are viewed and accepted. In some communities, children with disabilities are considered a blessing from God. In communities in which disabilities are more accepted, clinicians may find clients less willing to consider clinical intervention. When working with clients and families from cultural communities in which disorders are generally concealed, clients may be reluctant to respond to any questions that focus on the origins, nature, or course of a disorder. In communities in which adults have become wary of how society labels children with disabilities, clinicians may also find that terms such as *language disorder, handicap, disability,* or *impairment* are not readily accepted and, in some cases, may be offensive. Terms such as *problem* may be associated with a more serious condition such as mental retardation (Roseberry-McKibbin, 1995). Clinicians should use neutral terms and phrases such as *communication difficulties* rather than *communication disorder,* or *special language needs* rather than *language impairment.*

Clients may have different views of the underlying cause of the disorders or disability. For example, Maestas and Erickson (1992) studied Mexican American mothers' perceptions of the cause of their children's disability. Fifty percent or more of the mothers cited one of the following reasons for their child's disability: (1) mother had a *sustos* (big fright) during pregnancy, (2) punishment for bad behavior, (3) mother is too old, (4) mother has had too many children, or (5) someone cast a spell. In addition, 15% or more of the mothers attributed the disability to the following: (1) an earthquake, (2) an eclipse, (3) mother was too young, or (4) *mal ojo* (evil eye). Although these explanations are likely to differ from those that might be expected from mothers from mainstream American backgrounds, clinicians should not respond to such beliefs in a manner that suggests that they are inappropriate.

Familiarity and Degree of Experience with the Clinical Service Delivery Model

A client's degree of familiarity and experience with the clinical process should also be taken into account when working with clients from culturally diverse populations. In some cases, culturally diverse clients have had limited exposure to procedures used in speech-language pathology and other health-related fields. Clinicians should explain the evaluation process and documents that need to be signed, such as *confidentiality* and *informed consent,* because they may not be familiar to clients. When obtaining written consent for certain clinical procedures such as videotaping, clinicians should recognize that some clients may have religious or cultural belief systems that prohibit themselves or family members from being photographed or video-taped. Some traditional cultural beliefs equate the capturing of an individual's visual image in photographs with control over that individual's soul.

Diagnostic Testing Procedures

Selecting Appropriate Assessment Procedures: Standardized Testing and Test Bias

There are a number of factors that can have a negative impact on the collection and interpretation of test information and lead to a possible error in diagnosis of communicative impairment. These factors can include various forms of test bias, including, but not limited to, (1) situational bias, (2) format bias, (3) value bias, and (4) linguistic bias (Chamberlain & Medeiros-Landurand, 1991; Goldstein 2000; Taylor & Payne 1983; Vaughn-Cooke, 1986). *Test bias* occurs whenever clinicians attempt to use tests or other assessment procedures that have been normed or developed for use with populations that differ culturally, socially, or linguistically from those with whom the procedure is being used.

Situational Bias

Situational bias can occur in testing situations in which there is a mismatch between the communicative style of the client and the communication style of the mainstream. For example, differences in the interpretation of eye gaze may lead to the inappropriate diagnosis of a pragmatic disorder. The client may be from a culture in which diverted eye gaze during listening serves as a sign of respect. Clinicians must therefore be careful in using pragmatic language profiles and protocols that include culture-specific behaviors, such as sustained eye gaze, as a form of communicative competence.

Situational bias can also occur when a client has differing conversational roles from the mainstream norm. According to Battle and Anderson (1998), Heath (1982), Schieffelin and Eisenberg (1984), van Kleeck (1994), and others, children in some cultural communities are encouraged to initiate conversations with adults and are viewed as appropriate conversational partners in exchanges with adults. In contrast, there are other cultural communities in which children are rarely viewed as co-conversationalists and in which child-initiated conversation with adults is not encouraged.

The extent to which verbal elaboration is encouraged can also differ across cultural communities. According to Heath (1982) and Ward (1971), in southern and lower working class African American communities, children are not expected to initiate conversation with adults. They are generally socialized to speak only when spoken to. Heath (1982) and Ward (1971) noted that children tended to respond to adult requests for information by using the absolute minimum response. This has implications for the elicitation of a conversation from children from similar communities. The children may say very little during the evaluation process, not initiate conversation, and not elaborate in their verbal descriptions of test stimuli. Clinicians must once again be careful not to interpret these types of responses as evidence of expressive language difficulties.

Format Bias

Format bias can also be a factor in the testing performance of some clients. Format bias involves the use of testing formats or procedures, or both, that are less familiar to certain test takers. For example, in her study of

Southern working-class African American communities, Heath (1982, 1983, 1986) found that adults rarely asked children known-information questions. Heath (1986) noted that Mexican American children in more traditional communities are rarely asked known-information questions (e.g., about pictured objects within the view of the speaker and listener). When observing interactions between African American mothers and their children, Anderson-Yockel and Haynes (1994) found that African American mothers were less likely than white mothers to ask their children *wh-* and yes-no questions while reading stories. These differences in exposure to certain language performance tasks put some children at a disadvantage when tested using tasks that elicit information through picture labeling and story retelling. Similar differences may be seen with children who are raised in communities in which adults do not talk about the obvious or are rarely asked to respond to questions about known information (Wyatt, 1999).

The same concerns apply to the use of certain pictures and test prompts. Clinicians should not use pictures, topics, or vocabulary that are unfamiliar to the client owing to differing life experiences. For example, clients who live in desert areas may not have had experience with objects associated with the ocean (e.g., certain marine life, anchors, harbors). Clients who live in urban areas may be unfamiliar with camping or farming scenarios. Similarly, clients who live in warm climates may be unfamiliar with objects associated with cold-climate activities (e.g., toboggan). Clients who have newly arrived from other countries or who have not assimilated well into the mainstream culture may have had less exposure to objects, events, and items that are particular to American culture. Examples include household objects commonly found in American kitchens and homes (e.g., certain cooking utensils, such as blenders; furniture items; vehicles rarely seen in the client's home community, such as fire engines; American sports; musical instruments, such as banjos and harmonicas; clothing; historical events and important people, such as Abraham Lincoln; buildings, such as the Empire State Building; and certain items associated with holidays and celebrations, such as jack-o-lanterns or valentines) (Cheng, 1991).

Value Bias

Value bias results when test items are based on a given cultural group's values, beliefs, attitudes, opinions, or social norms. Value bias may occur with some logical or problem-solving test questions such as "What should you do if . . . ?" For example, if a client who lives on a farm is asked, "What should you do if you run out of milk?" then the most logical response might be to "go to the barn to get more milk from the cow." For clients with more urban experiences, the most logical response might be "go to the store." This type of bias can also occur on items for which clients are asked to provide explanations for "why" questions such as "Why do you brush your teeth?" which can be found on the *Preschool Language Scale-3* (*PLS-3*) (Zimmerman, Steiner, & Pond, 1992). It is common for African American children in some communities to respond to the question, "Why should you brush your teeth?" with "'Cause my momma tell me to." This response is considered incorrect according to standard *PLS-3* scoring guidelines. However, it may be rooted in daily home practices in which children are expected to follow through on the requests of adults simply because they have been asked to do so. Explanations are less likely to be given by parents to their children in communities in which adults are more directive versus explanatory in their verbal exchanges with children. Children reared in these communities may not give the response listed as "acceptable" in the *PLS-3* manual ("Because you might get cavities if you don't.").

Linguistic Bias

Linguistic bias occurs when the tests used are based on a language system different from that used by the client. This is an important issue for nonstandard English as well as nonnative English speakers. For example, many of the grammatical and phonologic rules and features of African American English (AAE) (e.g., the variable absence of the copula, past tense *-ed*, marker and final consonant sounds) serve as signs of disorder in Standard American English (SAE)–speaking populations (Wyatt, 1996). As a result, tests that assess grammatical, phonologic, and vocabulary forms that occur consistently in SAE but not in AAE can be problematic when attempting to identify disorder in AAE-speaking clients. If clinicians are not careful, they may diagnose typically developing AAE speakers who do not consistently produce certain grammatical forms, such as the copula, as having a speech or language disorder.

Linguistic bias also occurs when clinicians use English tests to assess the language skills of non-English or limited English-proficient speakers. As discussed in Chapter 7, it is not uncommon for native Spanish speakers to produce the final /z/ as /s/. As discussed in Chapter 3, Mandarin speakers do not use final past tense *-ed* and plural *-s*. As a result, when using English tests with non-English or limited English-proficient speakers, clinicians should be careful not to interpret omissions of these grammatical forms as evidence of disorder.

Other Sources of Test Bias

There are several other factors that contribute to test bias. These factors include, but are not limited to, (1) the use of standardization samples that fail to adequately reflect the diversity of test users and (2) the development of tests using frameworks designed for or based on research involving other test-taker populations.

Bias from Using Standardized Tests

Many of the tests developed for assessing speech and language are normed on populations that match the distribution of racial groups in the United States according to the latest census reports. With this approach, however, middle-class SAE-speaking individuals from white backgrounds continue to make up the majority of the normative sample. In addition, the scores of individuals from other socioeconomic, ethnic or racial, and dialect backgrounds are often grouped with those of white, middle-class SAE speakers. As a result, group differences can be masked. This results in a set of normative test scores that do not accurately represent the performance of any one subgroup within test standardization samples.

Even when individuals from other ethnic and racial backgrounds are included in the standardization sample, test developers provide little or no information about their dialect or language background. Clinicians have difficulty determining the language or dialect used by the subjects. In response to these concerns, many test developers are beginning to use a more linguistically diverse normative sample and are delineating the dialect or language backgrounds, or both, of individuals within the normative sample. Some test development companies are also beginning to use test bias review panels and differing standardization procedures such as over-sampling to control for possible test bias influences and subgroup performance differences (Flores, 2000). Finally, there is also a growing number of researchers and test developers who are attempting to develop speech and language screening or test procedures, or both, that are primarily developed for and standardized on clients who speak dialects other than SAE and languages other than English.

Bias from Using Tests Based on Inappropriate
Theoretical Frameworks

In some cases, standardized tests do not adequately meet the needs of clinicians serving diverse populations, because they are primarily based on theories of language, language development, and use that are derived from research on SAE-speaking populations. This is significant when one considers the language use patterns of bilingual individuals who may have labels for some concepts in one language but labels for other concepts in another language. To date, there are no tests that allow bilingual speakers to receive credit for responses obtained in a language other than that being targeted within a test (e.g., English or Spanish). This reveals a bias toward a monolingual view of language development and use. In addition, there are no tests of English grammar or phonology that take into consideration the variable nature of feature use in certain dialects such as AAE. Most tests of syntax target grammatical forms, such as the copula, in sentence environments in which the forms are required in SAE but can be variably absent in AAE. This approach reveals a theoretical view of language that is biased toward one dialect of English (SAE). The problem with using biased theoretical frameworks is that they fail to accurately consider differences between languages and language populations that are normal. The consequence is the inappropriate diagnosis of disorders in individuals whose language systems are not addressed by these frameworks.

Minimizing Test Bias

There are a number of strategies that have been proposed for determining and reducing test bias influences. They include, but are not limited to, the following:

- Determine the composition of the standardization sample
- Review the performance of subgroups within the standardization sample
- Review test items, picture stimuli, test administration instructions, and procedures for evidence of potential bias

Another method for identifying and minimizing potential test bias is to administer the test to parents, normally developing peers, or other individuals from the same cultural and language background as the client. This can be particularly useful with clients who speak a relatively unfamiliar language for which an interpreter is not available. Terrell, Arensberg, and Rosa (1992) provide an excellent example of how this approach was used with a child client who spoke Ibo-influenced English and who had a suspected communication disorder. After administering tests to the Ibo-English–speaking parent of the child, the clinician was able to better identify those English grammatical and speech sound production patterns used by the child that were used by other Ibo-English speakers and could thus be interpreted as normal first language–influenced productions. An examination of speech sound and grammatical patterns that deviated from adult speaker productions was then conducted to identify patterns that did not appear to be the result of normal Ibo language or developmental influences.

Alternative Assessment Procedures

When a clinician has determined that there are no available tests that can be used with a given client, owing to cultural or linguistic test bias issues, strong consideration should be given to the use of alternative assessment procedures such as language sampling, observation, interview, dynamic assessment, and nonstandardized criterion-referenced probes. These represent the best methods for overcoming the inherent problems of using standardized tests.

Obtain Parent, Teacher, or Family Report

One of the most effective ways for identifying persons with true speech and language disorders is to interview the client or family members, or both, regarding their perceptions of the client's communication difficulties and abilities. For example, parents know when their child's communication skills seem to be developing differently from those of other children in their home community who are from similar age and cultural and language backgrounds as their child. Spouses and other significant family members can also provide information on the communicative abilities of adult clients with suspected communication disorders. They can provide information on how the communication difficulties impact relationships and interactions with family, friends, and significant members of the client's community. They can also help identify those patterns of communication that would be considered "different" from the perspective of the family and community of the client.

Teacher reports can also provide information about the communication ability of children. When the teacher has had experience working with children from the ethnic, cultural, or language background of the client, the teacher will have a basis for identifying normal communication ability for the community or age group.

Observe Peer and Family Interactions
in Naturalistic Communication Contexts

Observation of peer and family interactions is another useful tool clinicians can use to identify children with true communicative impairments. According to Mattes and Omark (1991), children with communication impairments (1) rarely initiate verbal interactions with peers, (2) generally use gestures rather than speech to communicate, and (3) produce utterances that appear to have little or no effect on the actions of peers. In addition, clinicians should also look for evidence that peers (1) rarely initiate verbal interactions with the client and (2) use facial expressions or actions, or both, that indicate that they have difficulty understanding the child's communication. This strategy can also be used with adult clients involved in communicative interactions with other adults from similar cultural and language backgrounds.

When making observations of client and family interactions, clinicians must be sensitive to the fact that relevant conversational partners may differ across cultural communities. African Americans may have extended family and community networks that are likely to expand the range of important conversational partners (Huer & Wyatt, 1999). It is also not uncommon for African American clients to have multiple caretakers within and outside of the home. Therefore, when attempting to observe interactions with significant communication partners, clinicians need to consider individuals outside of the nuclear family. By focusing on the most familiar communication partners, clinicians can be assured of obtaining the most reliable assessment of authentic communication skills.

Collect Conversation and Language Sample Data in Naturalistic Contexts

The assessment of communication abilities during normal conversation is a very effective approach for avoiding many of the pitfalls associated with the use of standardized tests (Stockman, 1996). The value of language sampling is that key assessment data are obtained in a variety of different authentic communication situations. Language sampling also allows clinicians to evaluate conversational abilities with a variety of different language partners. This helps a clinician not only to identify possible communication concerns but also to obtain important information on a client's relative language proficiency level in all languages spoken. Language sampling in a variety of contexts with different individuals provides clinicians with the opportunity to examine language use patterns and the code-switching behavior of individuals who are bilingual or bidialectal and gives a more comprehensive view of a client's communicative repertoire.

Use Criterion-Referenced Testing

One additional alternative assessment approach advocated by Seymour (1986) is the use of criterion-referenced and nonstandardized elicitation probes for obtaining an individualized profile of a client's relative language strengths and weaknesses. A criterion-referenced framework serves as an alternative strategy for reporting standardized test results. Test results are reported in terms of the percentage of items passed, instead of using the normative, standard, and percentile-rank scores. The information can then be used to identify and describe relative language strengths and weaknesses across a number of different tasks and can be used to establish appropriate intervention goals.

Use Dynamic Assessment

Dynamic assessment is based on the use of a test-teach-retest paradigm for evaluating an individual's learning potential. Information gained from the use of this approach enables clinicians to distinguish between those individuals who do not perform well on a test as a result of culturally or linguistically based differences and those with underlying communication or cognitive deficits, or both.

In their study of African American and Puerto Rican preschool children, Peña, Quinn, and Iglesias (1992) showed that children who demonstrated a significant improvement in test performance after a brief mediated learning experience were individuals who most likely were tested due to limited experience or familiarity rather than due to a disorder. Findings from Peña, Quinn, and Iglesias (1992) suggest that dynamic assessment measures can help identify clients with communicative difficulties that cannot simply be attributed to differences in exposure, experience, or environment.

Modified Test Administration and Scoring Procedures

As a last resort, clinicians can use modified test administration procedures to minimize potential test bias (Goldstein, 2000; Kayser, 1998; Mattes & Omark, 1991; Roseberry-McKibbin, 1995; Roseberry-McKibbin & Hedge, 2000). Modified administration or scoring, or both, of standardized tests, however, rarely eliminate the problems of format bias. Test modification procedures include the following:

1. Reword test instructions. The wording of certain test prompts or instructions, or both, may be a subtle form of test bias. With certain clients, clinicians may find it more effective to use a prompt such as "Put your finger on the _____ " or "Point to the _____" instead of "Show me the _____ " or "Can you show me the _____?" Whenever rewording test instructions and prompts, however, clinicians should attempt to make sure that the changes in wording do not affect the primary goal of the task being administered or provide any cueing that might invalidate a client's response.

2. Change to a more familiar test format. Changing to a more familiar test format can also reduce the effects of format bias. When giving a test item designed to assess a child's categorical knowledge, such as "Wagon, doll, ball, puzzle—these are all . . . " on the *PLS-3*, the clinician may find it useful to change the format of the prompt if the child seems to be having difficulty understanding the requirements of the task (e.g., simply repeats the stimulus items instead of completing the sentence). Some children may understand the task better if it is presented in the form of a question, such as "What are these things . . . a wagon, doll, ball, and puzzle?" By using an elicitation prompt or format that is more familiar to the client, the clinician may obtain a more valid assessment of client knowledge. Peña and Quinn (1997) found this to be true when they compared African American and Puerto Rican children's performance on a description versus a single word–labeling task. The children per-

formed better on the description task than on the single word–labeling task. Any rewording or changes of test format, however, must be clearly detailed in the report of test findings. In addition, test performance should be described qualitatively with a caution statement regarding the interpretation of test scores.

3. Increase the number of practice items. Increasing the number of practice items can also help reduce format bias by providing clients more experience with testing formats that may be rarely used in a client's home community (e.g., label quests that involve naming pictures within the view of the examinee and examiner). Whenever format bias is suspected, clinicians should proceed with the administration of actual test items only after they are sure that the client fully understands the demands of a given test.

4. Allow extra time for responses. Allowing clients extra time to respond to test items is another modification that is useful with clients with limited English proficiency who need additional time to process items on English-language tests. Clinicians should not view delays in responding as receptive language difficulties in clients who are limited English proficient. Allowing extra time for response may also be useful with tests that have an unfamiliar test format. If task familiarity is the only concern, then the client's test performance should improve with the administration of subsequent items.

5. Continue beyond the test ceiling. Continuing to test beyond the ceiling can be used when a client's inability to correctly answer items is at least partly related to cultural exposure rather than an underlying linguistic or cognitive deficit. This is particularly useful when administering an English-language test to individuals who have recently immigrated from other countries or who may not be familiar with items not found in their homeland.

6. Ask clients to explain incorrect responses. Asking clients to explain incorrect responses is a useful means for minimizing test bias. For example, a clinician observed that one of her adult clients with aphasia repeatedly failed to identify a sandwich as a food item during therapy probe tasks. When the clinician asked the client why she did not include the sandwich on her list of foods, the client responded, "Honey, a sandwich ain't food. Food is things like greens, chicken, potato salad. Now that's real food." The client's response reveals the cross-cultural differences that can occur in how category membership is defined in different communities.

7. Record all responses. Recording clients' verbatim responses to all test items can also be helpful in minimizing test bias. Recording the entire response enables the clinician to later review the response and verify the appropriateness of the client's response with someone who is familiar with the client's cultural and language community and who can help the clinician more accurately determine the appropriateness of the response.

8. Use alternative scoring procedures. Clinicians may use an alternative scoring approach when responses are determined to be appropriate based on

the culture or language of the client. For example, if in response to "Mom is reading the newspaper and Dad is sitting in the chair" (as found on the *PLS-3* [Zimmerman et al., 1992]) an AAE speaker responds "Mom, she readin' the newspaper and Dad, he sittin' in the chair," the clinician should score the response as correct, because it corresponds to expected features of AAE. If, on the other hand, the child responds "Mom, she reading newspaper and Dad, he sittin' chair" with the preposition *in* and article *the* omitted, the clinician should score the response as incorrect, because the omission of these forms would not be considered acceptable forms of AAE.

Culturally Appropriate Report Writing

The diagnostic evaluation is not complete without a final written report of evaluation findings. It is important that clinicians not only provide an accurate and comprehensive report of important case history information and evaluation findings but also that they present findings using culturally sensitive and appropriate language.

Provide a Comprehensive Profile of Client Communication Abilities

To provide the most comprehensive picture of a client's communicative abilities, all diagnostic reports should also provide sufficient information about the client's language history, language-use patterns, and level of language proficiency in all languages used. These should be determined from the case history interview, observations of language use during language sampling, as well as from formal and informal tests. As a balanced description of test performance, it should provide communicative strengths as well as weaknesses for all languages used.

Report All Test Modifications

It is essential that all testing or scoring modifications be fully described. The communication behavior of the client should be presented without reliance on normative test data. A statement should be included that cautions against using the scoring norms provided with any standardized test when any part of the test or procedure was modified. Clinicians should also report whether the services of an interpreter or translator were used.

It is also useful to describe client performance using qualitative rather than quantitative descriptions of test performance. Qualitative descriptions include types of items missed, the nature of errors made, and examples of correct and incorrect responses. Quantitative test scores should be reported with a caution statement and with a wide confidence interval (e.g., 90% confidence interval) to highlight and adjust for the possible error in test performance associated with test bias.

Use Caution Statements

In cases in which standardized test scores and testing procedures are potentially biased, a caution statement about the validity of the test results must be included. This will alert the reader to be cautious in using the test findings to make a clinical diagnosis or an intervention decision. Clinicians must include reference to any sources of concern about the possible bias in the test or the procedure or any other observation that may have had an impact on the results.

Use Culturally Sensitive Language

When discussing speech sound and language "errors," clinicians should ensure that those productions related to normal first language development or dialect influences are clearly differentiated from those related to language disorders. Intervention goals and benchmark objectives should focus on difficulties directly related to an underlying disorder rather than to features of dialect or to first language. Communication difficulties resulting from normal first language or dialect should only be addressed as part of elective instruction programs, rather than clinical intervention (American Speech-Language-Hearing Association [ASHA], 1985). Furthermore, any productions associated with normal first language or dialect should be described using nondeficit or nondisorder terminology. Examples include using phrases such as *speech sound/grammatical differences* instead of *articulation and language errors.*

Reporting a Client's Ethnic or Racial Background

According to the California Speech-Language-Hearing Association's (1996) position statement on the delivery of services to culturally and linguistically diverse populations, only those findings directly related or relevant to the presenting case should be presented in clinical reports. References to race or ethnicity should only be reported if they have a direct bearing on the nature of the disorder, outcome of the assessment, or intervention planning. Additionally, in those rare instances in which such references are deemed appropriate, the client or responsible party should be fully informed of the rationale supporting the use of such references.

It is not important to delineate the racial or ethnic background of the client (e.g., "Jose is a 4-year-old Latino boy . . ."). It is more important to describe the client's language background if it is relevant to the diagnosis (e.g., "Jose is a 4-year-old bilingual Spanish and English speaker."). If the client is a recent immigrant, then delineating the country of origin can also provide useful and relevant information to understanding the nature of the client's communication behavior. Focusing on a client's cultural or language background versus racial or ethnic background helps clinicians minimize the possibility of conveying subtle stereotypes about a client's communicative abilities or cultural orientation. Examples of least-biased report writing samples can be found in Appendix 13-1.

Assessment of Bilingual and Limited English-Proficient Clients

Case History

The case history is important for obtaining important information about the language history of the client. By obtaining a comprehensive review of communication concerns in all languages used by a client, clinicians are able to distinguish between normal development, differences, and disorders. A true disorder can only be diagnosed when there is evidence that the disorder exists in the client's first language, as well as later-learned languages. Information about communicative abilities in all languages is essential for making appropriate clinical decisions.

Specific topics that should be addressed as part of the diagnostic interview with clients who speak more than one language include the following: (1) the age at which the client was exposed to each language; (2) conditions under which each language was acquired; (3) the course of development in each language; (4) the level of proficiency in both languages; (5) current language use patterns; (6) the nature of communicative difficulties in each language; (7) current level of proficiency in each language, including speaking, understanding, reading, and writing; and (8) client and family attitudes toward the language of intervention, if necessary.

Use of Interpreters and Translators

An *interpreter* "conveys information from one language to the other in the oral modality," whereas a *translator* "conveys information in the written modality" (Langdon, 1992, p. 202). When communicating with clients who have limited English proficiency, clinicians should be certain that the clients understand the information requested. All documents requiring the client's signature should be translated into the client's language. If documents are to be translated, then it is important to give the translator sufficient time to prepare the translation so that the information can be reviewed by the clinician before presentation to the client to ensure that the translation correctly presents the intent of the item (Kayser, 1995; Roseberry-McKibbin, 1995).

If the clinician is not a competent speaker of the client's primary language, then it is always advisable to use an interpreter. Interpreters are individuals who assist with the transmission of information between the clinician and client when the two parties use different languages. A properly trained interpreter can help clinicians explain the diagnostic process, clinical forms (e.g., informed consent), and other legal documents. Many interpreters can also translate informed consent forms or written reports, or both, into the language of the client or family, or both.

When the family or client indicates that they are comfortable being interviewed in English, the clinicians may still want to have an interpreter present in the event that the questions are not understood or require fairly elaborate responses that the client may feel more comfortable expressing in his or her first language. Some families may refuse the services of an interpreter or prefer not to use an interpreter, because they perceive a social stigma associated with the use of their native language in English-language settings. Clinicians should therefore discuss the role of the interpreter in a manner that conveys acceptance of their language and that does not imply an English-language bias.

Training Interpreters

Interpreters must be properly trained (Goldstein, 2000; Kayser, 1995, 1998; Mattes & Omark, 1991; Roseberry-McKibbin, 1995). They must have good oral and written language skills in English and in the language of the client. They must also have the following: (1) a solid understanding of professional ethics, (2) the ability to relate culturally to the client, and (3) the minimum educational standards and clinical competencies outlined by ASHA for the support personnel (ASHA, 1995).

There are several problems that can occur when the interpreter has not been properly trained (Cheng, 1991; Kayser, 1995; Roseberry-McKibbin, 1995). The interpreter may hide or minimize the extent of the client's communicative problems or fail to share information with the clinician that is perceived as being sensitive or personal. The interpreter may make errors during the oral transmission of information such as omitting, adding, or substituting words, phrases, or sentences. Errors can occur when the interpreter believes that a word, phrase, or sentence is not important; when concepts are difficult to translate into the language; or there is confusion about a term. Interpreters may have difficulty retaining the original message or keeping up with the pace of the speaker. There may be a desire to editorialize or be more elaborate (Cheng, 1991;

Kayser, 1995). These problems can be avoided by providing interpreters with adequate training and preparation before the diagnostic testing session. Clinicians can also facilitate accurate interpreting by doing the following: (1) speaking in short units with frequent pauses, (2) providing the client with sufficient time to respond to and ask questions, (3) providing the interpreter with the opportunity to ask for clarification when needed, (4) encouraging the interpreter to interpret the client's words and meaning, (5) looking at the client rather than the interpreter when speaking, and (6) avoiding any unnecessary side conversations with the interpreter in the client's presence (Roseberry-McKibben, 1995).

Establishing the Need for Testing in More Than One Language

When evaluating the speech and language skills of bilingual clients, it is very important to conduct at least part of the speech and language evaluation in the client's dominant language. The Individuals with Disabilities Education Act Amendments of 1997 mandate that a child be tested in his or her native or strongest language or mode of communication used most in addressing the child at home. In addition, ASHA supports the position that "assessment and intervention of speech and language disorders of limited English-proficient speakers should be conducted in the client's primary language" (ASHA, 1985, p. 30). Initial impressions of language dominance can be established from information provided during the case history interview. Issues such as patterns of language use in both languages, the language most frequently spoken at home, and the language first learned can be investigated during the case history interview. Preliminary determinations of language proficiency from the case history interview, however, should be validated by observations of language use during language-sampling procedures. Observations of a client's ability to respond to questions and to express him- or herself in English can be compared with his or her ability to accomplish these same tasks during conversational exchanges with family members or peers in any other languages spoken. Clinicians should also observe the number of times the client needs to have questions repeated in each language, the length of sentences produced in each language, evidence of more word-finding difficulties in either language, and evidence of code switching or mixing. These observations should provide the clinician with an intuitive sense of the client's strongest language.

Testing in Both Languages

Once the need to conduct an assessment in two or more languages is determined, it is beneficial to observe as much as possible in each language to determine their relative language strengths and weaknesses. The goal of this procedure is to identify weaknesses across both languages. Such weaknesses could include word-retrieval difficulties, reduced sentence length, and articulation patterns that occur in the first as well as the second language and cannot be explained solely on the basis of first-language influences or normal development. This procedure can yield information that allows the clinician to identify those areas of communication difficulty that may be a true disorder rather than a language difference. Once it has been determined that the client is more proficient in a language other than English, English tests should not be used exclusively to diagnose a disorder. Information obtained from English tests can be used to provide information about a client's degree of English-language proficiency. When using English tests as measures of proficiency, however, clinicians should report findings using descriptive analyses of performance rather than test scores.

Clinicians should collect language samples in all languages used by the client in a variety of different speaking situations with different conversational partners. For example, the clinician should observe or sample language in at least one context in which the client interacts with parents, siblings, or other family members. This will provide the clinician with information on typical language use patterns in a communicative context that will help to highlight language strengths and weaknesses. The clinician should observe the client's use of English and the native language. The collective use of information from all sampling contexts will yield the most comprehensive overview of language strengths and weaknesses in all languages used and establish a profile of relative language proficiency across all language domains.

Using Interpreters or Translators to Assist with Testing

If the clinician is not proficient in the language of the client, an interpreter or translator should be used to assist not only with the elicitation of the sample but also with the written transcription. Interpreters and translators can also assist with the administration of standardized tests in the native language of the client if the clinician is not fluent in that language. Interpreters and translators can help identify test items that are potentially difficult for individuals from that community. These individuals can serve as cultural informants in helping clinicians identify those test items that may present some form of cultural or linguistic bias.

Dialectal Variations

When evaluating information obtained in another language, clinicians should be aware of the dialectal differences that can occur within languages, particularly with respect to vocabulary and pronunciation. Language differences or dialects can exist within any language, just as they do in English. The variety of Mexican American Spanish spoken in New Mexico is not exactly the same as the varieties spoken in Puerto Rico, Southern California, and Texas. For example, in Puerto Rican Spanish, the medial /r/ can be produced as /l/ as in *puelta* or as an /r/ as in *puerta*; the final /s/ can be omitted, aspirated, or produced as an /h/ as in *dos* (Goldstein, 1993, 2000; Merino, 1992). *Naranja* or *china* can be used to refer to an *orange*, depending on the Spanish dialect. When administering Spanish tests normed on Mexican Spanish-speaking clients to Puerto Rican Spanish-speaking clients, it is appropriate to replace a word such as *naranja* (orange) with *china*.

Examining Patterns of Code-Switching and Code-Mixing

Although it is common for all bilingual speakers to switch between languages during conversation and even within the same sentence, it is possible that an analysis of bilingual code-switching patterns may help to identify some individuals with underlying communication disorders. Although code mixing and switching are natural and normal patterns of language use in bilingual clients, a substantial increase in code-mixed utterances after onset of the disorder can be evidence of an expressive language disorder. Reyes (1995, p. 167) stated that "although certainly not all lexical switches are indicative of lexical unavailability, switches of single words may be a red flag to clinicians that perhaps the patient is experiencing word-retrieval difficulties." An increased frequency of code switching could have clinical implications. Frequent code switching may signal a lack of competence in either language (Cheng & Butler, 1989; Langdon & Merino, 1992). To determine whether code-switching patterns have changed in frequency or nature, Reyes (1995) emphasizes the importance of inquiring about a patient's premorbid code-switching abilities and patterns and making comparisons to post-insult code switching.

Audiologic Assessments

When working with individuals who are native speakers of languages other than English, clinicians also need to be aware of some of the problems that can occur with certain audiologic assessment procedures, such as speech reception and discrimination testing. Non-English speakers can be at a significant disadvantage when speech discrimination testing is conducted using English-word stimuli (Danhauer, Crawford, & Edgerton, 1984). In a study comparing the performance of monolingual English, monolingual Spanish, and bilingual Spanish-English speakers on a 25-item nonsense syllable test originally designed for English-speaking populations, Danhauer and colleagues (1984) found that monolingual Spanish subjects performed considerably more poorly than the other two groups. The nonnative English speakers had difficulty discriminating between sound contrasts that did not exist in their native language. Furthermore, as Mattes and Omark (1991) point out, the use of English spondee word lists may be inappropriate for assessing the speech reception abilities of individuals who speak languages other than English because of the ways in which typical word-stress patterns vary across languages. For example, trochaic stress patterns (words with stressed first syllables and unstressed second syllables) may be more appropriate to use with native Spanish speakers than spondee words, because trochaic word stress patterns occur more frequently in Spanish.

Evaluating Bilingual Clients with Aphasia, Voice, and Fluency Disorders

When working with clients who exhibit voice, fluency, or a neurologically based disorder, a key indicator of a true communicative disorder is the existence of the problem in both languages. Clients who demonstrate speech apraxia or dysarthria, or both, in one language exhibit evidence of the same problem in any other languages spoken. Clients with a fluency disorder have similar patterns of dysfluency in each language. In a study of a bilingual Spanish-English speaker's dysfluency patterns, Bernstein-Ratner and Benitez (1985) found the subject to stutter more on verbs than nouns in both languages. This client also tended to be more dysfluent on sentence initial constituents in Spanish than English. The higher frequency of dysfluent sentence initial constituents in Spanish compared to English can most likely be attributed to the fact that a greater number of sentences in Spanish begin with verbs. In essence, the loci of stuttering were the same in both languages; however, the frequency of dysfluencies was higher in Spanish than in English because of language-specific grammatical differences.

The rate of dysfluencies in bilingual speakers may be higher in one language than the other as a result of the normal second language learning process. Specifically, when learning a second language, it is normal for a speaker to exhibit a number of phrase revisions, hesitations, and interjections in the second language until they become more proficient in that language. Clinicians, therefore, must look carefully at the nature of dysfluencies in both languages before making a definitive diagnosis of stuttering.

Clinicians should also be aware that there can be cross-cultural differences in the use of prosody and fluency patterns during narrative assessment tasks (Gutierrez-Clellen & Quinn, 1993; Hyter & Westby, 1996). Prosody and fluency must therefore be evaluated in light of culturally based criteria, as well as other aspects of narrative ability such as topic, content, structure, and organization.

As previously discussed, information on pre- as well as post-onset bilingual language abilities are important in evaluating the language and speech abilities of bilingual clients with aphasia. It is important to determine how current code-switching and code-mixing patterns compared to those exhibited before a client's stroke. Knowing this information will help the clinician better discern those patterns of language use that are the result of the neurologic disorder rather than from second language use.

As discussed in Chapter 10, when working with clients with voice disorders, clinicians must consider the possible cross-cultural variations that can occur in voice productions. Awan and Mueller (1996) and Salas-Provance (1996) cite findings from studies suggesting that the average fundamental frequency of African American men, women, and children may differ from that generally reported for their white counterparts. Cross-cultural differences in voice use patterns can occur for clients from other cultural backgrounds as well. As a result, when working with bilingual clients from other cultural backgrounds, clinicians should be mindful of the differing perceptions of voice that may exist across communities. What is acceptable in one community may not be acceptable in another.

Special Considerations for Accent Modification, English as a Second Language, and Dialect Instruction

When assessing the English-language abilities of clients desiring to improve their English pronunciation or grammar, or both, clinicians should ask many of the same questions as those asked of other bilingual or limited English-proficient clients with respect to language history and use. Issues such as current language use, current perceived level of proficiency in each language, and history of communication difficulties in the native language allow the clinician to rule out disorder-based communication difficulties in the client's first language as the basis for difficulties in the second. Knowing something about the client's language exposure history also enables the clinician to determine the extent to which first language influences are likely to impact on second language abilities.

When working with non-native English speakers, it is also helpful to elicit information on the following: (1) the perceived impact of English communication difficulties in social interactions; (2) the nature, duration, and perceived effectiveness of any previous pronunciation training or English language instruction, or both; and (3) current and future occupational or educational aspirations. Questions regarding the client's perceived nature and social impact of communication differences as well as future occupational goals and educational aspirations should also be addressed with clients interested in second dialect instruction. In addition, with both groups of clients, the clinician should also consider cross-cultural differences in communication style, values, and beliefs that may impact on the success of the instruction program. This information can be used in the design of an English communication instruction or second dialect instruction program that effectively meets the social, educational, and vocational needs of the client.

One last consideration is the goals of the evaluation process. Evaluation goals for English communication instruction clients differ from those for clients with possible speech-language disorders. For English communication instruction (e.g., accent modification, English as a second language) and Standard English as a second dialect clients, the primary focus is on learning to effectively use a second communication system. As a result, clinicians must approach the diagnostic evaluation process with a nondeficit orientation that does not consider differences as deficient or disorder based.

Differential Diagnosis: Distinguishing Development, Difference, and Disorder

Perhaps the most important aspect of the evaluation process is the interpretation and analysis of diagnostic findings. It is at this stage of the evaluation process that clinicians must apply what they know about normal language development, second language acquisition, language, and cultural differences to distinguish between those behaviors associated with normal language, language differences, and disorders.

Identifying Disorders in Nonstandard English Dialect Speakers

When evaluating the speech and language abilities of clients who speak a dialect of English the clinician should focus on the following: (1) non–dialect-specific aspects of speech and language production; (2) those aspects of communication that are universal such as early developing semantic and pragmatic functions; and (3) dialect-specific forms within linguistic contexts considered to be obligatory in the dialect. For example, when attempting to ascertain whether speech sound differences are the result of phonologic delay in speakers of AAE, clinicians should determine whether the speaker is delayed on the phonologic features that do not differ from SAE

(Stockman, 1996). Stockman (1996) refers to these shared phonologic features as *minimal core competencies*. The competencies include the speech sounds that occur similarly in the speech of African American and white children aged 0–3 years in initial word position: /m/, /n/, /p/, /k/, /g/, /h/, /j/, /t/, /f/, /b/, /s/, /f/, /w/, /l/, and /r/ (Stockman & Settle, 1991). Stockman and Settle (1991) noted that this minimal core of sounds was produced by 80–100% of African Americans, as well as by white English speakers by the age of 3 years. Bleile and Wallach (1992) compared the speech productions of African American preschoolers identified by their teachers as having "trouble speaking" or "no trouble speaking." They suggest that clinicians should focus more on sounds in initial and medial positions of words rather than the final word positions.

Haynes and Moran (1989) suggest that children using AAE do not differ from children using SAE in developmental patterns of phonologic process use. They found, however, that the deletion of final voiced sounds seemed to persist longer in African American subjects. These findings suggest that the examination of final consonant use patterns cannot be used exclusively to identify AAE speakers with true phonologic disorders. However, it is also important to recognize that some final sounds found in SAE are never absent in AAE. The AAE speaker who frequently fails to produce voiceless final stops and fricatives such as /p, k, s, f/ is most likely exhibiting a speech production pattern that is associated with a true underlying disorder. When evaluating use, the concept is the same. By focusing on those minimal core or non–dialect-specific or non-contrastive features of English (grammatical forms that occur in all dialects of English), clinicians are more likely to accurately identify AAE speakers with underlying language impairments. Examples include complex syntactic constructions—for example, infinitive clauses such as "He don't need *to stand up*" and "The bus driver told the kids *to stop*," noun phrase complements such as "I told you *there's a Whopper*," relative clauses such as "That's the noise *that I like*," and gerunds and participles such as "It get *rainy*"—which are less likely to be influenced by the morphosyntactic differences between AAE and SAE (Craig & Washington, 1994; Washington, 1996). Similarly, clinicians should focus on articles such as *a* and *the* (Seymour, Bland-Stewart, & Green, 1998) and adjective-noun word ordering which are used in the same manner in AAE and SAE. Clinicians should also be concerned about speakers older than 4–5 years of age who do not use complex sentence constructions, who frequently omit articles, or who use inappropriate sentence word order (e.g., say "kittens three" for "three kittens").

Clinicians should also consider AAE speakers' productions of dialect-specific grammatical and phonologic forms in contexts that have been identified as being obligatory for grammatical feature use. Several copula verb contexts have been identified as obligatory for AAE and SAE (e.g., after *what/that/it* subject pronouns and in first person singular, as well as past tense contexts) (Labov, 1969; Labov et al., 1968; Wolfram, 1969). Typically developing AAE child speakers display knowledge of these obligatory rules (Stockman et al., 1982; Wyatt, 1991, 1995, 1996). By using knowledge of these variable rule patterns, clinicians can effectively identify copula production patterns in child as well as adult speakers that appear to be atypical (e.g., frequent absence of the copula in contexts in which it should always be present).

In speakers who are younger than the age of 3 years, clinicians should focus on semantic and pragmatic aspects of language that are universal. According to Stockman and Vaughn-Cooke (1982) and Bridgeforth (1987), AAE-speaking children acquire the same semantic and pragmatic categories at the same stages of development and in the same sequence as SAE-speaking children. The only difference is the linguistic code AAE or SAE used to code these meanings and functions. Therefore, clinicians should be concerned with children who use a fairly restricted range of semantic meanings or language functions when compared to age peers. Concerns about possible delay should be based, of course, on reliably obtained language sample data.

One final note on the issue of distinguishing between development, disorder, and normal dialect differences is the range of linguistic variability that exists in a given ethnic group. For example, not every African American uses AAE, even within working-class African American communities in which AAE is presumed to be most widely spoken (Wyatt, 1995). It is important to first determine whether an individual is a predominate user of a dialect or is a bidialectal (AAE + SAE) speaker before identifying certain grammatical and phonologic patterns. One of the best ways to determine the dialect-status client is to examine dialect use patterns in a variety of different communicative settings, with a variety of different communicative partners who use different dialects of the language. During the interactions, the clinician should look for the use of distinctive dialect markers such as the habitual "be," negative "ain't," and the remote time "been" that are clearly associated with dialect but are not developmental or disorder error patterns.

Identifying Disorders in Bilingual and Limited English-Proficient Clients

Just as clinicians must understand something about the rules of various English dialects when working with AAE and other non–Standard English speakers, they must also be knowledgeable about the grammatical and phonologic structure of languages other than English when evaluating the communicative abilities of bilingual or monolingual non-native English speakers. References such as those listed in Additional Resources can be helpful for accomplishing this goal. Knowledge of these language differences enables a clinician to determine whether any differing productions of English sounds or grammatical structures can be attributed to normal first-language influences, normal dialect differences, universal second-language errors, or (in the case of children) developmental influences. Clinicians must rule out each of these factors when attempting to determine whether apparent English "errors" are the result of normal language differences or true disorder. When attempting to rule out normal first-language influences as the explanation for observed differences in a second language, clinicians should try to identify those speech sounds or grammatical omissions and substitutions that can be explained by the absence of that linguistic feature in a client's native language. It is common, for example, for many non-native English–speaking clients to substitute some other sound for /θ/ in English, because this sound does not exist in many non-English languages, including Spanish, several Asian languages, Polynesian languages, and the majority of Arabic dialects (Adler, 1993; Cheng, 1998; Kayser, 1995; Langdon & Merino, 1992; Roseberry-McKibbin, 1995; Ruhlen, 1975). As explained in Chapter 3, it is also common for native Chinese speakers to omit several English inflectional markers such as past tense -ed, plural -s, and possessive -s markers, because these forms do not exist in their native language. Although a sound may be present in English and the client's native language, it may never occur in a certain word position. Even though /b/, /p/, /g/, /m/, /t/, /k/, /tʃ/, and /f/ are sounds that exist in Spanish and English, it would be normal for Spanish speakers to omit these sounds in the final position of English words, because they never occur in final word positions in Spanish.

In some cases, it is not always possible to clearly attribute certain English grammatical or phonologic productions to first language influences. There are a number of English grammatical forms that have been found to be universally difficult for individuals acquiring English as a first language, regardless of their native language background. For example, according to Dulay and Burt (1974) and Dulay, Burt, and Krashen (1982) all second-language English learners have difficulty with the copula and auxiliary *be*, irregular past tense verbs, possessive -s, and the third person singular -s regardless of their first language background. In addition, it is common for second-language learners to go through a transitory stage of second-language acquisition (*interlanguage*) in which attempts at the production of target sounds and grammatical structures in the second language can change over time. The attempts of individual second-language learners, even from the same language background, can also be rather unique or idiosyncratic in nature. As the second-language learner gains more experience with the second language, however, these productions may change in nature, eventually becoming more similar to the target language structure. On the other hand, it is also possible for these productions to become fossilized (become a permanent part of the speaker's communicative repertoire).

Many errors made by children acquiring English as a second language are similar to those made by children acquiring English as a first language who have had the same number of years of exposure to English. It is not unreasonable, therefore, for non-native English child speakers with fewer than 3 years of English-language exposure to not use grammatical forms such as the copula, which is not used by monolingual English-speaking children younger than the age of 3 years.

Clinicians must also recognize that the developmental sequence of acquisition for certain sounds in a child's native language can differ from English, even when those sounds occur in the native language and English. The order in which certain grammatical forms or sounds are acquired can also differ for monolingual and bilingual speakers of the same language. As a result, clinicians must be careful about the set of comparative norms used for establishing expected ages of mastery. In summary, the differing English language productions of nonnative speakers acquiring English as a second language can have many sources of origin. They can be the result of normal first language influences (interference patterns), universal second language learning patterns, interlanguage phenomena, or normal child language acquisition (developmental) factors. In some cases, it may not be possible for the clinician to clearly delineate the source of differences or isolate one single causal factor. It is important for the clinician to recognize when patterns of second language difference seem to occur more frequently or are drastically different from what one would expect from most second-language learners. Final diagnosis of a disorder must be based on an analysis of first language abilities, observation, alternative assessments, and information obtained during the case history interview.

As discussed in this chapter, clinicians must be aware of the numerous cultural and linguistic factors that can impact the diagnostic evaluation process. Being culturally sensitive, competent, and aware is to recognize when cultural and linguistic factors are likely to influence the assessment process as well as knowing how to address these various factors in the diagnostic evaluation. This chapter has provided a framework for accomplishing each of these objectives.

References

Adler, S. (1993). *Multicultural communication skills in the classroom*. Boston: Allyn & Bacon.

American Speech-Language-Hearing Association (1982). Position paper on social dialects. *ASHA, 25*(3), 29–32.

American Speech-Language-Hearing Association (1985). Clinical management of communicatively handicapped minority language populations. *ASHA, 27*(6), 29–32.

American Speech-Language-Hearing Association (1995). Task Force on Support Personnel. Position statement for training, credentialing, use and supervision of support personnel in speech-language pathology. *ASHA, 37*, (Suppl. 14), 21.

Anderson-Yockel, J., & Haynes, W. O. (1994). Joint book-reading strategies in working-class African-American and White mother-toddler dyads. *Journal of Speech and Hearing Research, 37*(3), 583–593.

Awan, S. N., & Mueller, P. B. (1996). Speaking fundamental frequency characteristics of White, African American, and Hispanic kindergartners. *Journal of Speech and Hearing Research, 39*(3), 573–577.

Battle, D. E., & Anderson, N. (1998). Culturally diverse families and the development of language. In D. E. Battle (Ed.), *Communication disorders in multicultural populations* (2nd ed.) (pp. 213–245). Boston: Butterworth–Heinemann.

Bernstein-Ratner, N., & Benitez, H. (1985). Linguistic analysis of a bilingual stutterer. *Journal of Fluency Disorders, 10*, 211–219.

Bleile, K. M., & Wallach, H (1992). A sociolinguistic investigation of the speech of African American preschoolers. *American Journal of Speech-Language Pathology, 1*(2), 54–62.

Bridgeforth, C. (1987). *The identification and use of language functions in the speech of 3- and 4 1/2 year-old Black children from working class families*. Unpublished doctoral dissertation, Georgetown University, Washington, DC.

California Speech-Language-Hearing Association (1996). Position statement on the delivery of speech-language-hearing services to culturally and linguistically diverse persons. *CSHA, 24*(5), 19–21.

Chamberlain, P., & Medeiros-Landurand, P. (1991). Practical considerations for the assessment of LEP students with special needs. In E.V. & J. S. Damico (Eds.), *Limiting bias in the assessment of bilingual students*. Austin, TX: PRO-ED.

Cheng, L. L. (1991). *Assessing Asian language performance* (2nd ed.). Oceanside, CA: Academic Communication Associates.

Cheng, L. L. (1998). Asian- and Pacific-American cultures. In D. E. Battle (Ed.), *Communication disorders in multicultural populations* (pp. 73–116). Boston: Andover Medical Publishers.

Cheng, L. L., & Butler, K. (1989). Code-switching: A natural phenomenon vs. language deficiency. *World English, 8*, 293–309.

Craig, H. K., & Washington, J. A. (1994). The complex syntax skills of poor, urban, African-American preschoolers at school entry. *Language, Speech, and Hearing Services in Schools, 25*(3), 181–190.

Danhauer, J. L., Crawford, S., & Edgerton, B. J. (1984). English, Spanish, and bilingual speakers' performance on a nonsense syllable test (NST) of speech sound discrimination. *Journal of Speech and Hearing Disorders, 49*(2), 164–168.

Dulay, H. C., & Burt, M. K. (1974). Natural consequences in child second language acquisition. *Language Learning, 24*, 37–53.

Dulay, H. C., Burt, M. K., & Krashen, S. (1982). *Language two*. New York: Oxford University.

Emmons, S. (1998, January 9). Emotions at face value. *Los Angeles Times*, pp. E1, E8.

Flores, N. (2000, April). *Controlling test bias in the development of PLS-4.* Paper presented at the annual meeting of the National Black Association for Speech, Language, and Hearing, Jackson, MS.

Goldstein, B. (2000). *Cultural and linguistic diversity resource guide for speech-language pathologists.* San Diego: Singular Publishing Group, Inc.

Goldstein, B. (1993). Spanish phonological development. In H. Kayser (Ed.), *Bilingual speech-language pathology: An Hispanic focus* (pp. 17–39). San Diego: Singular Publishing Group, Inc.

Gutierrez-Clellen, V. F., & Quinn, R. (1993). Assessing narratives of children from diverse cultural/linguistic groups. *Language, Speech, and Hearing Services in Schools, 24*(1), 2–9.

Harris, G. A. (1998). American Indian cultures: A lesson in diversity. In D. E. Battle (Ed.), *Communication disorders in multicultural populations* (2nd ed.) (pp. 117–156). Boston: Andover Medical Publishers.

Haynes, W., & Moran, M. (1989). A cross-sectional developmental study of final consonant production in southern black children from preschool through third grade. *Language, Speech and Hearing Services in Schools, 20*, 400–406.

Heath, S. B. (1982). Questioning at home and school: A comparative study. In G. Spindler (Ed.), *Doing the ethnography of schooling: Educational anthropology in action.* New York: Holt, Rinehart, & Winston, Inc.

Heath, S. B. (1983). *Ways with words: Language, life, and work in communities and classrooms.* London: Cambridge University Press.

Heath, S. B. (1986). Sociocultural contexts of language development. In California State University, Los Angeles (Ed.), *Beyond language: Social and cultural factors in schooling language minority students* (pp. 143–186). Los Angeles: Evaluation, Dissemination, and Assessment Center, California State University, Los Angeles.

Huer, M. B., & Wyatt, T. A. (1999). Cultural factors in the delivery of AAC services to the African American community. *Communication Disorders and Sciences in Culturally Diverse Populations, 5,* 5–9.

Hyter, Y. D., & Westby, C. E. (1996). Using oral narratives to assess communicative competence. In A. G. Kamhi, K. E. Pollock, & J. L. Harris (Eds.), *Communication development and disorders in African American children* (pp. 155–188). Baltimore: Brookes.

Individuals with Disabilities Act Amendments (1997) Sec. 20 U.S.C., 1400 et seq. (2000).

Kayser, H. (1995). Interpreters. In H. Kayser (Ed.), *Bilingual speech-language pathology* (pp. 207–222). San Diego: Singular Publishing Group, Inc.

Kayser, H. (1998). *Assessment and intervention resource for Hispanic children.* San Diego: Singular Publishing Group, Inc.

Kochman, T. (1981). *Black and white styles in conflict.* Chicago: University of Chicago Press.

Labov, W. (1969). Contraction, deletion, and inherent variability of the English copula. *Language, 45,* 715–762.

Labov, W., Cohen, P., Robins, C., & Lewis, J. (1968). *A study of nonstandard English of Negro and Puerto Rican speakers in New York City* (Final report, Cooperative Research Project No. 3288). Washington, DC: U.S. Office of Education.

Langdon, H. W. (1992). Language communication and sociocultural patterns in Latino families. In H. W. Langdon & L. L. Cheng (Ed.), *Hispanic children and adults with communication disorders: Assessment and intervention* (pp. 99–131). Gaithersburg, MD: Aspen Publishers, Inc.

Langdon, H. W., & Merino, B. J. (1992). Acquisition and development of a second language in the Spanish speaker. In H. W. Langdon & L. L. Cheng (Ed.), *Hispanic children and adults with communication disorders: Assessment and intervention* (pp. 132–167). Gaithersburg, MD: Aspen Publishers, Inc.

Maestas, A. G., & Erickson, J. G. (1992). Mexican immigrant mothers' beliefs about disabilities. *American Journal of Speech-Language Pathology, 1*(4), 5–10.

Matsuda, M. (1989). Working with Asian parents: Some communication strategies. *Topics in Language Disorders, 9*(3), 45–53.

Mattes, L., & Omark, D. (1991). *Speech and language assessment for the bilingual handicapped* (2nd ed.). Oceanside, CA: Academic Communication Associates.

Merino, B. J. (1992). Acquisition of syntactic and phonological features in Spanish. In H. W. Langdon & L. L. Cheng (Ed.), *Hispanic children and adults with communication disorders: Assessment and intervention* (pp. 57–98). Gaithersburg, MD: Aspen Publishers, Inc.

Peña, E. D., & Quinn, R. (1997). Task familiarity: Effects on the test performance of Puerto Rican and African American children. *Language, Speech, and Hearing Services in Schools, 28*(4), 323–332.

Peña, E., Quinn, R., & Iglesias, A. (1992). The application of dynamic methods to language assessment: A nonbiased procedure. *The Journal of Special Education, 26*(3), 269–280.

Reyes, B. A. (1995). Considerations in the assessment and treatment of neurogenic communication disorders in bilingual adults. In H. Kayser (Ed.), *Bilingual speech-language pathology* (pp. 153–182). San Diego: Singular Publishing Group, Inc.

Roseberry-McKibbin, C. (1995). *Multicultural students with special language needs: Practical strategies for assessment and intervention.* Oceanside, CA: Academic Communication Associates.

Roseberry-McKibbin, C., & Hegde, M. N. (2000). *An advanced review of speech-language pathology.* Austin, TX: PRO-ED.

Ruhlen, M. (1975). *A guide to the languages of the world.* Stanford, CA: Stanford University Language Universals Project.

Salas-Provance, M. B. (1996). Orofacial, physiological, and acoustical characteristics: Implications for the speech of African American children. In A. G. Kamhi, K. E. Pollock, & J. L. Harris (Eds.), *Communication development and disorders in African American children* (pp. 155–188). Baltimore: Brookes.

Saville-Troike, M. (1986). Anthropological considerations in the study of communication. In O. Taylor (Ed.), *Nature of communication disorders in culturally and linguistically diverse populations* (pp. 47–72). San Diego: College-Hill Press.

Schieffelin, B. B., & Eisenberg, A. R. (1984). Cultural variations in children's conversations. In R. Schiefelbusch & J. Pickar (Eds.). *The acquisition of communicative competence* (pp. 377–420). Baltimore: University Park Press.

Semel, E., Wiig, E. H., & Secord W. A. (1995). *Clinical evaluation of language fundamentals* (3rd ed.). San Antonio: The Psychological Corporation.

Seymour, H. N. (1986). Clinical intervention for language disorders among nonstandard English speakers of English. In O. Taylor (Ed.). *Treatment of communication disorders in culturally and linguistically diverse populations* (pp. 135–152). San Diego: College-Hill Press.

Seymour, H. N., Bland-Stewart, L., & Green, L. J. (1998). Difference versus deficit in child African American English. *Language, Speech, and Hearing Services in Schools, 29*(2), 96–108.

Stockman, I. J. (1996). The promises and pitfalls of language sample analysis as an assessment tool for linguistic minority children. *Language, Speech, Hearing Services in Schools, 27*(4), 355–366.

Stockman, I. J., & Settle, S. (1991, November). *Initial consonants in young black children's conversational speech.* Poster presented at the annual convention of the American Speech-Language-Hearing Association, Atlanta.

Stockman, I., & Vaughn-Cooke, F. (1982). Semantic categories in the language of working class Black children. *Proceedings of the Second International Child Language Conference, 1,* 312–327.

Stockman, I., Vaughn-Cooke, F., & Wolfram, W. (1982). *A developmental study of Black English—Phase I* (Final report). Washington, DC: Center for Applied Linguistics. (ERIC Document Reproduction Service No. ED 245 555).

Taylor, O. L., & Payne, K. (1983). Culturally valid testing: A proactive approach. *Topics in Language Disorders, 3*(3), 8–20.

Terrell, S. L., Arensberg, K., & Rosa, M. (1992). Parent-child comparative analysis: A criterion-referenced method for the nondiscriminatory assessment of a child who spoke a relatively uncommon dialect of English. *Language, Speech, and Hearing Services in Schools, 23*(1), 34–42.

Terrell, S. L., Battle, D. E., & Grantham, R. B. (1998). African American cultures. In D. E. Battle (Ed.), *Communication disorders in multicultural populations* (2nd ed.) (pp. 31–71). Boston: Butterworth–Heinemann.

van Kleeck, A. (1994). Potential cultural bias in training parents as conversational partners with their children who have delays in language development. *American Journal of Speech-Language Pathology, 3*(1), 67–78.

Vaughn-Cooke, F. B. (1986). The challenge of assessing the language of nonmainstream speakers. In O. L. Taylor (Ed.), *Treatment of communication disorders in culturally and linguistically diverse populations* (pp. 23–48). San Diego: College-Hill Press.

Ward, M. (1971). *Them children: A study in language learning.* New York: Holt, Rinehart & Winston, Inc.

Washington, J. A. (1996). Issues in assessing the language abilities of African American children. In A. G. Kamhi, K. E. Pollock, & J. L. Harris (Eds.), *Communication development and disorders in African American children* (pp. 35–54). Baltimore: Brookes.

Wolfram, W. (1969). *A sociolinguistic description of Detroit Negro speech.* Washington, DC: Center for Applied Linguistics.

Wyatt, T. A. (1991). Linguistic constraints on copula production in Black English child speech. *Dissertation Abstracts International, 52*(2), 781B. (University Microfilms No. DA9120958).

Wyatt, T. A. (1995). Language development in African-American English child speech. *Linguistics and Education, 7*(1), 7–22.

Wyatt, T. A. (1996). Acquisition of the African American English copula. In A. G. Kamhi, K. E. Pollock, & J. L. Harris (Eds.), *Communication development and disorders in African American children* (pp. 95–116). Baltimore: Brookes.

Wyatt, T. A. (1999). An Afro-centered view of communicative competence. In D. Kovarsky, J. Duchan, & M. Maxwell (Eds.). *Constructing (in) competence: Disabling evaluations in clinical and social interaction.* Mahwah, NJ: Lawrence Erlbaum Associates, Publishers.

Zimmerman, I. L., Steiner, V. G., & Pond, R. E. (1992). *Preschool language scale-3.* San Antonio: The Psychological Corporation.

Additional Resources

The following are useful resources and references on the grammatical and phonologic features of English dialects and non-English languages.

These California State Department of Education Language Books are available from the California State Dept. of Education, P.O. Box 271, Sacramento, CA 95802-0271:

- Handbook for teaching Portuguese-speaking students
- Handbook for teaching Vietnamese-speaking students
- Handbook for teaching Philippino-speaking students
- Handbook for teaching Korean-speaking students
- Handbook for teaching Japanese-speaking students
- Handbook for teaching Cantonese-speaking students

American Speech-Language-Hearing Association. (1983). Position on social dialects. *ASHA, 27,* 23–25.

American Speech-Language-Hearing Association. (1985). Clinical management of communicatively handicapped minority language populations. *ASHA, 31,* 93.

Campbell, G. L. (1995). *Concise compendium of the world's languages.* London: Routledge.

Kamhi, A. G., Pollock, K. E., & Harris, J. D. (1996). *Communication development and disorders in African American children: Research, assessment and intervention.* Baltimore: Brookes.

Kayser, H. (1994). *Bilingual speech-language pathology: A Hispanic focus.* San Diego: Singular Publishing Group, Inc.

Kayser, H. (1998). *Assessment and intervention resource for Hispanic children.* San Diego: Singular Publishing Group, Inc.

Langdon, H. W., & Cheng, L. L. (1992). *Hispanic children and adults with communication disorders: Assessment and intervention.* Gaithersburg, MD: Aspen.

Mufwene, S. S., Rickford, J. R., Bailey, G., & Baugh, J. (1998). *African-American English: Structure, history, and use.* London: Routledge.

Roseberry-McKibbin, C. (1995). *Multicultural students with special language needs.* Oceanside, CA: Academic Communication Assoc.

Ruhlen, M. (1975). *A guide to languages of the world.* Stanford, CA: Stanford University (Language Universals Project).

van Keulen, J. E., Weddington, G. T., & Debose, C. E. (1998). *Speech, language, learning and the African American child.* Boston: Allyn & Bacon.

□ □ □
□ □ □
□ □ □

Appendix 13-1

Least Biased Report Writing

Providing a Balanced and Comprehensive Overview of Language Background, Abilities, and Difficulties

Sample Report 1: Adult Bilingual Spanish English–Speaking Client with Fluency Disorder

According to Mr. C., he currently speaks and prefers to use Spanish and English at home. On a typical day, Mr. C. reportedly uses Spanish 60% of the time and English 40% of the time. Spanish is used primarily when attending social events, when running errands in the community, when at church, and when interacting with family members. English and Spanish are used with friends and when he's at work. Mr. C. reported that he uses only English, however, when communicating with his boss.

Sample Report 2: Adult Bilingual Japanese English–Speaking Client with Aphasia

According to Mrs. T., when her husband was younger, his parents used Japanese and English at home. Japanese, however, was the only language used during his elementary schooling. When Mr. T. returned to California where he completed his Junior High and High School education, instruction was conducted in English and Japanese. At present, Mr. T. communicates in both languages with friends, using primarily English with his American friends and Japanese with his Japanese friends.

Sample Report 3: Preschool-Aged Bilingual Spanish English–Speaking Client with Suspected Speech and Language Difficulties

According to Ms. L., F. went through the normal babbling and cooing stages as an infant and began saying his first words in Spanish (e.g., *teta*) before 1 year of age. He began putting two-word utterances together in Spanish shortly thereafter. At present, Ms. L. estimates the average length of her son's sentences to be four to six words in English and Spanish. However, she has noticed that he will sometimes leave words out of sentences in both languages, confuse his pronouns in English (e.g., say *her* for *she*), and occasionally confuse articles in Spanish (e.g., use *el* for *la* and vice versa).

Sample Report 4: Six-Year-Old Bilingual Arabic English–Speaking Client with Mild to Moderate Expressive Language and Articulation Difficulties

G. is exposed to Arabic and English at home, but Arabic is the primary language spoken. According to Mr. and Mrs. S., G. speaks mostly Arabic with family members but speaks English only at school and with friends. At present, they estimate his level of proficiency to be "about the same" in both languages, although sentences are slightly longer in English. When asked to describe G.'s communication difficulties, G.'s parents reported that he has problems producing the /r, v, l/ sounds and in using plurals, negatives, and past tense -*ed* in English. In addition, he often leaves words out of sentences and has difficulty using pronouns in both languages. Mr. and Mrs. S. estimate their son's overall intelligibility of speech to be approximately 75% in both languages.

Sample Report 5: Adult Bilingual Japanese English–Speaking Client with Aphasia

According to Mrs. T., her husband is able to "understand" but has difficulty "getting his words out" in both languages. When asked about his communication abilities before his stroke, Mr. T. stated that he spoke and understood Japanese "fairly good," read Japanese "very little," and only wrote in Japanese "sometimes." In contrast, he reported that his English reading skills were "very good" and that his English speaking, writing and comprehension skills were "good." Since his stroke, Mr. T. reports his reading, writing, and speaking skills in both languages to be "poor" and his understanding of both to be "fair."

Reporting the Use of Test Modifications or an Interpreter

Sample Report 1: Six-Year-Old African American Client with Significant Expressive Language and Phonologic Delays

The *Preschool Language Scale-3* (Zimmerman, Steiner, & Pond, 1992) was administered to obtain a general measure of expressive and receptive language skills. Test scores are not reported, because this test was standardized primarily on children from a different cultural background than A. In addition, testing was also continued below the basal on the first subtest ("Auditory Comprehension") to obtain a more comprehensive view of A.'s language strengths and weaknesses.

Sample Report 2: Adult Bilingual Arabic English–Speaking Client with Aphasia

Several subtests of the *Minnesota Test for Differential Diagnosis of Aphasia* and the *Western Aphasia Battery* were informally administered in English to assess M.'s auditory comprehension, expressive communication, reading, and writing abilities. Some of the items missed by the client during testing in English were translated into Arabic and re-administered by the bilingual Arabic English–speaking paraprofessional to gain a more accurate picture of M.'s language abilities.

Reporting the Results of Testing Conducted in Two or More Languages

Sample Report 1: Adult Bilingual Arabic English–Speaking Client with Aphasia

The "Naming" and "Sequential Commands" subtests of the *Western Aphasia Battery* were given in English and Arabic to assess M.'s expressive naming and auditory comprehension skills. M. had difficulty naming objects and following two to three step commands with less than 50% accuracy on both subtests in both languages. On the "Naming" subtest, M.'s level of accuracy improved from 13–46% when items were administered in Arabic. On the "Sequential Commands" subtest, she displayed similar levels of accuracy (48%) in both languages; however, a comparison of error patterns revealed a great deal of inconsistency, with some of the items missed in English passed in Arabic and vice versa. . . .

An informal conversational sample analysis was also conducted to assess M.'s expressive language and speech production skills in Arabic and English. During conversation, M. displayed observable difficulties retrieving words in both languages, with frequent pausing, hesitations, and false starts noted. M.'s speech attempts in both languages were slow and labored and characterized by visible and audible groping of articulatory postures. Verbal perseveration was also observed during moments of communication difficulty and hand gestures as well as head nods were used to compensate for verbal difficulties in both languages.

Criterion Reference and Descriptive Analysis of Test Performance

Sample Report 1: Eleven-Year-Old African American Client with Suspected Language Difficulties

D. followed 19 of 26 directions (73%) correctly on the "Concepts and Directions" subtest of the *Clinical evaluation of language fundamentals*, 3rd edition (*CELF-3*; Semel, Wiig, & Secord, 1995). She had the most difficulty with two-level commands with assumed left-right orientation. She also had a great deal of difficulty with directions containing inclusion or exclusion phrases. For example, when told to "Point to either the little squares or the white triangles," D. pointed to both the little squares and the white triangles.

Sample Report 2: Six-Year-Old African American Client with Significant Expressive Language and Phonologic Delays

Analysis of test results revealed that A. was able to successfully follow one- and two-step commands with 70% and 80% accuracy, respectively. Three-step commands were more difficult, with A. achieving only 50% accuracy. In addition, A. performed best on commands involving spatial concepts (75% accuracy) but demonstrated difficulty with commands containing coordination (*and*), inclusion or exclusion (*one, or, all, either*), temporal relation or order (*first, and then, after, before*), and quantitative (*all except, all, except*) vocabulary terms.

Reporting Standardized Test Scores Using the 90% Confidence Interval

Sample Report 1: Three-Year-Old African American Client with Suspected Autism

The "Expressive Communication" subtest of *Preschool Language Scale-3* (Zimmerman, Steiner, & Pond, 1992) was administered to assess T.'s general expressive language abilities. She received a raw score of 18, which corresponds to a standard score of 72 (64–80, 90% confidence interval), a percentile rank of 3% (first through ninth percentile, 90% confidence interval), and an age-equivalent score of 1–11 (1–4 to 2–9, 90% confidence interval) indicating significant delays in expressive language.

Citing Potential Test Bias Influences and Using Caution Statements

Sample Report 1: Three-Year-Old African American Child with Suspected Autism

Standardized test scores should be interpreted with caution, however, given the fact that the *Preschool Language Scale-3* (Zimmerman, Steiner, & Pond, 1992) is standardized on children who come, primarily, from other cultural backgrounds and communities. It is felt, however, that even when potential test bias influences are taken into account, standardized test results provide a fairly accurate profile of T.'s relative language strengths and weaknesses.

Sample Report 2: Eleven-Year-Old African American Adolescent with Suspected Language Difficulties

Even though scores appear to be a fairly accurate estimate of D.'s receptive and expressive language strengths, caution should be used when interpreting scores, because the *CELF-3* was primarily standardized on children from a different social-cultural background than D. As a result, test bias influences are possible and reported test scores should only be used as a general measure of D.'s receptive and expressive language abilities.

Distinguishing Difference versus Disorder

Sample Report 1: Eleven-Year-Old African American Client with Suspected Language Difficulties

When the *Photo Articulation Test* was administered to assess D.'s production of speech sounds, results revealed only occasional speech sound differences such as the devoicing of final /z, v/ substitutions of d/ð in all word positions, and vowel substitutions of I/ɛ, ɛ/æ, and I/eI. It is possible that some or all of these productions are the result of normal English dialect differences, because the pronunciation of /ð/, final voiced sounds, and vowels such as /ɛ/ can vary in different English-speaking communities.

Sample Report 2: Eight-Year-Old Bilingual English Vietnamese–Speaking Client with Diagnosis of Autism

Similar to observed English speech sound productions, it is possible that some of T.'s grammatical difficulties in English are related to his dual language exposure to English and Vietnamese. For example, T.'s omission of past tense *-ed*, third person singular *-s*, and copula and auxiliary *be* may be related to the fact that there is no grammatical equivalent for these morphologic markers in Vietnamese. In Vietnamese, tense is generally conveyed through the use of other temporal discourse markers with no changes in the grammatical structure of the root verb form.

Sample Report 3: Adult Bilingual Japanese English–Speaking Client with Aphasia

Many of Mr. T.'s word repetition errors involved the omission or substitution of final sounds. Some of final sound omissions, however, may be due to normal Japanese language influences since words in Japanese rarely end in final consonants.

Sample Report 4: Adult Bilingual Chinese English–Speaking Client Seeking Accent Modification and English as a Second Language Services

Many of Ms. L.'s substitutions of /r/ for /l/ and her difficulties with the production of English vowels /e, I, æ/ are typical of the speech sound differences produced by native Chinese speakers learning English as a second language.

Sample Report 5: Six-Year-Old African American Client with Significant Expressive Language and Phonologic Delays

A whole word transcription analysis of A.'s speech errors revealed the presence of several persisting phonologic processes, including. . . . Although A.'s productions seem to be influenced by the presence of several persisting phonologic processes, it is important to note that the majority of A.'s speech sound errors occurred on later developing sounds such as /tʃ, dʒ, ʃ, z, r, ð, θ/. These sounds typically emerge between the ages of 5 and 7 years. However, it is also important to note that the majority of A.'s speech errors, with the exception of those occurring on /ð/, /θ/, and final /ɔ/, occurred on nondialect-specific sounds (sounds found in all English dialects).

Using Neutral Language to Describe Communication Differences

Sample Report 1: Adult Chinese English–Speaking Client Seeking Accent Modification and English as a Second Language Services

In summary, results from testing revealed difficulties with the pronunciation of several English consonants and vowels. Differences in the use of English stress and intonation patterns and the production of certain English grammatical forms and structures were also noted. Most of Ms. L.'s English difficulties appear to be the result of normal first-language influences. Based on these findings, it is recommended that Ms. L. consider enrollment in an English as a Second Language or accent modification program with goals focusing on (1) improving her pronunciation of final voiced English consonants and nasals, (2) improving her pronunciation of vowels /e, I, æ/, (3) improving her use of appropriate English stress and intonation patterns, and (4) improving her use of the following English grammatical forms: copula *be*, articles *a* and *the*, prepositions, plural *-s*, past tense *-ed*, and third person singular *-s*.

Recommending Non-Dialect–, Non-Language–Specific Therapy Goals and Targets

Sample Report 1: Six-Year-Old African American Client with Significant Expressive Language and Phonologic Delays

Recommendation No. 1

Therapy using contrastive minimal word pair approaches should be considered for eliminating A.'s persisting use of inappropriate phonologic processes. Processes that should be targeted as a first priority include gliding, stopping of fricatives (with the exception of /ð, θ/), fronting and backing of sounds due to assimilation. . . . glottalization of final stops, and the insertion of the intrusive medial /t/. . . . Second priority should be given to omission of final voiced sounds and deletion of unstressed syllables. Because the use of these two processes can vary between different dialects of English, and A.'s dialect status is not clearly discernable at this time. . . .

Recommendation No. 2

Emphasis should be placed on increasing A.'s mean length of utterance and production of age-appropriate morphosyntactic forms through the use of naturalistic language activities conducted within a functional communication context. First priority should be placed on the stabilization of English grammar forms that are nondialect specific (obligatory in all dialects of English) such as the articles *a* and *the*.

Sample Report 2: Eight-Year-Old Bilingual English Vietnamese–Speaking Client with Autism

Recommendation No. 1

At this time, it is recommended that T. receive speech-language therapy services with goals focusing on (1) improving receptive and expressive vocabulary knowledge, (2) increasing speech intelligibility in connected speech, (3) improving social pragmatic skills, (4) increasing his average length of sentences, (5) increasing the use of more varied complex grammatical structures, and (6) producing sentences with appropriate use of object-noun phrases. Therapy should be conducted in English given that English is and always has been T.'s strongest language.

Recommendation No. 2

It is also recommended that T. continue to work on those English grammatical forms that may be the result of normal other language influences (e.g., third person singular -*s*, past tense -*ed*, and copula and auxiliary *be*) during normal classroom language arts activities.

14

Clinical Practice Issues

Priscilla Nellum Davis,
Betholyn Gentry, and
Pamela Hubbard-Wiley

To provide more effective service to multicultural clients, speech-language pathologists and audiologists have recognized the need to become more knowledgeable about various cultural groups. According to Taylor (1987), the clinical practice setting should be perceived as a social setting. Taylor (1987) has voiced consistent and constant concern over the neglect of the multicultural issues in clinical training and service delivery. The cultural views of clients and clinicians influence every aspect of the clinical setting. Clients engage in the therapy process based on their cultural beliefs and values. The activities, materials, and clinical procedures that professionals have been trained to use may be sources of cultural conflict for some clients from various cultural, ethnic, religious, and geographic backgrounds. As a result of these conflicts in the clinical setting, high absenteeism, tardiness, and termination of clinical services may occur. This chapter discusses cultural factors that affect the therapy process. It also provides a list of technologic resources available to assist the speech-language pathologist in providing culturally appropriate clinical services. *Ethnography* is the study of culture, the work of describing culture (Spradley, 1979), or the recording and description of the life ways of a people (Werner, & Bernard, 1989). The main purpose of ethnography is to understand a person's way of living and how it is alike or different from other cultures. Ethnography makes it possible to learn from other cultures. The people clinicians help have a way of life and a culture of their own. Ethnography offers the educator a way of seeing a school through the eyes of the students; it offers health professionals a way of seeing health and disease through the eyes of patients from a myriad of different backgrounds. Ethnography offers a pathway into understanding the cultural differences that make us what we are as human beings. Perhaps the most important force behind ethnography is the realization that cultural diversity is one of the greatest resources of the human species.

Religious Practices and Clinical Practice

Religious beliefs are cultural factors that have an impact on the delivery of clinical services. They influence what clients eat, what they wear, and how they participate in the clinical program. Clinical services are often given from the point of view of the religion of the clinician, with little attention to the religious views of the client. Our educational and clinical practices are based on a European-Christian model that may have been appropriate when most of the people living in this country were Christian descendants of Europeans. Demographic changes that have occurred, however, have made the United States a land of many peoples. The country is becoming more culturally diverse with many recent immigrants coming from non-European countries. Cultural diversity means an increase in religious diversity.

Little has been written about the impact of religious practices on clinical practices. Davis (1992) obtained information about the religious practices and belief practices of various religious groups and how they affect the delivery of clinical services, by using an ethnographic interview format. In this study, cultural informants were interviewed to obtain information about the impact of recognized religions on clinical service delivery. All informants were familiar with speech-language-hearing services and some of the activities used in the clinical setting. The informants stated that they were aware of some practices in mainstream America that were different from practices in their culture. The information that was given was based on experiences and opinions of the respondents to a hypothetical situation that showed the effect their religion could have on the delivery of clinical services.

A questionnaire format adapted from Taylor (1986) called *Cultural Identities, Values, and Rules of Interaction* was used in each interview for uniformity. Questions were asked concerning family structure, interpersonal relationships, decorum and discipline, foods, holidays and customs, values, and beliefs about health care. Questions included the following:

1. Who is considered part of the "family"?
2. What are the rights, roles, and responsibilities of the members of the family?
3. How do people greet each other?
4. Who may disagree with whom?

5. How are insults expressed?
6. How do people behave at home and in public?
7. What means of discipline are used?
8. Who has authority over whom?
9. What is eaten?
10. What foods are taboo?
11. What holidays are observed?
12. What are the concerns about medicine and health care?

The interviews also addressed how these factors could influence clinical services.

Information from the interviews with religious groups indicated a wide range of beliefs and practices that directly affected the delivery of clinical services. The religious preferences of the groups interviewed were shown to influence scheduling, test and therapy materials, interpersonal communication, and nonverbal interactions. Some of the major practices for each of the groups interviewed and the implications for speech-language therapy are discussed in the following sections.

Hinduism and Buddhism

Hinduism and *Buddhism* are among the most prominent religious or moral systems among Southeast Asian cultures. Many of their basic beliefs and principles are in conflict with clinical practices. Hinduism, or Brahmanism, is the major religion of India and is also found in Cambodia and Laos. It is the oldest religion still practiced in the world, with its roots dating to prehistoric times. Although most Hindus live in India, their literature and philosophy have influenced people throughout the world. Hinduism was not founded on the beliefs of one man but, rather, developed gradually over thousands of years and was shaped by many cultures, races, and other religions. It is associated with Indian philosophy, deities, and traditional worship of Brahma, the Supreme Being who is at once the Creator, the Preserver, and the Destroyer, with a different wife for each form he manifests. The views of Hinduism, or Brahmanism, are often combined with animism, in which it is believed that spiritual and supernatural powers are present throughout the universe and that all natural phenomena and things animate and inanimate possess an innate soul.

Buddhism, one of the major religions of the world, was founded in India in approximately 500 BC by a teacher called *Buddha*. The nearly 200 million followers of Buddhism live or have their roots in Southeast Asia and Japan. More than 780,000 followers of Buddhism live in the United States (*The World Almanac*, 1997).

At various times, Buddhism has been a dominant religious, cultural, and social force in most of Asia. There are two branches of Buddhism: (1) Mahayana, or Great Vehicle, is prominent in Vietnam, China, Japan, and Korea and (2) Hinayana, or Little Vehicle, flourishes in Cambodia, Laos, Burma, Thailand, and Sri Lanka. Buddhist doctrine is summarized in the four noble truths:

1. All life is suffering.
2. Suffering is caused by desire or attachment to the world.
3. Suffering can be extinguished and attachment to all things can be overcome by eliminating desire.
4. To eliminate desire, one must live a virtuous life (Chan, 1992).

The Buddhist goal is to be released from the wheel of life, or circle of reincarnation, and reach *nirvana*. Nirvana is a state of complete redemption wherein all suffering is transcended and one's soul is merged into the cosmic and only true reality.

Buddhism, together with the teachings of Confucius, Lao-Tzu, and the tenet of ancestral worship, has a profound influence on the lives of Asians. Confucius founded Confucianism in 551 BC. Its major beliefs involve individual virtue and the moral fabric of a society. Believers of the teaching of Confucius embody five virtues that are embodied in the duties owed to parents and ancestors and reverence for ancestors whose spirits must be appeased. Ancestral worship is characterized by three basic assumptions: (1) All living people owe their fortunes to their ancestors, (2) all departed ancestors have needs that are the same as the living, and (3) departed ancestors continue to assist their relatives in the world, just as their descendants can assist them. With such belief in the connection of all things living and dead, it is not surprising that there are many clinical practices that conflict with Buddhist beliefs.

Among the populations that speech-language pathologists and audiologists serve are three general ethnicities in the Asian community: (1) Pacific Islander, mostly Hawaiians, Samoans, and Guamanians; (2) Southeast Asians, largely comprised of Indo-Chinese from Vietnam, Thailand, Cambodia, Laos, and Burmese and Filipino; and (3) East Asians, including Chinese, Japanese, and Korean.

The following factors are important in the delivery of clinical services to those who practice Confucianism, Buddhism, or the Hinduism beliefs. They are not meant to be all inclusive nor are they meant to apply to all persons who observe these religions. They are intended as a guide to assist the clinician in determining the most culturally appropriate mode of service delivery.

1. Most Buddhists and Hindus are vegetarians and eat diets of vegetables and grains. Meats are not included in the diet. Meat should be avoided in

activities, especially beef, because cows are thought to be sacred. Scenes and stories that depict the killing of animals should be avoided. Hindus believe that all life is sacred; therefore, they do not eat fish, chicken, shellfish, or any animal that is killed and eaten. Additionally, stories commonly used in children's books such as monkeys and snakes should be avoided. Monkeys and snakes are also thought to be sacred.

2. Knowledge of kinship terms is important. There is a strong belief in the importance of ancestors. The birth of a child and the death of an elder are significant events.

3. No photographs or videotapes should be taken of some female Hindu clients. Photographs of women are to be looked at only by male family members or other women. Care must be taken to obtain permission before audiotaping, videotaping, or photographing female clients. Male clinicians should exercise caution and ask for permission before photographing or videotaping.

4. Strict rules govern the relationship between the sexes for Buddhists and Hindus. Men and women are not permitted to work together and do not touch each other. Opposite-sex clinicians would not be permitted to work with some Hindus.

5. The head is the purest body part, because it contains the human spirit. Patting a child's or adult's head is a great offense. Explanations should be given when touching the head is required in speech-language therapy, audiologic testing, or oral peripheral examinations. Permission should be granted before engaging in any activity that involves touching the head.

6. It is considered rude to blow one's nose, talk loudly, or show one's teeth in public. This can have an impact on the client's willingness to participate in an examination of the oral mechanism or to increase vocal intensity as part of an evaluation for voice disorder. In addition, the clinician can mistake decreased vocal intensity for a pathology rather than a cultural behavior.

7. Show respect for elders. Never address elders by their first names unless given permission to do so. Use Mr., Mrs., Miss, or other appropriate titles with the family name for Chinese and Koreans to establish the connection with the ancestors (e.g., Tien Chang-Lin would be addressed as Mrs. Tien). For Cambodians, Laotians, and Vietnamese, use the first or given name. For example, Kamchong Laungpraseut would be addressed as Mr. Kamchong. Clinicians should refrain from addressing clients or their parents by their first name. This is especially important for elderly clients or new immigrants. Clinicians should also greet family members in order of age, beginning with the oldest man present. Samoans and other Asian groups allow older children to control young siblings, allowing parents the freedom to participate in religious, social, and cultural events. These siblings may

discipline and punish their younger brothers and sisters. Southeast Asians adhere to a strict social order and will consider the teacher or clinician an authority figure. Education is valued very highly, so these students or clients will be very cooperative. Sometimes they may be too polite to tell you they do not understand instructions or reports, but they will smile and nod. Do not take for granted that you are always understood. Pay particular attention to signs of hearing loss. The incidence of hearing impairment is high in this group. Difficulty in understanding is increased by this problem. Often Southeast Asians will not give eye contact as a sign of respect.

8. Conversations with clients and the family should begin with small talk before initiating the topic of the conversation or "getting to the point" for most Asian cultures. Some cultures take offense at brief exchanges using short declarative language. They may require more polite or indirect interactions. Direct or corrective feedback may embarrass some clients or students (Hites & Casterline, 1986).

9. Guests are welcomed warmly and invited to share in whatever meal the family has prepared. To decline the invitation to share the family meal or other food offerings is considered rude to the host or hostess.

10. Buddhists celebrate a special 3-day holiday in August. New Year's Day, the first day of the first month of the lunar calendar, is another holiday on which devout worshipers go to the shrine to pray.

11. The third, fifth, and seventh birthdays of children are important celebrations for Buddhists. Families travel to shrines on these birthdays to pray for the development of the young child.

12. Red is the color of good luck and represents life for most Asian cultures. White is the color of mourning and represents death. Wearing white medical smocks may be seen as a sign that the client is approaching death.

Islam

Islam was founded in the seventh century in the Empire of the Caliphs, which stretched from Spain and Morocco across the Middle East to central Asia. People who practice the religion of Islam are called Muslims or Moslems. There are nearly 500 million Muslims in the world today. They form the majority of the population in the Middle East; North Africa; and Southeast Asian nations such as Pakistan, Malaysia, and Indonesia. Islam is the fastest-growing religion in the United States, largely because of the increase of immigration of people from the Middle East and the conversion of many African Americans to Islam.

Followers of Islam believe that God gave his final revelation to the prophet Mohammed, who they believe to be the last in a succession of prophets, including Moses and Jesus. The *Koran*, the holy book containing

Mohammed's revelations, is believed to be the full expression of the divine will for human life (Sharifzadeh, 1992). Followers of Islam believe in the strength of the family and children and that wealth and children are the ornaments of this life (University of Virginia, 1997).

Muslims follow the lunar calendar, which is based on the phases of the moon. Each New Year begins on the second new moon after the winter solstice or any time between January and March.

Ramadan is a month-long observance of dedication and self-control. Because the time of Ramadan is determined by the lunar calendar, it begins on a different date each year on a solar or a Christian calendar. During Ramadan, no food or drink is consumed from sunrise to sunset. Children are required to participate for specified periods of time until they are 8 or 9 years of age. Children from the age of 8 or 9 years through adolescence are expected to participate from sunrise to sunset. Those who are ill or who have medical concerns are permitted to not observe Ramadan at all or to participate on a limited basis. A large feast is held on *Eid-al-Feter* to mark the end of the month of Ramadan.

The following practices have been suggested for consideration by speech-language pathologists by Muslims from India, Kuwait, Saudi Arabia, Pakistan, and Africa currently living in the United States. Because many Muslims are from different cultural and geographic regions, some of the following information may be based on culture rather than on religion:

1. No pork or food products containing pork should be used in clinical activities. Items such as bacon and sausage should not be included when discussing breakfast foods.

2. Religious and secular activities related to Christian holidays, such as Easter and Christmas, should be avoided.

3. Adult clients may observe Ramadan and may refuse food or water during the month-long observance. Although those with health problems are excused from the practice, many may wish to observe the fast on a limited basis. Children are not required to participate in the observance, but some alteration in family patterns during the holiday period may still exist.

4. Activities using violence or advocating hunting for sport should not be used. Animals are killed only for food, and religious teachings dictate how animals should be killed. Giving animals humanlike characteristics and other forms of anthropomorphism is discouraged by some Muslims. For example, stories that use animals, such as a talking cat, may be taboo. Stories such as *The Three Little Pigs* should never be used.

5. Activities about dressing and clothing should be used carefully. Devout Muslim women do not wear revealing clothes and often cover their faces. Activities involving dressing or bathing dolls should be avoided, unless previously discussed with parents and clients. Teaching body parts using

anatomically correct dolls should be avoided. The use of cosmetics in language lessons is discouraged (i.e., lessons teaching face parts by using lipstick and eye shadow with female clients should be avoided).

6. Friday is the Muslim Sabbath; it is called *Jum'a*. Some Muslims have restricted *Jum'a* celebrations to 1:00 PM on Friday afternoons. Others may celebrate *Jum'a* at a different time, depending on the time zone. Some Muslims agree to diagnostic and intervention sessions on Friday and others do not. Devout Muslims pray five times daily, with special prayers at sunrise, noon, and sunset. This can affect scheduling options.

7. Islamic religions allow no physical contact between men and women in public. Women do not give orders or instructions to men. If services for a female client by a male clinician are accepted, strict rules would require that a parent or a family member be present at all times.

8. Elders are considered authorities. Older clients may not comply when younger clinicians, especially female clinicians, give instructions or use direct requests with imperatives. Indirect requests and suggestions are more desirable methods.

9. Extended families are common. Family members other than the parents may be included in conferences. Fathers or the oldest males make the decisions regarding members of the family. Their presence is essential to the service-delivery process (i.e., at family conferences, individualized education program and individualized family service plan conferences, and whenever decisions are made about scheduling and treatment techniques).

10. Knowledge of kinship terms is important. For example, different names may be used for the maternal or paternal grandparent. In addition, because polygamy is still practiced in some Muslim cultures, children may have more than one mother. Terms such as *senior mother* and *natural mother* may be used.

11. Touching, hugging, and gazing are considered overly familiar behavior, especially among members of the opposite gender. Men do not establish eye contact with women. To show respect for women, men avert their gaze. To show respect for adults, children do not look adults directly in the eyes. In conversational discourse and the clinic setting, lack of eye contact from the client is considered respectful. In Ghana, when children are verbally reprimanded, the child is supposed to kneel at the feet of the elder. A child from Ghana would not look a teacher or clinician in the eye as he or she was being corrected.

12. Home visits are not encouraged. Because some Muslims view the home as private, business activities are not to be conducted in the home by outsiders. Some parents prefer to come to the clinic rather than have the clinician visit them at home. Friends, usually people of the same religion, may

make unannounced visits. Outsiders, people who are not Muslims, are expected to wait for an invitation or to make an appointment.

13. Because it is thought that the Koran is carried in the head, touching, hitting, or patting the head should be avoided.

14. Devout Muslims believe that only *Allah* knows the future. Muslims, therefore, do not plan more than a few weeks ahead. Discussing long-term educational plans for infants may not seem important to parents and caregivers.

15. Use of the left hand to pass items is considered rude. When handing items to someone, place the item in the person's hand, not on the table or counter. To place materials, papers, and instrumentation on the counter is considered rude and offensive.

Judaism

Judaism is the religion of approximately 15 million people worldwide. There are more than 5 million Jews in the United States. Judaism is the oldest religion of the Western world and the first to teach monotheism. It is founded on the laws and teachings of the Hebrew Bible, or Old Testament, and of the Talmud. Christianity and Islam are both derived from Judaism, even though they both differ in many basic beliefs and practices. Because Jews do not recognize one single authority, they have found it possible to differ about their religion and still remain Jews. Today these differences are expressed through four major religious groups: Hasidic, Orthodox, Conservative, and Reformed.

Orthodox Judaism and Hasidic Judaism are two distinct branches of Judaism. Theologically, Orthodox Jews strictly adhere to the teachings of the Written Law (the Torah) and Oral Law (the Talmud). In practice, they can be modern or more traditional. Orthodoxy, in part, defined itself in light of the growing Reform movement in Germany in the eighteenth century (Chosen Peoples Ministries, 2001).

Hasidic Judaism was founded in Poland in 1760 by a charismatic revivalist leader named Eliezer Ba'al Shem Tov. He inspired a popular movement among the Jewish people of Eastern Europe by stressing that God and the Torah (the five books of Moses) were accessible, not only to rabbinic scholars but also to all. Today, Hasidic Judaism is like Orthodoxy in that it places great stress on the study of the Torah and Talmud.

Orthodox Jews represent a branch of Judaism that resists most change. They believe that they are observing the law as handed down to Moses on Mount Sinai. Orthodox Jews are the most devout. They observe all Jewish laws, including kosher dietary restrictions such as not eating pork or shellfish. They do not allow meat and dairy products to be served on the same dishes or to be served in the same meal. Many Orthodox Jews maintain two separate sets of dishes: one for meat meals and one for dairy meals.

Orthodox Jews observe all Jewish holy days. Jewish holidays are Rosh Hashanah, Yom Kippur, Succoth, Shemini Atzeret, Simchat Torah, Hanukkah, Passover, and Shavuoth. Each holiday begins at sunset of the day before the holiday. Orthodox Jews observe the Sabbath starting at sundown on Friday. Restrictions on the Sabbath include all forms of work, including riding in automobiles or pushing elevator buttons.

Conservative Jews accept Jewish law as the primary Jewish expression of all time. They observe many, but not all, Jewish holy days and may observe the dietary restrictions only during periods associated with the major holy days (e.g., Hanukkah, Yom Kippur, and Rosh Hashanah).

Reformed Jews are the largest and fastest-growing Jewish movement (Hoffman, 1993). They are the most assimilated into American society. They believe that Jewish tradition constantly changes. They emphasize the need to interpret tradition from the perspective of individual conscious and informed choice. They may not follow all kosher dietary restrictions or strictly observe the rules of the Sabbath. They observe only the major Jewish holy days, such as Hanukkah, Rosh Hashanah, and Yom Kippur. The following information may not apply to all Jewish groups but should serve as a guide during clinical services.

1. Judaism has strict dietary rules. Pork and shellfish should not be discussed as a part of a therapy session. Mixing or serving food dishes that include meat and dairy products are forbidden. Orthodox and Conservative Jews strictly observe all dietary rules. Reformed Jews may or may not observe the dietary rules in accordance with their religious convictions. Activities and foods used in the therapy setting should be selected with these considerations in mind.

2. Orthodox and Reformed followers of Judaism observe Jewish holidays and nonsectarian American holidays.

Guidelines for Culturally Relevant Intervention

Furst (1971) and Bull, Montgomery, and Kimball (2000) identified teaching guidelines for working with culturally diverse populations in classrooms. They are applicable to clinicians as well. These guidelines can be adapted for the multicultural clinical setting. For successful intervention, the following guidelines should be observed:

1. *Present clear explanations of objectives.* The clinician should make sure the client understands the objective of the assessment and treatment pro-

gram. Asians prefer that the professional assume authority and provide clear and full information, such as what will be provided by and what is expected from each person attending the meeting, therapy session, or conference.

2. *Use methods and procedures that do not violate the beliefs of the client.* A cultural informant could be used to assist the clinician in selecting culturally appropriate methods and materials. Clinicians should respect a client's religious and spiritual beliefs and values, including taboos. Many Asians have difficulty accepting disabilities, school failure or mediocre performance, and speech and language disorders, because they think of these disorders as bringing shame to the individual and the family. Be sensitive in reporting diagnostic findings. Special effort should be taken to explain to the family that cognitive, language, speech, and hearing impairments are not a source of shame, and cooperation between the family and the professionals can resolve or reduce the impact of many of them.

3. *Be flexible in selecting materials and activities.* Clinicians should be willing to vary the therapy content and teaching style as needed. The learning environment should allow the client to be creative and motivated to take communication risks in the setting. Although an organized training program is desired, clinicians should be willing to change the content and activities as the situation dictates. Clinicians should adapt materials to the needs of the particular client. Learning style differences may provide significant information about how the client learns. Several inventories are available to help a client determine his or her learning style. A comprehensive list of learning styles is provided by the Arizona State University website. For information about learning styles, see http://www.asu.edu/upfd/online_resources/student_styles.html. Another website from San Jose State University (http://www.engr.sjsu.edu/nikos/courses/me111/resourc.htm) provides instruments and surveys that can be taken by you or by your students or clients. Note that teachers usually teach the same way that they learn. If you learn a certain way, then be careful not to teach only to students who learn the way you do. Learning resources from the University of Toronto website can be found at http://snow.utoronto.ca/Learn2/resources/stylelinks.html.

4. *Be flexible in scheduling.* Avoid scheduling therapy on a Sabbath or on religious holidays, when possible. Some absenteeism will be unavoidable when therapy falls on holidays. American Indians, African Americans, and some Hispanic groups have an elastic concept of time (e.g., they believe they have kept the appointment if they arrive 5–15 minutes after the scheduled appointment time or any time within a flexible time period; they may consider it permissible to arrive between 2:00 and 3:00 PM for a 2:30 PM appointment). Therefore, they may arrive late for an appointment without apologizing. Some Asians and Pacific Islanders view time as a solution to

some problems. In due time changes will occur whatever the outcome was meant to be. If a person has too many obligations for a particular time period, then whatever goal was obtained was meant to happen. Therapy sessions and conferences may be missed for these reasons. Some Asian and Pacific Islanders, such as the Hmong, believe time itself can solve problems better than human intervention and, therefore, do not like to move quickly to solve problems (Schwartz, 2001).

5. *Interact with clients according to their perception or expectation.* In some cultures, the clinician's showing enthusiasm, vigor, or confidence is a sign of competence. In other cultures, touching, showing enthusiasm, using elevated pitch, and "gushing" over babies may be offensive. Some Native Americans do not permit hugging, kissing, and excessive handling of their babies by strangers. Hugging and patting children on the head are forbidden in some Asian cultures.

6. *Be businesslike and task oriented.* Clients need to feel that the clinician has a purpose for activities and lessons. Examples from real-life situations could show the importance of the lesson and how to use the new information appropriately. Some individuals need to be shown how certain activities fit into their lifestyles and how they relate to the intervention process. When selecting play-based assessment and intervention, parents should be made aware of the value of play and the information that can be gained by the clinician while using this style. Some cultures such as African American consider play as "just messing around."

7. *Use praise and encouragement.* Criticism should be used wisely and sparingly. Too much negative criticism is not good. Some criticism, however, is desirable, in that it reinforces and encourages the flow of communication. The clinician can never give too much praise and encouragement. In some groups, a negative report of progress can result in punishment of the child. Some Asian and Pacific Islanders are embarrassed when praised before their peers. Praise and comments should be given in private (Huang, 1993).

8. *Provide opportunities to learn.* In the therapy setting, the clinician should create a warm environment that enriches the social interaction and accepts the client's culture and communication style. The client should have many opportunities to communicate. Activities should relate to the client's cultural patterns, customs, values, and holidays. Parents from various ethnic groups such as African American, Native American, and Hispanic have reported how initially they were "flattered" when asked to share information about their culture to becoming "empowered" and politically active to make sure that their culture is included and that their needs are met.

9. *Preview and review lessons.* Repetition and variety have been suggested as key factors to aid learning. Tell the clients what the lesson is about

and why it is important. Review concepts discussed. The review may help clarify any concepts that are not clear. Clients from some cultures are taught to review by repeating material themselves. Including the client as a participant in the review process can reinforce main points and give an opportunity for feedback where clarification is needed.

10. *Use multiple levels of questions or cognitive discourse.* Knowledge and use of different styles is important to increase the client's repertoire of useful language. Simplification of adult speech, repetition of phrases, expansions, and filling in omissions are ways that adults interact with young children. Knowledge of cultural activities and various speaking needs should be used to demonstrate different pragmatic aspects of language. The clinician should teach concepts in different settings and different ways. Clients should be taught according to learning styles (Dunn & Dunn, 1999).

The inclusion of multiculturalism into intervention is a concept that has gained widespread support. According to the Individuals with Disabilities Education Act (1997), knowledge of various cultures is necessary to provide more effective service delivery. Cultural competence is a goal for individuals as well as organizations. Therapy techniques, as well as environment, should create a feeling of inclusion that reflects the recognition and appreciation of diversity in America. By using a culturally competent approach to service provision, therapy becomes more relevant and interesting to clients (Lynch & Hanson, 1992; Tiedt & Tiedt, 1990). Additionally, this approach promotes understanding of other groups and reduces potential racial conflicts. Addressing every possible source of cultural conflict that could occur in the therapy process is beyond the scope of this chapter. The following sections, however, provide additional suggestions that the clinician can refer to when serving a client from a different culture. In the clinical setting, the actual physical environment, activities, food, music, play, literature, toys, animals, holidays, and parental involvement are important considerations in the therapy setting.

Physical Environment

Waiting rooms and therapy rooms should be inviting and inclusive, reflecting an appreciation for multiculturalism. Signs and leisure reading materials should be available in the languages of the clients served by the clinical program. Informational materials such as developmental charts, videos, and other educative literature should also be available in the language of the clients in the community. Therapy rooms should be decorated with culturally relevant and appropriate pictures that reflect a multicultural society. Large pictures and posters are available that depict persons with various racial and ethnic backgrounds, genders, and disabilities living in varied communities and performing a variety of activities. Pictures should show nuclear families, extended families, multigenerational families, families with a person with disabilities, and families with mixed races. These pictures can be used to elicit language, as well as to make the therapy room appear inclusive. Pictures that may be culturally offensive, such as animals depicted as humans, should be avoided.

Clinic forms, signs, and documents should be available in languages common to the community. Intake forms could be developed to provide information on the client's country of origin, ethnic affiliation, the family and community support system, languages spoken in the home, food preferences and prohibitions, preferred toys and leisure activities, and names and roles of persons in the home and family. Many children are being reared or cared for by grandmothers who may be called *mommy* or a very young mother who may be called by her first name. Clarifying family roles avoids confusion, particularly when considering the genetic history of the client.

Therapy Activities

Knowledge of cultural differences and similarities can enhance clinical service delivery. Clients can be encouraged to share information about their culture with the clinician and other clients. Clients, students, and parents who participate in culture-sharing activities report that they no longer feel invisible and that they feel empowered and a part of the process. Information from various cultural groups can be found at http://www.plazaco.com/communities and used in the therapy setting.

Food

Culture can be incorporated into intervention programs by introducing food items likely to be found in the client's household while teaching basic vocabulary. For example, many Japanese families consume noodles as a staple for breakfast, lunch, and dinner. Likewise, many Hispanic families consume beans (*frijoles*) as a staple (Baedeker, 1993). Hawaiian children eat *musubi* for a snack. An increasing number of families rely on fast-food establishments for breakfast, lunch, and dinner. Actual food items can be tasted and experienced in the therapy setting. Permission should first be obtained from the parents, however, to determine whether there are any types of foods that are not permitted. Attention also should be given to family dining patterns. In some homes, meals are served as a formal family event with established routines. In others, food is consumed when individuals are hungry or in less formal situations. Culturally relevant therapy facilitates carryover of the speech and language objectives into the home.

Play

All children engage in some form of play. Differences may occur with the type of play exhibited by children from different cultures. Swick (1987) discusses how children in New Guinea play games in which neither side wins. A game will end only when both sides achieve equality. This can be contrasted with Western games that strongly encourage competition and winning. Shigaki (1991) observed that Japanese child care providers communicate different cultural values to children than American child care providers and encourage the children to engage in shared or group activities promoting the importance of the group and interdependence of the group, as opposed to independence and self-reliance. Schwartzman (1983) found that children from poor working-class families engage in very creative and imaginative play using items from the environment. Symbolic play is also discouraged in some cultures. For a clinician to encourage it could be a potential conflict. This is found with some African Americans and Europeans from the United Kingdom who discourage imaginative play and view it as an overactive imagination. Some parents stated that imaginary play led to lying and deceitful behavior. Play is essentially a way for young children to practice the roles and skills they will need as adults, and the behaviors will vary from culture to culture. In a therapy setting, a dramatic play area or an opportunity to engage in different types of play will enable the clinician to accurately assess the levels of play or to enhance cultural awareness through play. Kendall (1983) suggests that the materials in the dramatic play area be changed periodically to reflect different styles of living, such as providing different types of food and clothing. The objectives for these sessions should be explained.

Music

Music is an integral social construct to all groups and can be incorporated into therapy activities. Popular styles of music such as rap have been found to be effective in teaching different language concepts. This is often the music listened to by many African American and non-African American children and young adults in the home. Producers who specialize in educational music for children have replicated this style of music in formats easy for children to comprehend. Popular music is an excellent way to promote language and include culture in therapy. The clinician could encourage children to write their own songs about assigned concepts or topics.

Literature

Culturally relevant literature can provide an excellent introduction for reinforcing culture while teaching various aspects of language. There are many books available that teach and promote culture while providing interesting stories for all ages. Concepts taught include nouns, verbs, sequencing, retelling stories, predicting outcomes, discussing feelings, inferences, idiomatic expressions, and so on. Resources for literature are presented in Appendix 14-1.

Toys

Toys are an integral component of therapy when working with children. Although many toys are appropriate, culture differences and preferences in the selection process should be taken into consideration. Animals and dolls are probably used more frequently than other types of toys. There are many dolls and other playthings that reflect various racial and cultural groups. Dolls should look like the clients of various races and skin tones, and forms of dress are available. For example, many African American dolls have braids and wear colorful clothing, whereas others are more mainstream in appearance. Many doll makers produce dolls that distort and magnify facial and physical characteristics of African Americans and other racial groups. They may be offensive to some clients and their families. Time should be taken to select dolls that are appealing to children and create an accurate reflection of the racial group for which they are intended.

Animals

The use of animals to stimulate language is appropriate for all groups. However, culture again influences the types of animals used in therapy. Some Muslim groups consider it an anthropomorphism taboo to give animals humanlike characteristics. Animals such as the cow that is held sacred by Hindus should not be included in therapy. Some American Indian tribes consider the owl to be a bad omen or evil force. Some groups do not have cats or dogs as pets. Asians and Arabic cultural groups are more likely to have birds as pets.

Holidays and Special Celebrations

Most cultural groups have holidays and special celebrations, such as *Cinco de Mayo*. Clinicians can use these events and celebrations to incorporate a multicultural theme into the clinical program. However, care should be taken to avoid focusing on religious holidays. It is also important to note that some fundamental and religious groups such as Jehovah's Witnesses do not celebrate any holidays, including birthdays. Halloween, for example, is a religious holiday celebrated by many people as a secular celebration. Some groups forbid the celebration of Halloween because of the frequency of "devil" themes. Many Native Americans link misfortune and etiology of disabilities to witchcraft, spirit loss, spells, and other supernatural causes. A witch on a broom or a clinician pretending to be a witch in the clinical setting may be perceived as offensive. Clinicians should refrain from Halloween decorations, which could be offensive to others. Instead, themes of fall can be used, including, for example, harvest themes, pumpkin pies, and leaves instead of jack-o-lanterns.

New immigrants may not understand holidays with a connection to American History. Regardless of the holiday that the clinician emphasizes, it should be kept in mind that newly arrived immigrants might be unfamiliar with many of the American holidays. It should not be assumed that clients are familiar with the concepts of American history and historical figures such as George Washington, Abraham Lincoln, or even Martin Luther King, Jr. The therapy session can be used to instruct new immigrants in the cultural icons of the country. A Thanksgiving meal can be provided with foods representing the various cultures. A culturally competent therapist would ensure that all cultural groups and their contributions to America are included.

The following are holidays and celebrations important to several cultural groups:

> *Kwanzaa* is an African American cultural celebration that was started in 1966 by Dr. Ron Maulana Karenga. This celebration begins on December 26 and ends on January 1. It celebrates cultural tradition, the strength of the family, and unity. It is neither a religious holiday nor a substitution for Christmas.
>
> *Cinco de Mayo* is a widely commemorated Mexican holiday, celebrated in honor of the Mexican army's victory over the French in the Battle of Puebla in 1867. Although properly a Mexican celebration, it has become increasingly popular in the United States, especially in areas bordering Mexico.
>
> The *Lunar New Year* is the principal holiday for many Asians. The Chinese usually celebrate this day in February, depending on the moon. Cambodians and Laotians celebrate their New Year's Day in the fifth month of the lunar calendar, which usually occurs in mid-April, shortly after harvest time (Tijero, 2001).

There are many cultures in the United States. Thematic units can be developed that incorporate multiculturalism in everyday activities. The clinician should be careful not to take culturally specific information and apply it to every member of a cultural group. The value of cultural knowledge is that it raises or poses questions that should be considered and underscores our desire to respond sensitively and competently to our clients.

Parental Involvement

Some cultures view parental involvement differently from what some professionals expect. Some groups may not feel comfortable participating in planning individualized education plans or articulation or phonologic exercises for practice at home. In general, some groups such as Asian and Pacific Islanders see the clinician as the utmost authority over the child's education or intervention program. They believe that parents are not supposed to interfere with this process and may regard clinicians who seek parental involvement as incompetent (Schwartz, 2001). It is important to explain that parental involvement is important in the treatment program. However, because the level of parental involvement varies with cultures, parents and caretakers should be involved in the clinical process according to their cultural values.

Learning Styles

Not all people learn in the same way. There are many styles of learning. Dunn and Griggs (1988) described learning styles in terms of how the individual's ability to learn new or difficult material is affected by the following variables: (1) the immediate environment (noise level, temperature, amount of light, and furniture design); (2) emotionality (degree of motivation, persistence, responsibility, and need for structure); (3) sociological needs (learning alone or with peers, learning with adults present, and learning in groups); (4) physical characteristics (auditory, visual, tactile, and kinesthetic strengths; best time of day for learning; need for food and drink while learning; and mobility requirements); and (5) psychological inclinations (global and analytical strengths).

Most Americans have been educated using one teaching style. There is no one teaching style that is best for all people. It is important to determine what teaching style works best for a particular individual. Carbo and Hodges (1988) determined that many children with behavioral impairments and at-risk children have been taught using teaching styles that are at odds with their learning styles. In the clinical setting, a communication gap can exist between the teaching style of the clinician and the learning style of the client.

Anderson (1988) determined that there are different learning styles across multicultural groups. White children do best on analytic tasks—that is, they learn material that is inanimate and impersonal more easily, and their performance is not greatly affected by the opinions of others. Many Mexican American, Puerto Rican, and African American children are thought to be more global in their learning styles.

In the clinical setting, cultural and cognitive conflicts occur when a client is asked to perform in a manner and setting that is different from the style that he or she prefers. Using therapy techniques based on an analytical learning style in the clinical setting can place some clients at a disadvantage. According to Anderson (1988), what is a valuable and valid communication process under one cognitive style becomes a deformed example of cognitive or linguistic deficits under another.

Clinicians should be aware of cultural differences in learning styles. Carbo and Hodges (1988) suggested that instruction should be based on learning styles. For example, for the global learner, the following approaches should be used: (1) listening to and reading good literature, (2) acting in plays, (3) creating models, (4) drawing pictures and writing about them, and (5) using puppets as characters in storytelling activities.

Some professionals incorporate information about learning styles into their clinical programs. Others question the appropriate use of these models. Caution should be taken when using and interpreting the information. The following strategies, adapted from Carbo and Hodges (1988), are suggestions for considering the preferred learning styles of clients in clinical intervention:

1. Determine what learning style the client uses most often during the assessment or intervention program. Most information available on the different ethnic groups, with the exception of the Asian group, suggests that analytic styles are not preferred. Many inventories are available online and available for downloading. The following inventory can be submitted and automatically scored on the Internet (Soloman & Felder, 1999).

2. Explain the purpose or goal of the treatment session. Share the results of the assessment with the client. If an ethnographic interview is performed, then the clinician should discuss how cultural views differ and make every effort to include the cultural views of the client in decisions about therapy and materials. Objectives should be structured, flexible, and clearly stated. Provide clear and full information, such as what will be provided and what is expected from each person in the meeting. Deal with immediate needs and give concrete advice.

3. Incorporate action involvement with clear objectives that relate to real life in therapy sessions. Act out situations, model, use pantomime, and use songs and chants to help the client relate therapy to real life. Demonstrations and motor and kinesthetic approaches that involve the hands and the whole body should be used rather than drills, work sheets, and board games.

African American students seem to prefer motor and kinesthetic approaches rather than sitting quietly listening to stories. Variety and action are the key words for successful intervention sessions.

4. Allow clients to work in a cooperative style with peers, friends, or adults. Some school-age clients may want a friend or buddy to accompany them to the therapy session. Other may not. Most individuals from non-Western countries prefer to work with others in groups and to help others in a cooperative style. Competitive activities should not be used.

5. Use stories, storyboards, and picture stories rooted in the client's culture whenever possible.

6. Structure real-life situations to teach pragmatic skills. These situations can be set up, for example, in group settings, special field trip assignments, role playing, films and videotapes, and storytelling.

7. Be sensitive when asking groups for information. Some adults have had negative experiences with authoritarian or social systems and may resist attempts to reveal personal information.

References

Anderson, J. (1988). Cognitive styles and multicultural populations. In L. Cole (Ed.), *Communication sciences and disorders: Marketing careers to minority students*. Rockville, MD: American Speech-Language-Hearing Association.

Baedeker, K. (1993). *Baedeker's Mexico*. Englewood Cliffs, NJ: Prentice Hall.

Bull, K. S., Montgomery, D., & Kimball, S. L (2000) Working with culturally diverse students. In Oklahoma State University (Ed.), *Quality University instruction: A teaching effectiveness training program*. Stillwater, OK: Oklahoma State University.

Carbo, M., & Hodges, H. (1988). Learning styles and strategies can help students at risk. *Teaching Exceptional Children, 55,* 55–56.

Chan, S. (1992). Families with Asian roots. In E. W. Lynch & M. J. Hanson (Eds.), *Developing cross-cultural competence: A guide for working with young children and their families* (pp. 181–257). Baltimore: Brookes.

Chosen Peoples Ministries (2000). http://www.chosen-people.com.

Davis, P. (1992). Clinical practice issues. In D. Battle (Ed.), *Communication disorders in multicultural populations* (pp. 306–316). Boston: Andover Medical Publishers.

Dunn, R., & Dunn, K. (1999). *The complete guide to the learning styles inservice system*. Boston: Allyn & Bacon.

Dunn, R., & Griggs, S. A. (1988). The learning styles of multicultural groups and counseling implications. *Journal of Multi-Cultural Counseling and Development, 17,* 146–153.

Furst, N. (1971). *International analysis in teacher education: A review of studies.* Washington, DC: Washington Association of Teacher Education in Collaboration with ERIC Clearinghouse of Teacher Education.

Hites, J. M., & Casterline, S. (1986). *Adapting training for other cultures.* Paper presented at NSPI Annual Conference, San Francisco (ERIC Document Reproduction No. ED 274 879).

Hoffman, L. (1993). *What's a Jew?* New York: Macmillan.

Huang, G. (1993). *Beyond culture: Communicating with Asian American children and families* [On-line]. Available: http://www.ed.gov/databases/ERIC_Digests/ed366673.html.

Individuals with Disabilities Education Act. (1997). (20 U.S.C.) [Sec. 1400, 1411–1420 and 1471–1485]. Available: http://www.ed.gov/offices/OSERS/IDEA/the_law.html.

Kendall, F. E. (1983). *Diversity in the classroom. A multicultural approach to the education of young children.* New York: Teachers College Press.

Lynch, E., & Hanson, M. J. (1992). *Developing cross-cultural competence: A guide for working with young children and their families.* Baltimore: Brookes.

Palacios, A. (1993). *VIVA MEXICO! A Story of Benito Juarez and Cinco de Mayo.* New York: Steck-Vaughn Company.

Schwartz, W. (2001). *A guide to communicating with Asian American families* [On-line]. Available: http://eric-web.tc.columbia.edu/guides/pg2.html.

Schwartzman, H. B. (1983). Child-structured play: A cross-cultural perspective. In F. Manning (Ed.), *The world of play* (pp. 25–33). West Point, NY: Leisure Press.

Sharifzadeh, V. (1992). Families with Asian roots. In E. W. Lynch & M. J. Hanson (Eds.), *Developing cross-cultural competence: A guide for working with young children and their families* (pp. 319–352). Baltimore: Brookes.

Shigaki, I. (1991). An examination of social interaction and play activities of infants and toddlers in Japanese day care. (ERIC Document Reproduction Service No. ED 338419).

Soloman, B. A., & Felder, R. M. (1999). *Index of learning styles questionnaire* [On-line]. Available: http://www2.ncsu.edu/unity/lockers/users/f/felder/public/ILSdir/ilsweb.html.

Spradley, J. P. (1979). *The bilingual child.* New York: Academic.

Swick, K. (1987). *Perspectives on understanding and working with families.* Champaign, IL: Stipes.

Taylor, O. (1986). *Treatment of communication disorders in culturally and linguistically diverse populations.* San Diego: College Hill.

Taylor, O. (1987). Communication as a social process. In G. Cole & V. Deal (Eds.), *Communication disorders in multicultural populations.* Unpublished manuscript. Rockville, MD: American Speech-Language-Hearing Association.

Teidt, P. L., & Tiedt, L. M. (1990). *Multicultural teachings: A handbook of activities, information and resources* (3rd ed.). Boston: Allyn & Bacon.

Tijero, K. (2001). *New Year's around the world* [On-line]. Available: http://www.proteacher.com.

University of Virginia. (1997). *The* Koran *at the Electronic Text Center, University of Virginia* [On-line]. Available: http://etext.lib.virginia.edu/koran.html.

Werner, O., & Bernard, H. R. (1989). Short take 13. *Ethnographic Sampling Cultural Anthropology Methods, 1*(1), 461.

World almanac and book of facts, The. (1997). New York: Press Publishing (The New York World Almanac, 1997, p. 463).

Additional Resources

ADL: A World of Difference Institute: http://www.adl.org/frames/front_awod.html.

ADL Education Department Front Page: http://www.adl.org/frames/front_education.html.

Blackburn, J. (1992). *Hispanic play*. Minisession within the session, "Multicultural Play," at the American Association for the Child's Right to Play. Denton, TX.

Ebbeck, F. N. (1971). Learning from play in other cultures. *Childhood Education, 48*(2), 69–74.

Electronic Magazine of Multicultural Education: http://www.eastern.edu/publications/emme.

Hinduism Today: http://www.HinduismToday.kauai.hi.us/ashram/.

Lundsteen, S. (1997). *Multicultural play awareness* [On-line]. Available: http://www.earlychildhood.com/articles/multplay.html.

Multicultural Art Lessons for K-12: KinderArt: http://www.kinderart.com/multic.

Multiculturalism: http://www.fortunecity.com/millenium/garston/49/multi.html.

Preschool Activities for Small Groups: http://www.preschoolrainbow.org/activities-small.htm.

Swick, K. (1991). *Teacher-parent partnerships to enhance school success in early childhood education*. Washington, DC: National Education Association (ERIC Document Reproduction Service No. ED 339 516).

Swick, K., & Graves, S. (1993). Empowering at-risk families during the early childhood years. Washington, DC: National Education Association (ERIC Document Reproduction Service No. ED 360 093).

World Community Access: http://www.plazaco.com/communities.

Appendix 14-1

Resources for Information on Cultural Awareness

In addition to the therapy activities listed in this chapter, there are many resources available to the clinician that provide information, instruction, and education about cultural awareness. With the availability of information on the Internet, clinicians have a wealth of information at their disposal. The following list of resources includes books and website addresses for more information.

Books

Buchman, D. (1994). *Family fill-in book: Discovering your roots.* New York: Scholastic. *A book that provides an opportunity for children to engage in discussions with parents about family history and roots.*

Hudson, W. (1993). *I love my family.* New York: Scholastic. *A book for primary-age children that talks about family pride.*

Lynch, E., & Hanson, M. (1992). *Developing cross-cultural competence: A guide for working with young children and their families.* Baltimore: Brookes. *A landmark resource that provides strategies for effective cross-cultural interactions with families of young children who may be at risk for speech-language and hearing problems. Each of eight chapters describes a particular cultural group, including Anglo-European, Native American, African American, Latino, Asian, Filipino, Native Hawaiian and Pacific Islander, and Middle Eastern. Chapters describe geographic and historical origins, values, beliefs, and language and provide recommendations for effective cross-cultural interaction.*

Randall-David, E. (1989). *Strategies for working with culturally diverse communities and clients.* Baltimore: Association for the Care of Children's Health. *A guide to train project participants in learning principles applicable to working with families caring for children from diverse cultures. Exercises are provided that are designed to increase cultural awareness of the importance cultures play in shaping attitudes, values, and practices. Cultural awareness should lead to more culturally appropriate community outreach and culturally sensitive health care.*

Multicultural Websites

The following is a list of websites providing information about more than 20 languages and cultures. The information provided in these websites may be of interest to people learning a language or looking for more information about a specific country or culture. *Please keep in mind that many websites change, move, or are down or discontinued; however, at the time of this writing, the websites listed in this appendix are accurate.*

Languages

The Computer Clubhouse. http://www.computerclubhouse.org/about1.htm. *"An after-school learning environment where young people explore their own interests and become confident learners through the use of technology." Contains games and activities for children for a variety of cultures.*

Honouring Diversity—A cross-cultural approach to infant development for babies with special needs: A handbook from the Centennial Infant and Child Centre. http://cicc.on.ca/pub.htm.

Internet resources for Latin America. http://lib.nmsu.edu/subject/bord/laguia/.

Multicultural education resources. http://www.udel.edu/sine/educ/mult-cult.htm. *"Presents resources available on the Internet to support Multicultural Education."*

Multicultural pavilion: Defining multicultural education. http://curry.edschool.virginia.edu/go/multicultural/initial.html. *This website provides resources on multiculturalism to educators.*

Multicultural studies—Selected Asian, Latino, and Native American resources on the web. http://www.lib.umich.edu/rrs/classes/multicul-as-lat-nat.html.

Resources in area & ethnic studies. http://www.swarthmore.edu/Library/Interdisc/area.html. *Provides links to World Wide Web, gopher, and Telnet resources of ethnic interest (African American, Asian, Latino, Native American, multicultural).*

Voice of the shuttle: Minority studies page. http://vos.ucsb.edu/shuttle/minority.html. *Provides links to general resources websites and to African American, Asian American, Chicano, Latino, Hispanic, immigrant/refugee, Jewish, Native American and Native Alaskan (also includes world indigenous and aboriginal cultures), Pacific, and other (minority cultures in Europe) websites.*

Bilingualism

Baharona Center for the Study of Books in Spanish for Children and Adolescents. http://www.csusm.edu/campus_centers/csb/index.html.

Bilingual Education Resources on the Internet. http://www.edb.utexas.edu/coe/depts/ci/bilingue/resources.html.

Bilingual families web page. http://www.nethelp.no/cindy/biling-fam.html. *A place for bilingual parents to find information and resources to help them raise their children bilingually.*

Estrellita: accelerated beginning Spanish reading. Bilingual education resources on the net. Links readers to other Web pages that have information on bilingual education. http://www.estrellita.com/bil.html.

National Clearinghouse for Bilingual Education (NCBE). http://www.ncbe.gwu.edu/. *Used to collect, analyze, and disseminate information relating to the effective education of linguistically and culturally diverse learners in the United States.*

When English is the foreign language. http://www.overlode.com/net1.html. *Teacher training for ESL students—multicultural classrooms.*

Hispanic Culture

Index search of Latino websites. http://latino.sscnet.ucla.edu/.

Resources for Spanish language and literature. http://www.library.vanderbilt.edu/central/span.html.

African American Culture

African and Asian languages program. http://www.registrar.northwestern.edu/nucatalog/catalog9799/cascourses/afrasilanguage.html.

African Studies Center at the University of Pennsylvania. http://www.sas.upenn.edu/African_Studies/AS.html.

Melanet's Watoto World. http://www.melanet.com/watoto/watoto.html. *Website for children, parents, and educators of African descent.*

The Universal Black Pages. http://www.ubp.com.

Asian American Culture

African and Asian languages program. http://www.registrar.northwestern.edu/nucatalog/catalog9597/cascourses/afrasilanguage.html. "*Offers an opportunity to explore through language study some of the fascinat-*

ing cultures that are most vital for Americans to understand: those of Africa, China, Japan, Korea, and the Middle East."

Asian American Internet sites. http://latino.sscnet.ucla.edu/Asian.links.html. *Provides links to listservs, websites, and newsgroups.*

Asian American resources. http://www.mit.edu:8001/afs/athena.mit.edu/user/ i/r/irie/www/aar.html.

AsiaRain automated translators. http://sg.jobstreet.lycosasia.com/jobs/2000/ a/asrinsga3.htm. *"Specializes in large-scale translation for technical documents and software messages from English to Chinese and other Asian Languages."*

Translation, Theory, and Technology home page. http://www.ttt.org. *Simple notices and communications can be sent to parents who need messages in their own language.*

Native American Culture

American Indian Heritage Foundation. http://www.indians.org/.

Beaded Lizard web designs. http://www.kstrom.net. *American Indian arts page.*

The Flags of the Native American People of the United States. http:// users.aol.com/Donh523/navapage/index.html.

General Resources

Cecelia Bard Multicultural Library for Peace. Adults and children and adolescents. http://www.buffalostate.edu/library/collect/bardadult.html; http:// www.buffalostate.edu/library/collect/bardchild.html. *These sites provide resource and reference material for African American, Asian, Gay and Lesbian, General reference, Latino, Native American, religious, and women's issues.*

15 □□□
□□□
□□□

Research Involving
Multicultural
Populations

Theodore J. Glattke

The history of research addressing communication disorders in multicultural populations is short, sparse, and confounded by many conceptual and methodological issues. In 1994, the American Speech-Language-Hearing Association's (ASHA) Multicultural Institute entitled *Challenges in the Expansion of Cultural Diversity in Communication Sciences and Disorders* sought to address issues relevant to culturally sensitive and appropriate research design. The Institute participants could not find evidence of a tradition of research regarding multicultural issues in the mainstream scholarly publications that addresses communication sciences and disorders. A negligible proportion of the literature (25 of more than 1,000 citations) relevant to communication disorders in multicultural populations could be traced to referred scholarly journals that focused on communication sciences or disorders (Glattke, 1994). The vast majority of the literature in communication sciences or disorders seemed to be in the form of books, editorials, or articles in professional magazines, few of which were archived and few of which were indexed and available through search engines. This stood in contrast to sources of information from scholarly journals dealing with medicine, public health, counseling, psychology, linguistics, special education, early intervention, and related fields.

Improvements have occurred in the past few years: Work addressing multicultural issues is only beginning to find its way into the ASHA scholarly journals. An Ovid (Copyright 2000–2001, Ovid Technologies, Inc., New York, NY) search of the *Journal of Speech-Language-Hearing Research* in the 4-year period of 1997–2000 reveals that only 10 of 413 (2.4%) manuscripts contained words or phrases such as *ethnic, minority,* or *African American.* No abstract contained words or phrases such as *multicultural, Hispanic,* or *Chinese American.* An important improvement is that electronic indexes include many more publications than were available previously. A decade ago, publication of new data in a chapter in an edited series or book was equivalent to consigning the information to outer space: It was difficult to locate without reading the source completely, and such contributions are rarely cited by other authors who make later contributions to edited series or books. Improvements in the scope of electronic search engines such as the PsychINFO Database Record (Copyright 2000, Washington, DC: American Psychological Association) have helped to make this literature more accessible to consumers.

There is no single source of information that will provide a map to enable an investigator to anticipate all of the issues that must be addressed to conduct research in an unbiased manner. There is a dynamic, changing understanding of the interplay among issues of cultural and language diversity and obtaining accurate health and related history information, performance of individuals on standardized tests, approaches to intervention, and many other facets of communication disorders (e.g., Alberts, Davis, & Prentice, 1995; Corson, 2001; Gonzalez-Calvo, Gonzalez, & Lorig, 1997; Wilkinson & King, 1987). Among the most common challenges is the need to account for demographic variability that can confound studies that attempt to isolate race or culture as a variable (Sue, 1983). Stated another way, if race is used as an "independent variable" in research, then often there is an underestimation of within-group variation (Wyatt, 1991).

Another less obvious complication can emerge. As Wilkinson and King (1987) noted, any definitions of participant groups on the basis of racial, ethnic, or cultural features carry the risk that interpretation of the data will reflect the beliefs of the dominant culture or, at least, the culture of the investigators. Buchanan, Moore, and Counter (1993) cited a 1964 investigation that explained differences in hearing sensitivity between African American and white men in terms of the "natural habitats" of the African Americans, as well as their closer relationships with "animal predators." If the studies had been conducted within a more rigorous framework, then interpretation of the findings in terms of noise exposure, diet, medical condition, and many others might have brought the interpretation of the study to a better conclusion. Sue (1983) provides a thoughtful discussion of the process of comparing white and nonwhite that may lead to interpretation of differences as deficiencies.

Culture is not static. The characteristics of all people are products of their histories and experiences in their countries of residence, as well as the values and beliefs that are kernel to their traditional cultures (Sue, Chun, & Gee, 1995). *Acculturation*, or the modification of beliefs and behavior of persons from one culture as the result of exposure to a different culture, confounds efforts to identify groups of subjects solely on the basis of ethnicity, even when attempts are made to control for variables such as income and education levels (dela Cruz, Padilla, & Agustin, 2000). The very concept of race also can be challenged. Sue, Kuraski, and Srinivasan (1999) identify several issues that stem from attempts to designate race or ethnicity: (1) Differences in physical characteristics are often matters of degree; (2) recognition of any number of races is arbitrary; (3) behavioral researchers rely on self-identification rather than biological markers to categorize study participants; (4) members of the same racial group may have markedly different ethnic backgrounds; and (5) members of an ethnic group may be from more than one race.

Creating a Representative Sample

Historically, research community in the United States had systematically ignored large portions of the population since the founding of the National Institutes of Health (NIH) in the 1950s. Factors such as the prevalence of coronary artery disease in women, differential rates of hypertension in African Americans and people of European origin, and many other major health issues drove a political process that led to passage of Section 492B of the Public Health Service Act, aided by the NIH Revitalization Act of 1993, Public Law 103-43. In response, the NIH developed guidelines for insuring that women and members of federally designated, underrepresented minority populations were included in research supported by the NIH.

The *NIH Guide* (National Institutes of Health, 1994) contains regulations regarding the inclusion of women and members of underrepresented minority groups in research supported by the NIH. The regulations include the following introductory comments:

> Since a primary aim of research is to provide scientific evidence leading to a change in health policy or a standard of care, it is imperative to determine whether the intervention or therapy being studied affects women or men or members of minority groups and their subpopulations differently. To this end, the guidelines published here are intended to ensure that all future NIH-supported biomedical and behavioral research involving human subjects will be carried out in a manner sufficient to

elicit information about individuals of both genders and the diverse racial and ethnic groups and, in the case of clinical trials, to examine differential effects on such groups. (National Institutes of Health, 1994, p. 2)

The *NIH Guide* also states:

> While the inclusion of minority subpopulations in research is a complex and challenging issue, it nonetheless provides the opportunity for researchers to collect data on subpopulations where knowledge gaps exist. (p. 16)
>
> It would also be appropriate for researchers to test survey instruments, recruitment procedures, and other methodologies used in the majority or other population(s) with the objective of assessing their feasibility, applicability, and cultural competence/relevance to a particular minority group or subpopulation. This testing may provide data on the validity of the methodologies across groups. (p. 17)
>
> An important issue is the appropriate representation of minority groups in research, especially in geographical locations, which may have limited numbers of racial/ethnic population groups available for study. The investigator must address this issue in terms of the purpose of the research, and other factors, such as the size of the study, relevant characteristics of the disease, disorder or condition, and the feasibility of making a collaboration or consortium or other arrangements to include minority groups. (p. 17)
>
> NIH interprets the statute in a manner that leads to feasible and real improvements in the representativeness of different racial/ethnic groups in research and places emphasis on research in those subpopulations that are disproportionately affected by certain diseases or disorders. (p. 18)

NIH guidelines underscore the importance of proactive sampling to insure that research results are generalized appropriately. As reviewed by Walders and Drotar (2000), investigators who wish to create samples that are representative of the population must address several challenges. Traditional methods of developing a sample were created for the convenience of the investigator (Foster & Martinez, 1995). One common example involves obtaining normative data from children enrolled in a large school district. Reliance on this method may define the sample in terms of social, economic, and other factors that will bias the outcome. In addition, it excludes individuals who have dropped out of school or who have poor attendance (Walders & Drotar, 2000). Often, research that appears to be inclusive on the surface cannot be applied generally. For example, an investigation involving American Indians that sampled only individuals living in urban settings would not be representative of persons living in rural areas of reservations. Comparisons of American Indians in the southwestern United States with white people living in the northeastern United States will be compromised by environmental factors. Investigations of Hispanics must include Mexican Americans, Puerto Ricans, and immigrants from Cuba and Central and South America or be limited in their interpretations. An investigation of Asian and Pacific Islander participants cannot ignore historical, political, economic, cultural, and other factors that contribute to the diversity among immigrants from those regions of the world. Sasao and Sue (1993) observe that representative sampling requires considerable effort and will probably increase the cost of the investigation. Sue, Kuraski, and Srinivasan (1999) argue that investigators should receive training in techniques such as ethnography, and the research team should include individuals who are familiar with the population so that viewpoints of cultural "insiders" can be represented.

The regulations and guidelines spawned by the legislation and responses of federal agencies are producing tangible results that have a positive impact on communication sciences and disorders. For example, persons interested in studying speech, hearing, or language disorders can adopt strategies used by epidemiologists to orchestrate formal investigations and guide individual clinical practice. Lubker (1997) and Antoniadis and Lubker (1997) describe the principles of epidemiology and illustrate how those principles can create a lattice to support steps designed to describe and prevent communication disorders. Various facets of the discussion address topics such as: (1) descriptive versus experimental investigations, (2) perceptions of populations, (3) efficacy of treatment, (4) identification of new disorders, (5) surveillance issues, (6) risk factors, and (7) contrasts between affected and nonaffected populations. In one example of the application of those principles, Tomblin, Smith, and Zhang (1997) investigated prenatal and perinatal risk factors associated with specific language impairment. They studied the speech and language status of 7,218 monolingual English-speaking children in three Iowa population centers. Their findings suggested that factors associated with the parents of children with specific language impairment had a greater association with the occurrence of specific language impairment than factors occurring during fetal development or the perinatal period.

More recently, Shriberg, Tomblin, and McSweeny (1999) conducted an investigation of speech delay in children that is an example of an excellent response to the NIH sampling requirements. They obtained data from a large (more than 1,300) group of children who were a subset of the larger population studied by Tomblin, Smith, and Zhang (1997). The subjects represented a range of socioeconomic, racial, and cultural backgrounds and were selected to reflect the 1990 census. For example, the distribution of African American and white participants in the sample was 11.6% and 88.5%, respectively. Other factors such as gender, education level, income per capita, and ratio of income to poverty threshold were also used to make the sample representative of the census data. The care used in construction of the sample allowed the authors to report the prevalence of speech delay in 6-year-old monolingual English-speaking children. Their findings can be generalized to the larger population because of their sampling methods.

Moore (1999) explored relationships among ethnicity and conductive hearing loss in a large-scale (more than 3,000 people) investigation of American Indian, Inuit, and nonnative individuals distributed across the age range of preschool to adult. Because of her sampling techniques, she was able to parcel out the relative contributions of ethnicity, relevant medical history, age, and gender. Moore (1999) suggests that the study results cannot be generalized to the population at large, but her findings indicate that the Inuit patients are at higher risk for development of hearing loss resulting from chronic otitis media than the other groups. Although all participants lived in the Canadian Arctic, Moore (1999) notes that environmental factors such as wind conditions in various settlements, sunlight (and resultant activity), and smoking habits could have contributed to the results. In spite of their limitations, the investigations of Shriberg and co-workers (1999) and Moore (1999) have tremendous strength because of the representative sampling and large numbers of participants that were included.

Protection of Human Subjects

Another area that has received renewed attention in recent years is the protection of human subjects. In 1974, the NIH created an expert panel to develop recommendations regarding the ethical treatment of humans who participate in research. The experts met at the Belmont Conference Center of the Smithsonian Institution between 1976 and 1979 and created the *Belmont Report* (U.S. Department of Health, Education, and Welfare, 1979). The *Belmont Report* addresses differences between practice and research, basic ethical principles, and applications of the general principles to issues related to obtaining informed consent, costs and benefits to participants, and selection of subjects. The principles articulated in the *Belmont Report* stem from the Nuremberg Code, developed after the trials involving medical personnel who were responsible for experimentation on concentration camp prisoners. The code, adopted in 1947, provides the framework for basic protection and includes provisions requiring (1) informed consent, (2) participation of volunteers without coercion, and (3) avoidance of physical and mental suffering.

The ethics of researchers in the United States have been brought into question on a number of occasions in which individuals were denied proper medical treatment or exposed to risk without their consent. Regrettably, the most notorious of these actions involved racial or ethnic minorities or individuals who were not competent. For example, an experiment used African American men to study the course of syphilis while depriving them of effective treatment in order not to interrupt the project, long after such treatment became generally available (Jones, 1993). As Dunn and Chadwick (1999) note, development and adoption of the Nuremberg Code had no impact on the study, which continued until 1973. Dunn and Chadwick (1999) review other investigations conducted in the 1960s, such as the Jewish Chronic Disease Hospital Study, in which patients were injected with live cancer cells and the Willowbrook studies that involved the intentional infection of children in a mental hospital with hepatitis. Parents who wished to have their children accommodated in the Willowbrook facility were coerced into giving their permission.

In the vast majority of instances, research involving communication sciences and disorders will not pose a great risk to the health of the participants. Nonetheless, investigations that address development or disruption of communication skills involve two vulnerable populations: children and older individuals. The *Belmont Report* states,

> Respect for Persons—Respect for persons incorporates at least two ethical convictions: first, that individuals should be treated as autonomous agents, and second, that persons with diminished autonomy are entitled to protection. The principle of respect for persons thus divides into two separate moral requirements: the requirement to acknowledge autonomy and the requirement to protect those with diminished autonomy. An autonomous person is an individual capable of deliberation about personal goals and of acting under the direction of such deliberation. To respect autonomy is to give weight to an autonomous persons' considered opinions and choices while refraining from obstructing their actions, unless they are clearly detrimental to others. To show lack of respect for an autonomous agent is to repudiate that person's considered

judgments, to deny an individual the freedom to act on those considered judgments, or to withhold information necessary to make a considered judgment when there are no compelling reasons to do so.

However, not every human being is capable of self-determination. The capacity for self-determination matures during an individual's life, and some individuals lose this capacity wholly or in part because of illness, mental disability, or circumstances that severely restrict liberty. Respect for the immature and the incapacitated may require protecting them as they mature or while they are incapacitated.

There are many concerns that emerge from these ethical considerations. For example, is it sufficient to have the spouse of a patient who has had a stroke give permission for the patient to participate in research on aphasia? If an investigator wishes to obtain a family history from a study participant, then should all members of the family give their permission? Should an Asian American child for whom English is a first language agree to involve his or her parents who do not speak English in an investigation?

The *Belmont Report* continues by stating that it is the responsibility of the researcher to "learn what is harmful" and to avoid harming the people who are recruited into investigations. In the study of human communication, this translates to developing an understanding of the impact of the experimental situation on the participant. Members of various ethnic groups may view offering an "incorrect" answer on a test as anything from inconsequential to devastating. Using individuals who can guide the investigators in determining the impact of test situations on participants is essential (Hughes, Seidman, & Williams, 1993; Sturm & Cahagan, 1999). In addition, there is a significant risk that test protocols may not be valid when used in multicultural situations.

Obtaining a Valid Measure

Validity of a measure refers to its conformity with truth. Measures of human performance that are based on data collected from "normal" members of a mainstream population pose particular difficulties if one wishes to apply them to diverse populations. As Sue, Kuraski, and Srinivasan (1999) state, the adaptation of such measures requires demonstration of equivalence in terms of (1) concept, (2) language, (3) socioeconomic factors, and (4) metric outcomes.

A fundamental obstacle to the conduct of bias-free research in a multicultural environment is the fact that concepts are not equivalent across cultures

(Brislin, 1993). For example, reaction time is thought to be a manifestation of competency—that is, rapid responses are desirable in the mainstream population of the United States. Other cultures that place a value on reaction time may believe that a pensive, articulate, and delayed response to a question or other stimulus is the preferred way to respond. American Indian participants may prefer to delay a response for a longer period of time than that used by white participants or expected by white experimenters (Tharp, 1989). Test requirements that appear to emphasize autonomy or competition among participants will create a conflict for persons such as American Indians or Asians whose orientation is toward community cooperation rather than accomplishments of an individual (Sue, Kuraski, & Srinivasan, 1999).

Related to the transfer of a concept between cultures is the significance (or lack thereof) that may be attributed to a behavior. As Finn and Cordes (1997) have reviewed, the rich history of studies of cultural perspectives on stuttering provides a lesson in this area. Wendell Johnson's assertion that "The Indians have no word for it" fueled a debate that spanned four decades (Johnson, 1944; Zimmermann, 1985; Zimmerman, Liljeblad, Frank, & Cleeland, 1983). The debate provides an excellent chronology of the slow death of a bias and a snapshot of the diversity of views among "one" group of people (American Indians).

Establishing equivalency of language also poses a difficult challenge. If the concepts incorporated in the test instrument can be transferred between cultures, then, according to Herrera, Delcampo, and Ames (1993), the investigator should (1) translate the instrument into the second language, (2) arrange for a retranslation into the original language, and (3) conduct field tests to insure that both forms are equivalent. Sue, Kuraski, and Srinivasan (1999) point out that the back translation should be undertaken by individuals in the target population group to help insure that ambiguous portions of the test instrument are interpreted consistently and accurately. They argue that translators who are highly skilled and experienced may be able to interpret translations that are very poor, whereas members of the target population would have difficulty with the same material.

The influence of socioeconomic factors on the applicability of a test instrument is complicated and is affected by the status of the ethnic groups that are included. For example, a vocabulary test that uses pictures of modern plumbing fixtures would probably not produce valid results among members of a group that has no indoor plumbing. Similarly, images of sophisticated consumer appliances are unlikely to elicit "correct" answers from persons who have no commercial electrical service.

Finally, the numerical or metric outcomes of standardized tests that have been translated or otherwise modified to try to improve their application across cultural boundaries must be considered with great care. A classic overview of the application of numbers to measurement in the field of experimental psychology was provided by Stevens (1951) approximately 50 years ago. Nicholas Schiavetti and Dale Metz provide a modern overview of the same issues (Schiavetti & Metz, 1997). Following Stevens' (1951) lead, we categorize numbers according to how they can be applied to measurements or by the arithmetic power that characterizes each category. The scales are: *nominal, ordinal, interval,* and *ratio.* Standard scores on behavioral tests, such as vocabulary tests, and scaling of features of speech (e.g., intelligibility, fluency) are examples of interval scales. Because the choice of a starting point for an interval scale is arbitrary, a researcher can only add and subtract numerical outcomes. Just as adding 50 degrees to 50 degrees will produce a sum of 100 degrees, so will adding standard scores produce a valid sum. What *cannot* be done with interval data is arrive at mathematically valid conclusions about the products or quotients, on one hand, and the observed behavior on the other. It is common practice to submit interval data to statistical analyses that involve multiplication and division (e.g., the mean score was 1,000, the standard deviation was 100). It is not logical to conclude that someone with a score of 1,000 is twice as intelligent (fluent, hoarse, intelligible, and so on) as a person with a score of 500 on the same test. Perhaps more importantly, the examiner must decide whether an interval increase has the same meaning along the entire scale and whether the interval has the same meaning on a translated test as on the original version. The numbers that represent the outcomes of such tests are often put into play as variables in statistical analyses with little thought about how they should be interpreted.

The two general types of statistical analyses are called *parametric* and *nonparametric* (Schiavetti & Metz, 1997; Siegel, 1956). Nonparametric analysis is appropriate for nominal and ordinal data. The nonparametric analysis techniques allow an investigator to compare the frequency with which scores, or differences in scores, occurred among the participants of the investigation with outcomes that might be expected by chance. Alternatively, scores may be compared through a correlation procedure that is based on rank order. Parametric analysis is the most powerful and requires that the information submitted to analysis be interval or true ratio data. The data should be distributed according to a so-called "normal" distribution in which the scores that occur most frequently are located in the middle of the range between low and high scores. Parametric analysis also requires a relatively large group of participants so that inferences may be made with respect to the population at large. Many of these requirements are difficult to address adequately because of the lack of true interval or ratio power in the numbers produced by the measurements. For example, if an examiner believes that a change in intelligence quotient score of 50–60 is equivalent to a change from 95 to 105 or from 140 to 150, then he or she might apply parametric statistics to such scores. If the examiner does not believe that the 10-point changes reflect equivalent shifts in intelligence, then the application of parametric analysis to such scores would be questionable. The interpretation of test outcomes is confounded when "standard" tests are translated into other languages. Individuals that produce the translated versions must demonstrate that the distribution of responses to the translated test items mirror the distribution of responses on the first edition of the test. Without that evidence, the equivalence of the translated form remains undemonstrated. Many lines of evidence demonstrate that members of linguistic minority groups perform differently on standard tests as a byproduct of test norms that were not inclusive and not due to any disorder, impairment, or disability (Cole & Taylor, 1991; Stockman, 1996; Taylor & Payne, 1983). Hence, a standard test may incorporate a bias that creates a numerical difference that may be "significant" in a statistical sense but leads the investigator and the consumers of research information down the wrong path.

General Investigation Design

Investigations reported in professional and scholarly literature in communication disorders are usually descriptive in nature. The title of the work often takes the form "The effect of *this* on *that*" in which "this" and "that" are so-called variables. The typical investigation incorporates one or more participant characteristics selected by the investigator. Participants may be grouped according to such factors as age, gender, grade in school, handedness, medical condition, race, culture, or ethnicity, and the groups represent the investigator's attempt to account for the independent variable that is of interest. Each participant then undergoes some sort of measurement (e.g., hearing test, vocabulary test, intelligence quotient test), and the results are sorted according to the participant's position within the independent variable classifications. The test outcome is presumably influenced by the independent variable. During a typical investigation, a set of observations is made, often based on norm-referenced test materials, and the outcomes are described in the context of characteristics of the participants. Or, the observations may be repeated after the participants have been allowed to receive a treatment, attend a class, reach a certain age, or undergo some other intervention. The addition of the intervention or other control for the participant characteristic adds an experimental component.

In practice, many investigations are blends of descriptive and experimental strategies. Experimental studies, or combinations of descriptive and experimental strategies, are usually designed to test a set of assumptions or a hypothesis. Developing a research strategy that allows one to address a significant question related to participant characteristics seems easy, but the task is very difficult.

Ethnographic investigations, long accepted in anthropology and related fields, are appearing in increasing numbers in journals related to communication (e.g., Aoki, 2000; Sanger, Creswell, Dworak, & Schultz, 2000; Young, Ackerman, & Kyle, 2000). An ethnographic study involves the systematic description of a particular group of persons. Under ideal circumstances, an ethnographer will obtain data by using techniques that do not alter or intrude on the typical behavior of the persons who are studied. Sue, Kuraski, and Srinivasan (1999) note that issues related to the "objectivity" and efficiency of ethnographic studies often pose challenges for investigators.

The anthropology and related literature carries frequent references to *emic*, as in phon*emic* versus *-etic*, as phonetic studies. The former are characterized as "qualitative" and the latter as "quantitative" investigations. Sue, Kuraski, and Srinivasan (1999) argue that emic or culture-specific research permits the investigator to "discover" concepts that might remain unrevealed by more structured quantitative approaches. Open-ended or structured interviews and the use of focus groups are two approaches that are currently popular. Using either of these techniques poses special challenges in many ethnic groups. For example, structured interview situations may be uncomfortable for members of cultures that rely on lengthy narratives to exchange information. Rules that govern speaking will affect the dynamics of members of a focus group.

Zane and Sue (1986) describe three ways to address research questions in a multicultural environment. These are called *point*, *linear*, and *parallel*. Most descriptive studies involve a point design in which an attempt is made to develop group comparisons on one set of issues. The issues are usually defined in terms of the majority culture, and care must be taken to insure that equivalent concepts are recognized in the other cultures. The linear techniques involve following up on the initial findings of a study by attempting to stratify the members of each cultural group according to a relevant criterion. For example, if the prevalence of some communication disorder seemed to be different when two groups were compared, then one would want to insure that the groups were matched for other factors that might influence the prevalence figures. Ideally, the linear approach would stem from concepts that emerge from the cultures that are studied, rather than from the majority viewpoint. The parallel approach encourages in-depth or linear studies of each of the cultures that is of interest, so that the opportunity for concepts peculiar to the individual cultures to emerge is maximized. The World Health Organization

(2000) is in the process of revising the *International Classification of Functioning, Disability and Health*, and the debate regarding the use of labels such as impairment, disability, and handicap, included in the 1980 version, may be helpful. In the draft document (World Health Organization, 2000), "activity limitation" replaces *disability*, "participation restriction" replaces *handicap*, and impairment is used in a context of a deviation in structure. The debate over terminology is driven by the desire to neutralize the terminology when it translates into languages other than English.

The individual chapters in this text provide the researcher with a rich fund of information regarding concepts, communication strategies, and assessment and treatment approaches for people whose beliefs, attitudes, and actions emerge from several different cultures. Individuals who wish to embark on nonbiased research must be mindful of the information that is peculiar to each and will find the type of information included in the text to be helpful when considering research involving groups that are not represented. Among the recurring suggestions are these:

1. Follow social customs regarding dress, forms of greeting, turn-taking, and questioning of study participants.
2. Ensure that the tasks requested of the study participants are appropriate for their life experiences and permissible within their cultures.
3. Determine whether the responses anticipated from the participants are compatible with their cultural norms in terms of verbal and non-verbal communication, timing, and other factors such as perceived competition.
4. Conduct the research in the first language of the participants, if possible; recognize that "literal" translations may not convey the meaning of the test items across languages.
5. Recognize that taking a risk is not valued in the same way by all cultures and that "guessing" to respond to a test item may be at variance with acceptable behavior.
6. Learn about and control for the interaction of the study participants with the experimenter based on such factors as gender, age, ethnicity, place of origin, and race.
7. Acknowledge that cultures vary in terms of the significance that is attached to differences in behavior or physical makeup.
8. Respect the definition of privacy that may be associated with a particular group of people, the autonomy of each individual, and individual value systems.
9. Construct a representative sample; sampling should be dictated by the research question, not by convenience.

10. Frame the research question by scientific and ethical considerations, not by availability of participants.
11. Do no harm.
12. Appreciate that people can be *wronged* but not *harmed*.

As Dunn and Chadwick (1999) note, the risks of biomedical research are often limited to the participants in the experiment, but the risks of behavioral research extend to others, including social groups, ethnic populations, and even entire societies.

Georg von Békésy received the Nobel Prize for Medicine and Physiology in 1961 for his work on the basic mechanisms of the auditory system (von Békésy, 1960). In the Introduction to *Experiments in Hearing*, von Békésy stated

> When a field is in its early stage of development the selection of good problems is a more hazardous matter than later on, when some general principles have begun to be developed. (von Békésy, 1960, p. 4)

von Békésy listed eight types of problems ranging from (1) the "classical problem" to (8) the "pseudo problem." In his view, investigators hammered away at the classical problem for years without reaching a solution (von Békésy, 1960). The lowest rank was reserved for the pseudo problem, which often is an assertion made in the form of a question (e.g., "Don't you think that . . . ?"). The pseudo problem usually provides a platform for the questioner to restate a set of beliefs, rather than sets the stage for a new research direction. Between the two end points, he cited problems that extend from premature to unimportant and earmarked a special category called the "embarrassing question, commonly arising at meetings in the discussion of a paper and rarely serving any useful purpose" (von Békésy, 1960, p. 5). von Békésy's (1960) view has as much currency today as it did 40 years ago. We must use care so that we identify important problems, frame questions in ways that allow answers to emerge, and exercise extreme caution to avoid pseudo problems. If we fail to exercise appropriate caution, then we not only risk arriving at conclusions that are incorrect but also may be responsible for placing misinformation in the public domain that will be used in an uncritical way by consumers of our scholarly and professional literature. The description, measurement, and interpretation of communication behaviors for research purposes must be guided by the sensitivities that should underlie the clinical diagnostic and treatment procedures used by our professions.

References

Alberts, F. M., Davis, B. L., & Prentice, L. (1996). Validity of an observation screening instrument in a multicultural population. *Journal of Early Intervention, 19*(2), 168–177.

Aoki, E. (2000). Mexican American ethnicity in Biola, CA: An ethnographic account of hard work, family and religion. *The Howard Journal of Communications, 11*(3), 207–227.

Antoniadis, A., & Lubker, B. B. (1997). Epidemiology as an essential tool for establishing prevention programs and evaluating their impact and outcome. *Journal of Communication Disorders, 30*(4), 269–284.

Brislin, R. (1993). *Understanding culture's influence on behavior.* New York: Harcourt Brace Jovanovich.

Buchanan, L. H., Moore, E. J., & Counter, S. A. (1993). Hearing disorders and auditory assessment. In D. E. Battle (Ed.), *Communication Disorders in multicultural populations* (pp. 256–286). Boston: Andover Medical Publishers.

Cole, P. A., & Taylor, O. L. (1991). Performance of working class African American children on three tests of articulation. *Language, Speech and Hearing Services in the Schools, 21*(3), 171–176.

Corson, D. (2001). *Language diversity and education.* Mahwah, NJ: Lawrence Erlbaum Associates.

dela Cruz, F. A., Padilla, G. V., & Agustin, E. O. (2000). Adapting a measure of acculturation for cross-cultural research. *Journal of Transcultural Nursing, 11*(3), 191–198.

Dunn, C. M., & Chadwick, G. (1999). *Protecting study volunteers in research.* Boston: CenterWatch, Inc.

Finn, P., & Cordes, A. K. (1997). Multicultural identification and treatment of stuttering: A continuing need for research. *Journal of Fluency Disorders, 22,* 219–236.

Foster, S. L., & Martinez, C. R., Jr. (1995). Ethnicity: Conceptual and methodological issues in children's clinical research. *Journal of Clinical Child Psychology, 24,* 214–226.

Glattke, T. J. (1994, January). *Cultural sensitivity and appropriate research designs.* Presented at ASHA Multicultural Institute: Challenges in the Expansion of Cultural Diversity in Communication Sciences and Disorders, Sea Island, GA.

Gonzalez-Calvo, J., Gonzalez, V. M., & Lorig, K. (1997). Cultural diversity issues in the development of valid and reliable measures of health status. *Arthritis Care & Research, 10*(6), 448–456.

Herrera, R. S., Delcampo, R. L., & Ames, M. H. (1993). A serial approach for translating family science instrumentation. *Family Relations, 42,* 357–360.

Hughes, D., Seidman, E., & Williams, N. (1993). Cultural phenomena and the research enterprise: Toward a culturally anchored methodology. *American Journal of Community Psychology, 21,* 729–746.

Jones, J. H. (1993). *Bad blood. The Tuskegee syphilis experiment.* New York: Maxwell McMillan International.

Johnson, W. (1944). The Indians have no word for it. *Quarterly Journal of Speech, 30,* 330–337.

Lubker, B. B. (1997). Epidemiology: An essential science for speech-language pathology and audiology. *Journal of Communication Disorders, 30*(4), 251–267.

Moore, J. A. (1999). Comparison of risk of conductive hearing loss among three ethnic groups of Arctic audiology patients. *Journal of Speech Language and Hearing Research 42*(6), 1311–1322.

National Institutes of Health (1994). NIH Guidelines on the inclusion of women and minorities as subjects in clinical research. *NIH Guide, 23*(11), March 18, 1994.

Sanger, D. D., Creswell, J. W., Dworak, J., & Schultz, L. (2000). Cultural analysis of communication behaviors among juveniles in a correctional facility. *Journal of Communication Disorders, 33*(1), 31–57.

Sasao, T., & Sue, S. (1993). Toward a culturally anchored ecological framework of research in ethnic-cultural communities. *Journal of Community Psychology, 21,* 705–727.

Schiavetti, N., & Metz, D. E. (1997). *Evaluating research in communicative disorders.* Boston: Allyn & Bacon.

Shriberg, L. E., Tomblin, J. B., & McSweeny, J. L. (1999). Prevalence of speech delay in 6-year-old children and comorbidity with language impairment. *Journal of Speech Language and Hearing Research, 42*(6), 1461–1481.

Siegel, S. (1956). *Nonparametric statistics for the behavioral sciences.* New York: McGraw-Hill.

Stevens, S. S. (1951). Mathematics, measurement and psychophysics. In S. S. Stevens (Ed.), *Handbook of experimental psychology* (pp. 1–49). New York: John Wiley & Sons.

Stockman, I. J. (1996). The promises and pitfalls of language sample analysis as an assessment tool for linguistic children. *Language, Speech & Hearing Services in the Schools, 27*(4), 355–365.

Sturm, L., & Cahagan, S. (1999). Cultural issues in provider-parent relationships. In D. Kessler & P. Dawson (Eds.), *Failure to thrive and pediatric undernutrition: A transdisciplinary approach* (pp. 351–374). Baltimore: Brookes.

Sue, S. (1983). Ethnic minority issues in psychology: A reexamination. *American Psychologist, 38,* 583–592.

Sue, S., Chun, C.-A., & Gee, K. (1995). Ethnic minority intervention and treatment research. In J. F. Aponte, R. Y. Rivers, & J. Wohl (Eds.), *Psychological interventions and cultural diversity* (pp. 266–282). Boston: Allyn & Bacon.

Sue, S., Kuraski, K. S., & Srinivasan, S. (1999). Ethnicity, gender and cross-cultural issues in clinical research. In P. C. Kendall, J. N. Butcher, & G. N. Holmbeck (Eds.), *Handbook of research methods in clinical psychology* (pp. 54–71). New York: John Wiley & Sons.

Taylor, O. L., & Payne, K. T. (1983). Culturally valid testing: A proactive approach. *Topics in Language Disorders, 3*(3), 8–20.

Tharp, R. G. (1989). Psychocultural variables and constants: Effects on teaching and learning in schools. *Journal of the American Psychological Association, 44*, 1–11.

Tomblin, J. B., Smith, E., & Zhang, X. (1997). Epidemiology of specific language impairment: Prenatal and perinatal risk factors. *Journal of Communication Disorders, 30*(4), 325–344.

U.S. Department of Health, Education and Welfare. (1979). *The Belmont report.* Available from the Government Printing Office. (DHEW Publication No. [OS] 78-0013 and No. [OS] 78-0014).

von Békésy, G. (1960). *Experiments in hearing.* New York: McGraw-Hill.

Walders, N., & Drotar, D. (2000). Understanding cultural and ethnic influence in research with child clinical and pediatric psychology populations. In D. Drotar (Ed.), *Handbook of research in pediatric and clinical child psychology* (pp. 165–188). New York: Kluwer Academic/Plenum Publishers.

Wilkinson, D. Y., & King, G. (1987). Conceptual and methodological issues in the use of race as a variable: Policy implications. *Milbank Quarterly, 65*, (Suppl. 1), 56–71.

World Health Organization (2000). ICIDH-2 *International Classification of Functioning, Disability and Health. Prefinal Draft, December 2000.* Geneva: World Health Organization.

Young, A. M., Ackerman, J., & Kyle, J. G. (2000). On creating a workable signing environment: Deaf and hearing perspectives. *Journal of Deaf Studies & Deaf Education, 5*(2), 186–195.

Wyatt, G. E. (1991). Examining ethnicity versus race in AIDS related sex research. *Social Science Medicine, 33*, 37–45.

Zane, N., & Sue, S. (1986). Reappraisal of ethnic minority issues: Research alternatives. In E. Seidman & J. Rappaport (Eds.), *Redefining social problems* (pp. 289–304). New York: Plenum Press.

Zimmermann, G. N. (1985). The Bannock-Soshoni still have terms for it: Whither Stewart. *Journal of Speech and Hearing Research, 28*, 315–316.

Zimmerman, G. N, Liljeblad, S., Frank, A., & Cleeland, C. (1983). The Indians have many terms for it: Stuttering among the Bannock-Shoshoni. *Journal of Speech and Hearing Research, 26*, 315–318.

Additional Resources

Aponte, J. F., Rivers, R. Y., & Wohl, J. (1995). *Psychological interventions and cultural diversity.* Needham Heights, MA: Allyn & Bacon.

Banks, J. A., & Banks, C. A., McGee (Eds.). (1995). *Handbook of research on multicultural education.* New York: Macmillan.

Braithwaite, D. O., & Thompson, T. L. (2000). *Handbook of communication and people with disabilities.* Mahwah, NJ: Lawrence Erlbaum Associates.

Canino, I. A., & Spurlock, J. (1994). *Culturally diverse children and adults: Assessment, diagnosis and treatment.* New York: Guilford Press.

Comunian, A. L., & Gielen, W. P. (Eds.). (2000). *International perspectives on human development.* Lengerich: Pabst Science Publishers.

Dana, R. H. (2000). *Handbook of cross-cultural and multicultural personality assessment.* Mahwah, NJ: Lawrence Erlbaum Associates.

Drotar, D. (Ed.). (2000). *Handbook of research in pediatric and clinical child psychology.* New York: Kluwer Academic/Plenum Publishers.

Gay, G. (2000). *Culturally responsive teaching: Theory, research and practice.* New York: Teachers College Press.

Gibbs, J. T., & Huang, L. (1998). *Children of color: Psychological interventions with culturally diverse youth.* San Francisco: Jossey-Bass.

Guerra, J. C., & Butler, J. E. (Eds.). (1997). *Writing in multicultural settings.* New York: Modern Language Association of America.

Herring, R. D. (1999). *Counseling with Native American Indians and Alaska Natives: Strategies for helping professionals.* Thousand Oaks, CA: Sage Publications.

Kendall, P. C., Butcher, J. N., & Holmbeck, G. N. (Eds.). (1999). *Handbook of research methods in clinical psychology* (2nd ed.). New York: John Wiley & Sons, Inc.

Macklin, R. (1999). *Against relativism: Cultural diversity and the search for ethical universals in medicine.* New York: Oxford University Press.

Newman, I., & Benz, C. R. (1998). *Qualitative-quantitative research methodology: Exploring the interactive continuum.* Carbondale, IL: SIU Press.

Samuda, R. J., et al. (1998). *Advances in cross-cultural assessment.* Thousand Oaks, CA: Sage Publications.

Schiavetti, N., & Metz, D. E. (1997). *Evaluating research in communicative disorders* (3rd ed.). Needham Heights, MA: Allyn & Bacon.

Silverman, F. H. (1997). *Research design and evaluation in speech-language pathology* (4th ed.). Needham Heights, MA: Allyn & Bacon.

Trawick-Smith, J. W. (2000). *Early childhood development: A multicultural perspective.* Upper Saddle River, NJ: Merrill.

Index

Note: Page numbers followed by *f* indicate figures; numbers followed by *t* indicate tables.